HORMONES AND CANCER

ADVANCES IN EXPERIMENTAL MEDICINE AND BIOLOGY

Recent Volumes in this Series

HORMONES AND CANCER

Edited by

Wendell W. Leavitt

Worcester Foundation for Experimental Biology
Shrewsbury, Massachusetts

PLENUM PRESS • NEW YORK AND LONDON

Library of Congress Cataloging in Publication Data

Symposium on Hormones and Cancer (1980 : Worcester Foundation for Experimental Biology)
    Hormones and cancer.

    (Advances in experimental medicine and biology ; v. 138)
    "Proceedings of the Symposium on Hormones and Cancer, held March 24-26, 1980, at the Worcester Foundation for Experimental Biology, Shrewsbury, Massachusetts" — T.p. verso.
    Bibliography: p.
    Includes index.
    1. Generative organs — Cancer — Congresses. 2. Hormones, Sex — Physiological effect — Congresses. 3. Hormone receptors — Congresses. I. Leavitt, Wendell W. II. Title. III. Series. [DNLM: 1. Genital neoplasms, Female — Etiology — Congresses. 2. Genital neoplasms, Male — Etiology — Congresses. 3. Hormones — Adverse effects — Congresses. 4. Neoplasms, Hormone dependent — Congresses. W1 AD559 v. 138 / WP 145 S99lh 1980]
RC280.G4S96   1980   616.99′46307   81-15743
ISBN 0-306-40831-7   AACR2

Proceedings of the Symposium on Hormones and Cancer, held March 24–26, 1980, at the Worcester Foundation for Experimental Biology, Shrewsbury, Massachusetts

PREFACE

The papers in this volume were presented at the Symposium on Hormones and Cancer held March 24-26, 1980, at the Worcester Foundation for Experimental Biology, Shrewsbury, MA. The meeting was organized to review recent advances in basic and clinical research work on hormone-responsive tumors of the reproductive system. The association between protracted hormone action and cancer of the reproductive system is now irrefutable. Yet we still do not know how hormones initiate and promote neoplastic transformation of their target cells. A major effort is currently being directed at understanding the hormonal regulation of neoplastic cells, especially those arising from the breast, uterus, pituitary gland and prostate. The symposium brought together leading experts whose research is focused on this important area of human health. Although many questions remain to be answered by future studies, the material covered in this volume provides an up-to-date overview of the current status of work in this area. The subjects range from the mechanism of hormone action to the treatment of hormone-dependent tumors, and topics include estrogen, progestin, androgen and glucocorticoid action; hormone receptors; specific protein responses; developmental effects of estrogens and antiestrogens; the DES syndrome; regulation of the cell cycle; therapeutic effects of antiestrogens, aromatase inhibitors, iodoestrogens, progestins on estrogen-dependent tumors; characterization of retinoid-binding sites; and the utility of various tumor markers. Our intent was to synthesize current information from basic and applied studies in the hope that this might clarify controversial areas and provide added impetus to the search for new approaches to cancer control. Although this book is intended primarily for oncologists, endocrinologists and cancer biologists, it is directed to all scientists and students with an interest in carcinogenesis.

The generous financial support of the following contributors is gratefully acknowledged: Beckman Instruments; Dupont Biochemical Division/Sorvall; Interlab Associates; Merrell National Laboratories; New England Nuclear Corporation; Packard

Instrument Company; The Upjohn Company; and the Mimi Greenberg
Cancer Fund, Worcester Foundation for Experimental Biology.

    The editor is indebted to Drs. James Clark, David Kupfer,
Mortimer Lipsett, Christopher Longcope and Helen Padykula for
their help in arranging the program. Special thanks go to William
Robidoux, Merilyn Glew, Janeth Flemming, Mina Rano, Lois Hager,
Carol Cutress, and many other members of the Worcester Foundation
staff for their exceptional assistance with the symposium and the
preparation of the proceedings for publication. Finally, I extend
my appreciation to the directors of the Worcester Foundation,
Drs. Mahlon Hoagland and Federico Welsch, for their continued
support and encouragement.

                                    Wendell W. Leavitt

                                    November, 1980

CONTENTS

THE POLYNUCLEOTIDE BINDING SITES OF ESTRADIOL RECEPTOR COMPLEXES

Herbert W. Dickerman[1] and S. Anand Kumar[2]

Division of Laboratories and Research, New York State
Department of Health, Albany, NY 12201; Department of
Biochemistry, Albany Medical College of Union University;[1] and Department of Chemistry, State University
of New York at Albany[2]

SUMMARY

As a model for interaction of steroid receptors with DNA, the
binding of estradiol receptor complexes (E_2R) to oligodeoxynucleotides, covalently linked to cellulose, was studied in detail.
Binding was optimal at concentrations of monovalent cationic salts
at, or near, isotonic levels and was selective for intracellular
receptors in contrast to extracellular steroid binding proteins.
Among the oligomers, the order of affinity was oligo dG>oligo dT≥
oligo dC>>oligo dA>>oligo dI. The binding to oligo dG was stable
to 37° C exposure and the processes of adsorption and desorption,
while reactivity with oligo dT, oligo dC and oligo dA was labile.
The decrease in binding following purification was restored by
histone 2B. Oligo dG binding was the most resistant to inhibition
by cibacron blue F3GA (CB) and pyridoxal-5-phosphate. On the basis
of these data, a hypothesis is proposed for the interaction of
mouse uterine cytosol E_2R with prevalent nonspecific and putative
specific sequences of DNA.

INTRODUCTION

Of the components involved in the nuclear binding of estradiol receptor complexes, DNA, alone or in cooperation with specific
chromosomal proteins, appears to be of prime importance. Cytosol
receptor complexes from various target tissues are DNA binding
proteins which contain at least two distinct domains: the binding
sites for steroid ligands and those for polydeoxynucleotides. These

1

two functionally distinct domains are spatially separated. Limited
proteolysis of steroid receptors results in a loss of DNA binding
without altering steroid binding (1, 2). More recent studies with
a series of inhibitors, including pyridoxal-5-phosphate (3, 4, 5)
aurintricarboxylic acid (6) and cibacron blue F3GA (7) have shown
losses of nuclear, DNA and oligodeoxynucleotide binding with little
effect on the binding of steroid. In the cases of pyridoxal-5-
phosphate and cibacron blue F3GA (CB), the inhibition was competitive with respect to DNA or oligodeoxynucleotide.

While these experiments indicate that a polydeoxynucleotide
domain exists in E_2R and other steroid receptors, they do not define
the components of DNA recognized by the receptor complexes. It is
well established that in the procaryotes, a limited number of unique
nucleotide sequences are the determinants in the productive binding
of gene regulatory proteins to DNA. The application of such a model
to account for the modulation of gene expression by steroid receptor
proteins has not been supported by experimental evidence, since the
binding to DNA of E_2R was neither restricted to a limited number of
high affinity sites nor was it specific for the source of the DNA.
Yamamoto and Alberts have argued that, due to the prevalance of
nonspecific binding, as many as 10^3 specific sites in DNA might be
masked by the methods of analysis which were used (8). Yet, even
with these methods, the binding was not random as preferences were
reported for DNA rather than RNA (9), double stranded DNA rather
than single stranded DNA, (10,11), BudR-substituted DNA rather than
unsubstituted DNA (12). In addition, Simons demonstrated by competition equilibrium that glucocorticoid receptors bound preferentially to natural DNAs rather than to synthetic polydeoxynucleotides
(13). These data suggest that differences in the primary and/or
secondary structure of nuclear DNA are recognized by steroid receptors which in turn may play a role in the alteration of transcription.

The biological relevance of the DNA-binding domains of steroid
receptors was demonstrated by the isolation of two mutant classes
of glucocorticoid-resistant S49-1 mouse lymphoma cells by Yamamoto
and his co-workers (14). One class was found to have depressed
nuclear binding (nt⁻), and the other increased nuclear binding (nt[i])
as compared to the wild type receptors. The alterations in nuclear
binding of the mutant receptor complexes were analogous to their
respective affinity for DNA cellulose. These results indicated
that a mutation affecting the polynucleotide binding domain of a
steroid receptor, including those which increase total binding to
DNA, resulted in a phenotype resistant to the action of the steroid
hormone.

Another method of examining the polynucleotide binding domain
of E_2R, as well as other steroid hormone receptor complexes, em-
ploys oligodeoxynucleotide celluloses, in which the oligomer is

covalently linked through the 5' phosphate to the supporting matrix
(15). Following the report of Thrower and his colleagues on the
partial purification of rat uterine cytosol E_2R with oligo(dT)-
cellulose column chromatography (16), our group undertook a study
of the properties of the interaction between the oligodeoxynucleotides and the estradiol receptor complexes of mouse kidney and
uterine cytosol. The results to be presented in the following report will include the effect of monovalent cations, the specificity
for intracellular steroid receptors, the inhibition of binding by
CB, the comparison of binding preferences to different oligodeoxynucleotide templates, and the effects of nucleosomal histones
on binding and preservation of holoreceptors. The basic conclusion
of these studies is that E_2R can discriminate between the nucleotide
bases. In addition, we propose a model for the interaction of E_2R
with the prevalent nonspecific and putative specific sequences
within DNA

Materials and Methods

The defined (dT) oligomers were purchased from Collaborative
Research, Waltham, MA. The remainder of the materials and all of
the methods are fully described in other publications (7,17,18,19)
and in the figure legends.

Results

E_2R binds to oligodeoxynucleotide celluloses. It became apparent from our initial studies that the binding to oligo (dT)-cellulose
provided an assay, as well as a probe for analyzing the polynucleotide domain of the receptor complexes. However, before the oligonucleotide cellulose binding assay was used, the effects of varying
experimental conditions were determined. Among the variables
examined, salt concentration had the most profound effect on the
extent of E_2R binding. Although some binding occurred at low ionic
strength, it was markedly stimulated by monovalent cationic salts
in the concentration range of 0.1-0.2M. In Fig. 1, the variations
in binding to oligo(dT)-and oligo(dG)-cellulose as a function of
KCl concentration are depicted. Optimal binding to the oligo-
pyrimidine occurs at a lower concentration than to the oligopurine
with little, or no effect, on binding to the blank cellulose. At
concentrations above 0.2M, there was a decrease in binding. Divalent
cation salts were also stimulatory but to a lesser extent and at
lower concentrations (1-3mM). With all the matrices, optimal binding was observed at/or near physiological ionic strengths, and there
was a lack of specificity with respect to the monovalent cation
used.

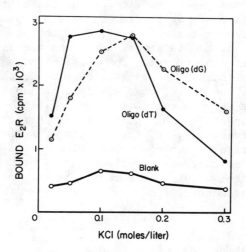

Fig. 1 Dependence on KCl of E_2R binding to oligo(dG)- and oligo(dT)-celluloses. E_2R binding to indicated celluloses were as described in an earlier publication (17) except that the concentration of KCl was varied. 34 fmoles of E_2R (158 cpm/fmole) were used in each binding assay.

One possible way in which isotonic salt concentrations could stimulate binding of receptor complexes would be to "activate" E_2R in a manner analogous to the activation of liver glucocorticoid receptors (20,21). However, when kidney cytosol E_2R was preincubated at 0.2M KCl and exposed to oligo(dT)-cellulose in 0.03M KCl only 9% of the input receptor complex was bound. This percentage was the same extent observed when both the preincubation and binding reactions were done at 0.03M KCl. However, if the binding mixture contained 0.2M KCl, 31% of the input E_2R was bound regardless of whether the preincubation KCl concentration was 0.03M or 0.2M. Prior exposure of the oligodeoxynucleotide cellulose had no effect on the subsequent extent of binding. This experiment indicated that the presence of salt was obligatory to the interaction between E_2R and the oligo(dT) ligand, not as a factor in alteration of the complex or ligand prior to binding.

The DNA binding activity of cytosol steroid hormone receptor complexes, including those for estradiol, appear to be a character-

istic of intracellular receptors differentiating them from other
types of steroid binding proteins. For instance, Mainwaring and
Irving (22) found that human serum β-globulin-5α-dihydrotestosterone
complexes did not bind to DNA cellulose under conditions where prostate androgen receptors did efficiently. The binding to oligo(dT)-
cellulose was examined with reference to the selectivity of the
steroid binding macromolecule. Neither free estradiol nor heat inactivated cytosol E_2R bound to oligo(dT)-cellulose. Bovine serum
albumin with estradiol in a low affinity, high capacity complex, was
inactive in binding. The specificity was further demonstrated with
the extracellular glycoprotein, α fetoprotein to which estradiol
binds with high affinity. As seen in Fig. 2, there was no binding
of α fetoprotein over the same input range in which kidney cytosol
E_2R was bound efficiently. Oligodeoxynucleotide binding is not restricted to E_2R as initial studies in our laboratory indicate that
mouse kidney androgen receptor complex, described by Bullock, Mainwaring and Bardin (23), actively binds to the oligomers (24). These,
and other, data indicated that oligodeoxynucleotide cellulose binding simulates the DNA-binding characteristics reported for intracellular steroid receptors.

    <u>Estradiol receptor complexes can recognize deoxynucleotide bases</u>.
Our initial reaction to the observed interaction of E_2R with oligo-
(dT)-cellulose was that it was nonspecific, probably solely controlled by electrostatic interactions between the polyphosphate
backbone of the oligomer and the cationic groups of the receptor
protein. Nonetheless, a comparison was undertaken of the capacity
of oligo(dT)- and oligo(dA)-celluloses to bind kidney cytosol E_2R
(Fig. 3). When crude cytosol was used, there was an apparent saturation in the extent of binding to oligo(dT)- and oligo(dA)-cellulose
at higher receptor inputs (Fig. 3A). But with a partially purified
0-30% ammonium sulfate fraction, the binding to oligo(dT)-cellulose
was linear (Fig. 3B). This result is consistent with the contention
that non-receptor factors in the crude cytosol interfere with the
DNA-binding properties of E_2R (25,26). Binding to oligo(dA)-cellulose
was however not linear even with the ammonium sulfate fraction.

    Of even more importance was the anomaly in the binding of E_2R
to oligo(dT)- and oligo(dA)-celluloses despite the fact that the
affinity matrices contained equal oligonucleotide concentrations.
A comparison was undertaken between uterine cytosol E_2R binding to
oligo(dT)-, oligo(dC)-, oligo(dA)-, oligo(dG)- and oligo(dI)-cellu-
loses. Of 54 fmoles of E_2R, the amount bound was as follows: oligo-
(dG)-, 20 fmoles; oligo(dT)-, 15 fmoles; oligo(dC)-, 11 fmoles;
oligo(dA)-, 2 fmoles and oligo(dI)-, <1 fmole. This experiment
was performed at equivalent oligodeoxynucleotide concentrations and
the ligands were of the same mean chain lengths. The difference in
binding between oligo (dG) and (dI) was surprising as the only chemical
difference between them is the side group at position 2 of the bases,
i.e. an amino group in oligo (dG) and a hydrogen in oligo (dI). The

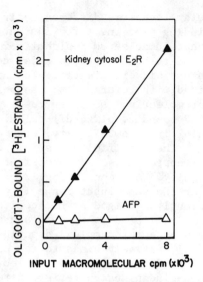

Fig. 2 Comparison of oligo(dT)-cellulose binding of E_2R and of estradiol-α-fetoprotein complex. The α-fetoprotein (AFP) was partially purified from mouse amniotic fluid and [^{3}H] estradiol was exchanged for α-fetoprotein-bound estrone. The kidney E_2R used was a 0-30% ammonium sulfate fraction of [^{3}H] estradiol-charged cytosol. Binding conditions were as described in an earlier publication (17).

relative binding over an extensive concentration range of uterine E_2R was done at limited oligonucleotide concentrations using a GF/C filtration technique which allowed full recovery of very small amounts of the affinity matrices. The results are shown in Fig. 4. The order of binding again was oligo(dG)->> oligo dT-> oligo dC and at low concentrations of E_2R, a distinct cooperative effect was observed when oligo(dG)-cellulose was the template.

So, rather than a general nonspecific interaction between kidney or uterine cytosol E_2R and oligodeoxynucleotides, it is apparent that the receptor complexes discriminate among the nucleotide base moieties of DNA, even to the point of recognizing the 2-amino group of oligo(dG). After this work was completed, we read a report of King in which, using polynucleotides affixed to filters, the order of binding for rat uterine nuclear E_2R was found to be poly rG> poly rC> poly rI (27). As both studies were done with immobilized ligands it was of interest to see if soluble oligonucleotides could

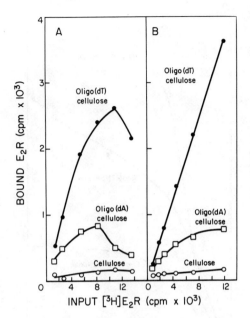

Fig. 3 Effect of receptor concentration on the extent of binding to modified and unmodified celluloses. The receptor preparations
used were [^{3}H] estradiol-charged kidney cytosol (A) and the 0-30%
saturated $(NH_4)SO_4$ fraction of that cytosol (B). The organic phos-
phorous content of the celluloses was 50-51 µg/mg of cellulose.
Assay conditions were as in Ref. 17.

interact with uterine E_2R. To test this, oligo(dT) of homogenous
chain length was preincubated with the receptor complex and their
binding to either oligo(dT)- or oligo(dG)-cellulose was assayed.
Significant inhibition of binding to oligo(dT)-cellulose was observed only when the competing oligomer exceeded 8 nucleotides in
chain length. Furthermore, inhibition by oligo(dT) was more pronounced with the homologous oligo(dT)-cellulose than with the
heterologous oligo(dG)-cellulose (Fig. 5). These findings confirmed
the nucleotide base recognition property of E_2R and, in addition,
suggested that a minimum chain length was required for a stable
interaction to occur.

Estradiol receptor complexes are inhibited at their polynucleotide binding domain by cibacron blue F3GA. The polysulphonated
aromatic blue dye, CB (Fig. 6) has been reported to act as an inhibitor or an affinity ligand for a number of enzymes of polynucleotide
metabolism such as: RNA polymerase (28), DNA polymerase (29), poly-

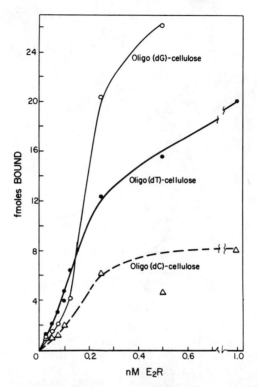

Fig. 4 Binding to oligodeoxynucleotide celluloses as a function of mouse uterine cytosol E_2R concentrations. Reaction mixtures (0.6 ml, total volume) contained indicated concentrations of E_2R with a suspension of oligonucleotide cellulose (representing 20 nmoles of oligonucleotide) in Tris-HCl pH 7.6 containing 0.15 M KCl, 1.5 mM EDTA and 1 mM DTT. The contents were mixed on a rotator at 4° for 60 min. The mixture was then filtered through GF/C filter discs, washed three times with 10 ml of 10 mM Tris-HCl pH 7.6, 1.5 mM EDTA and 1 mM DTT. E_2R bound to the oligonucleotide cellulose matrix was determined by measuring radioactivity retained on the filter discs.

nucleotide phosphorylase (30), polynucleotide kinase (31) and tRNA synthetase (32). In all cases, the interaction of the dye is at the polynucleotide binding site and not at the mononucleotide reactant site. These studies suggest that CB recognizes some feature common to the polynucleotide binding domains. We examined the effect of CB on the binding of mouse uterine cytosol E_2R to oligo(dT)-cellulose and DNA-cellulose (7) and found it was an effective inhibitor at micromolar concentrations. Conversely, at these and higher concentrations, CB had no effect on the association or dissociation of estradiol at the steroid binding site. CB not only blocked the uptake of E_2R by oligo(dT)-cellulose but released E_2R from preformed E_2R:oligo(dT)-cellulose complexes. When subjected to analysis, the

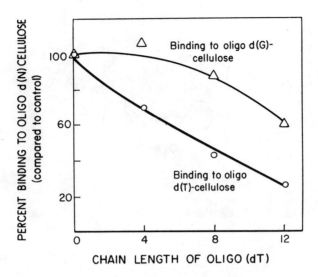

Fig. 5 Competition for E_2R binding between soluble and immobilized oligonucleotides. E_2R (94 fmoles) was incubated with 200 nmoles
of oligo(dT) of indicated chain length in 10 mM Tris-HCl pH 7.6
containing 1.5 mM EDTA, 0.15 M KCl and 1 mM DTT at 4° for 30 min on
a multipurpose rotator. Then, oligo(dT)- or oligo(dG)-cellulose
(representing 20 nmoles of oligonucleotide) was added and incubation
continued for another 30 min. Buffer and other components were also
added to obtain the same final concentrations as described above in
a total volume of 0.6 ml. The reaction mixture was filtered through
GF/C filter discs, washed three times with 10 ml each of 10 mM Tris-
HCl pH 7.6 containing 1.5 mM EDTA and 1 mM DTT. E_2R bound to the
oligonucleotide cellulose matrix was determined by measuring the
radioactivity retained on the filters, in a Beckman Scintillation
counter using Biofluor.

inhibition by CB was found to be competitive with the oligodeoxynucleotide cellulose, clearly implicating an interaction at the
polynucleotide binding domain of E_2R. The inhibition was not merely
a facet of the polyanionic character of the dye as its inhibition
was much more effective (on an equivalent anion basis) than heparin
or poly-1-glutamate.

These experiments indicate that an inhibitor with profound

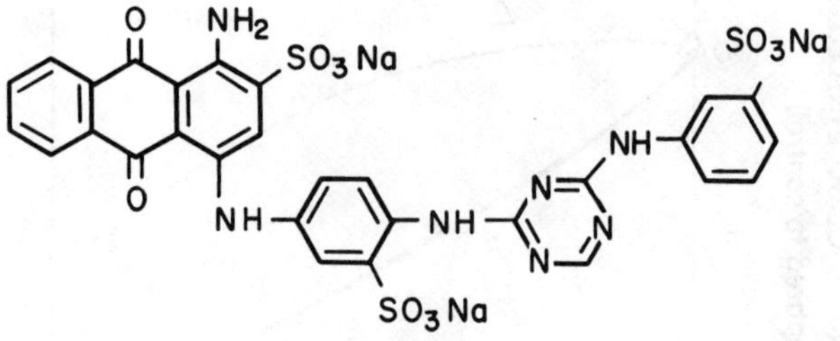

CIBACRON BLUE F3GA

Fig. 6   Structure of cibacron blue F3GA

effects on the template binding site of enzymes of DNA and RNA metabolism also interacts at the DNA binding site of E_2R possibly recognizing a structural component common to these proteins.

There are at least two types of subsites in the polynucleotide
binding domain of E_2R. Although the relative order of preferences
of E_2R binding to oligodeoxynucleotides was determined, the question
was asked if there were any differences in the interactions when
exposed to inhibitors of DNA binding and/or increase in ionic strength.
The relative effectiveness of CB inhibition was tested and 50% inhibition was seen in the binding of uterine cytosol E_2R to oligo(dT)-
cellulose at 1.7 µM, oligo(dC)-cellulose at 4 µM and oligo(dG)-
cellulose at 4.8 µM (Table I). Studies using oligo(dA)- or oligo-
(dI)-cellulose were not performed because of the low efficiency of
binding to these ligands. Pyridoxal-5-phosphage (PLP) has been
shown to be an effective inhibitor of hepatic glucocorticoid recept-
or and rat uterine estradiol receptor complexes to DNA (3,33). The
concentrations required for 50% inhibition of binding of mouse
uterine E_2R to oligo(dG)-, oligo(dT)- and oligo(dC)-celluloses were
determined. Again, oligo(dG) binding was more resistant to inhibition than the interactions with the oligodeoxypyrimidines. In this
case, the binding to oligo(dC)-cellulose was the most sensitive to
inhibition by PLP.

Not only were differential effects of CB inhibition of binding
observed but also on the dissociation of E_2R from preformed complexes
from the various oligodeoxynucleotide celluloses. As shown in Table

I, the concentration of CB required to displace 50% of the bound E_2R was 4.6 µM for oligo(dG)-cellulose, 1.5 µM for oligo(dT)-cellulose and 2.3 µM for oligo(dC)-cellulose. Similarly, the concentration of KCl required to disociate E_2R from preformed oligonucleotide complexes was higher for oligo(dG) than for the oligodeoxypyrimidine ligands. These comparisons using inhibitors of E_2R binding to polynucleotides, as well as alteration of ionic strength, indicate that the binding of mouse uterine cytosol E_2R to oligo(dG) is the most stable of the interactions. This is especially interesting in that PLP inhibits by forming a Schiff base with lysine residues in the polynucleotide binding domain while CB probably mimics some facet of the secondary structure of DNA in its non-covalent interaction with E_2R. Unlike oligo(dG) binding, there was variation in the effect of these reagents on the binding to the oligodeoxypyrimidines with no clear cut distinction possible.

Although prior experiments indicated more extensive and increased stability of binding of uterine E_2R to oligo(dG) than to the other ligands, there were no clear qualitative differences among the E_2R-oligonucleotide interactions. In order to detect such differences, the affinity of E_2R for different ligands was estimated after exposure of the complex to potential denaturing conditions. The change in temperature was the first perturbation which was studied. As published in our initial report (17) with kidney receptor complex and confirmed in our studies with uterine E_2R, there was no increase in the extent of binding to oligo(dT)-cellulose by increasing temperature to 20-30°C. In fact, with an increase to 37°C, there was a rapid loss of binding of uterine E_2R to oligo(dC)-cellulose, and to a slightly lesser extent, oligo(dT)-cellulose (Fig. 7). However, binding to oligo(dG)-cellulose remained unabated over the same time course. In this experiment, the amount of E_2R used in the binding reactions was normalized for the loss of macromolecular bound steroid which was approximately 60% over the 30 minute incubation and there was no indication of significant differential binding of estradiol to the ligands.

The stability of oligo(dG)-cellulose binding was echoed in a study of differential binding following partial purification of uterine E_2R. Mouse uterine cytosol was enriched seven-fold by adsorbtion to oligo(dT)-cellulose at low ionic strength and by subsequent elution with 0.5 M KCl. Following this procedure, binding to oligo(dT)-cellulose was reduced or eliminated but the activity could be restored by histone 2A, histone 2B or histone 3 derived from calf thymus (18). The differential stability of binding activities was tested in a similar fashion. Uterine E_2R was adsorbed onto either oligo(dT)- or oligo(dG)-cellulose and eluted with 0.5 M KCl. The partially purified complexes were then tested for binding to oligo(dG)-, oligo(dT)-, oligo(dA)- and oligo(dC)-celluloses in the presence and absence of histone 2B. The results shown

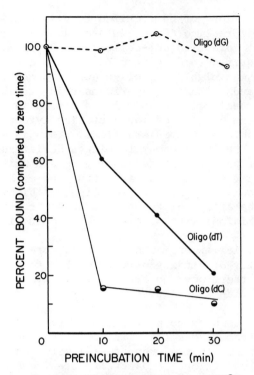

Fig. 7   Effect of preincubation of E_2R at $37^\circ C$ on binding to oligodeoxynucleotide celluloses. E_2R was incubated for times indicated at 37°. At the end of the incubation, free estradiol was removed by treatment with charcoal-dextran and binding assays with oligo(dG)-, oligo(dC)- and oligo(dT)-celluloses were carried out using aliquots representing equivalent quantity of E_2R. Incubations were at 4° for 90 min. In each case the amount of bound E_2R which had not been preincubated (0 min controls) represents 100%.

in Table II indicate that following salt induced elution, E_2R did not bind to any of the ligands except oligo(dG). This was completely different from the range of interactions seen with the initial cytosol. A partial restoration of binding to oligo(dT)-, oligo (dC)- and oligo(dA)-celluloses was observed in the reactions containing histone 2B. Histone 2B also stimulated the binding activity associated with oligo(dG)-cellulose.

The perturbations of the environment involved in heating or purification resulted in the observed qualitative differences in the oligodeoxynucleotide binding indicating that at least two subsites exist in the binding domain. They are the stable sites involved in oligo(dG) recognition and the more labile ones which interact with the other oligodeoxynucleotides.

Table I: Reagent Concentration Required for Half-Maximal Effect

	Oligo(dG)-Cellulose	Oligo(dT)-Cellulose	Oligo(dC)-Cellulose
Inhibition of binding by Cibacron Blue	4.8×10^{-6}M	1.7×10^{-6}M	4.0×10^{-6}M
Inhibition of binding by Pyridoxal-5-phosphate	3.1×10^{-3}M	1.5×10^{-3}M	0.8×10^{-3}M
Displacement of bound E_2R by Cibacron Blue	4.6×10^{-6}M	1.5×10^{-6}M	2.3×10^{-6}M
Displacement of bound E_2R by KCl	~ 0.5M	~ 0.3M	~ 0.35M

Table II: Rebinding of E_2R eluted from oligo(dT)- and oligo(dG)-cellulose complexes to oligodeoxynucleotide cellulose

	E_2R off oligo(dT)-cellulose		E_2R off oligo(dG)-cellulose	
Cellulose type	% bound	of input	E_2R	
	-H2B	+H2B	-H2B	+H2B
Oligo(dG)	18	33	21	32
Oligo(dA)	0	6	0	6
Oligo(dC)	0	12	0	14
Oligo(dT)	0	22	1	23

$E_2R \cdot$ oligo(dG)- or oligo(dT)-cellulose complexes were formed under standard binding assay conditions. Elution of bound E_2R was achieved using 0.5 M KCl. 0.2 ml aliquots of the elutes were used

in the rebinding assay with fresh oligodeoxynucleotide celluloses
in a total volume of 0.6 ml so that the final concentration of KCl
was 0.15 M. 50 µg of histone H2B were added to the rebinding assay
where indicated. The methods were as described in an earlier publication (17).

DISCUSSION

It is apparent from many lines of evidence, using a variety of
probes, that steroid receptor proteins are functionally multifaceted.
In the current study, immobilized oligonucleotides have been used
as probes to investigate the nature of one of the facets, namely,
the polynucleotide binding domain of estradiol receptor proteins.
In addition to the electrostatic interactions between cationic amino
acid side chains of the receptor protein and the polyphosphate anions
of the oligonucleotide backbone, the binding domain possesses structural features which are capable of discriminating between the
nucleotide bases. For mouse uterine cytosol E_2R there is a definite
order of preference for the nucleotide bases such that oligo(dG)>
oligo(dT)$\geq$oligo(dC)>>oligo(dA)>oligo(dI). The wide difference between the preferences of E_2R for dG and dI indicates the importance
of primary structure of DNA in the recognition process. The structural difference between dG and dI is only in the presence or absence
of an amino group at position 2 of the purine ring. It has been
shown by x-ray diffraction studies by Zimmerman and co-workers that
the secondary structures of the ribopolymers of these two nucleotides
are virtually identical (34).

In addition to the base discrimination properties of the polynucleotide binding domain, certain other topological features have
been characterized. Using immobilized and soluble oligo(dT) in a
competition assay, a requirement has been observed for a minimum
chain length needed for the formation of a stable complex between
E_2R and the oligomer. The polyaromatic dye, cibacron blue F3GA, a
"super secondary structure" probe for the polynucleotide binding
domains of a number of DNA and RNA binding proteins, has been shown
to be a powerful inhibitor of the interaction between E_2R and oligonucleotide celluloses. Thus, the base recognition properties, the
possible requirement for a minimum chain length and the inhibition
by cibacron blue F3GA, all suggest reciprocal features in the topol-
ogy of the polynucleotide binding domain of E_2R. The differences
in the sensitivities of the binding reactions to environmental
perturbations have suggested two classes of subsites within the
polynucleotide binding domain. Subsites which preferentially bind
dG are more stable to environmental perturbations such as temperature, ionic strength and inhibitors and are designated the G sites.
The less stable sites are designated N sites which have been thought
to be less discriminatory towards the structure of the nucleotide
bases.

These observations indicate some of the intricacies of one facet of the estradiol receptor protein. There are, however, two other equally intricate facets, thus making the allegorical three faces of Eve; the estradiol binding site which will not be discussed here and a site for binding to cationic proteins such as histones (Fig. 8). Dilute solutions of partially purified E_2R dissociate into aporeceptor and free estradiol, particularly more pronounced at elevated temperatures, which can be demonstrated by sedimentation analysis on sucrose density gradients. Preincubation of the receptor protein with histone 2A, 2B or to a lesser extent histone 3, reduced the dissociation of the holoreceptor. The stabilizing effect was shown to be localized in the N-terminal half-molecule of histone 2B which was obtained by cyanogen bromide cleavage (35). This half-molecule contained 1-58 residues, 32% of which were basic. In contrast, the C-terminal half-molecule had no such stabilizing effect.

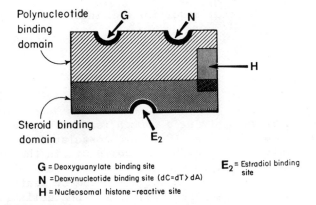

Fig. 8. A model for estradiol receptor complex - The three faces of Eve.

Based on our observations discussed in this report and other published papers, we propose a hypothetical model to describe the nature of the interactions between DNA and estradiol receptor. The model is illustrated in Fig. 9. In this model it is envisaged that the hormone receptor binds to the prevalent and the putative specific

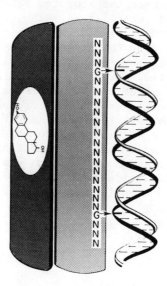

Fig. 9   A hypothetical model for E_2R interaction with DNA.

sites on the DNA by recognizing a common feature between the two
types of sites. Seeman et al. (36) have postulated that in lac
repressor, recognition of two GC base pairs within the DNA helix is
required for specific DNA:protein interaction. In analogy with this
postulate, we propose a model in which the common feature between
prevalent and putative specific sites on the DNA helix is the spatial
disposition of two dG residues. It is further envisaged that the
receptor protein interacts with one surface of the helix and hence
the two dGs could be derived from either of the two strands. This
postulate thus accomodates both the DNA double helix and the single
stranded oligonucleotide probes that we have used. The difference
between the prevalent and the specific sites are distinguished by
the differences in the sequence of nucleotides around the postulated "anchor" dG residues. The former is postulated to be non-
productive whereas the latter to be productive with respect to
steroid modulation of gene transcription. The proposed model is
amenable for further modifications to involve histone and nonhistone acidic proteins. A suggestion in this regard based on the
experiments shown in Table II is that the N subsites are malleable,
labile under potentially denaturing conditions yet restructured in

the presence of histone 2B. If this restoration is due to direct interaction at the cationic protein binding site, it might represent a form of allosterism in which the binding repertoire of the DNA binding domain is altered. Histones may not be the only effector molecules which can alter the deoxynucleotide preferences of E_2R but may include nonhistone proteins as well or even small molecular weight compounds. Regardless of the specific factors, our hypothesis suggests that recognition sites at the polynucleotide binding domain are not rigid but can be altered by interactions with nuclear components other than DNA. In addition, binding to juxtanucleosomal DNA in a location where the N-terminii of histone 2A and 2B might react with E_2R could facilitate preservation of the holoreceptor within the nucleus in a ternary complex (histone:E_2R: DNA).

ACKNOWLEDGEMENTS

     This work was possible only because of the efforts of Dr. Kantilal H. Thanki, Mrs. Thaisa A. Beach, Ms. Sharon Gross and Dr. Katherine P. Henrickson. Research from our laboratory was supported in part by research grants AM19253 and AM23075 REB awarded by the National Institute of Arthritis, Metabolic and Digestive Diseases, PHS/DHEW.

REFERENCES

1. André, J. and Rochefort, H. (1973) FEBS Lett. 32:330-334
2. Wrange, Ö. and Gustafsson, J.-Å. (1978) J. Biol. Chem. 253: 856-865
3. Cake, M.H., DiSorbo, D.M. and Litwack, G. (1978) J. Biol. Chem. 253:4886-4891
4. Nishigori, H., Moudgil, V.K. and Toft, D. (1978) Biochem. Biophys. Res. Commun. 80:112-118
5. Nishigori, H. and Toft, D. (1979) J. Biol. Chem. 254:9155-9161
6. Moudgil, V.K. and Weekes, G.A. (1978) FEBS Lett. 94:324-326
7. Kumar, S.A., Beach, T.A. and Dickerman, H.W. (1979) Proc. Natl. Acad. Sci., USA 76:2199-2203
8. Yamamoto, K.R. and Alberts, B. (1975) Cell 4:301-310
9. Yamamoto, K.R. and Alberts, B. (1974) J. Biol. Chem. 249:7076-7086
10. André, J., Pfeiffer, A., and Rochefort, H. (1976) Biochemistry 15:2964-2969
11. Kallos, J. and Hollander, V.P. (1978) Nature 272:177-179
12. Kallos, J., Fasy, T.M., Hollander, V.P. and Bick, M.D. (1978) Proc. Natl. Acad. Sci., USA 75:4896-4900
13. Simons, S., Jr. (1977) Biochim. Biophys. Acta 496:349-359

14. Yamamoto, K.R., Stampfer, M.R. and Tomkins, G.M, (1974) Proc.
     Natl. Acad. Sci., USA 71:3901-3905
15. Gilham, P.T. (1964) J. Am. Chem. Soc. 86:4982-4985
16. Thrower, S., Hall, C., Lim, L. and Davison, A.N. (1976) Bio-
     chem. J. 160:271-280
17. Thanki, K.H., Beach, T.A. and Dickerman, H.W. (1978) J. Biol.
     Chem. 253:7744-7750
18. Thanki, K.H., Beach, T.A., Bass, A.I. and Dickerman, H.W.
     (1979) Nucleic Acids Res. 6:3859-3877
19. Kumar, S.A., Beach, T.A. and Dickerman, H.W. (1980) Manuscript
     submitted for publication
20. Milgrom, E., Atger, M. and Baulieu, E-E. (1973) Biochemistry
     12:5198-5205
21. Kalimi, M., Colman,P. and Feigelson, P. (1975) J. Biol Chem.
     250:1080-1086
22. Mainwaring, W.I.P. and Irving, R. (1973) Biochem. J. 134:113-
     127
23. Bullock, L.P., Mainwaring, W.I.P. and Bardin, C.W. (1975)
     Endocrine Res. Commun. 2(1):25-45
24. Gross, S. Unpublished data
25. Chamness, G.C., Jennings, A.W. and McGuire, W.L (1974) Bio-
     chemistry 13:327-331
26. André, J. and Rochefort, H. (1975) FEBS Lett. 50:319-323
27. King, R.J.B. In: Eds. B.R. Rabin and R.B. Freedman. Effects
     of Drugs on Cellular Control Mechanisms; University Park Press,
     Baltimore (1972) p. 17
28. Kumar, S.A. and Krakow, J.S. (1977) J. Biol. Chem. 252:5724-
     5728
29. Brissac, C., Rucheton, M., Brund, C. and Jeanteur, P. (1976)
     FEBS Lett. 61:38-40
30. Drocourt, J-L., Thang, D-C. and Thang, M-N. (1978) Eur. J.
     Biochem. 82:355-362
31. Nichols, B.P., Lindell, T.D., Stellwagen, E. and Donelson,
     J.E. (1978) Biochim. Biophys. Acta 526:410-417
32. Moe, J.G. and Piszkiewicz, D. (1979) Biochemistry 13:2810-2814
33. Muldoon, T.G. and Cidlowski, J.A. (1980) J. Biol. Chem. in
     press
34. Zimmerman, S.B., Cohen, G.H. and Davies, D.R. (1975) J. Mol.
     Biol. 92:181-192
35. Iwai, K., Ishikawa, K. and Hayashi, H. (1970) Nature 226:
     1056-1058
36. Seeman, N.C., Rosenberg, J.M. and Rich, A. (1976) Proc. Natl.
     Acad. Sci., USA 73:804-808

ESTROGEN RECEPTOR AND THE DEVELOPMENT OF ESTROGENIC RESPONSES IN

EMBRYONIC CHICK LIVER

Catherine B. Lazier*, Susan A. Nadin-Davis*, Alex

Elbrecht*, Marie-Luise Blue** and David L. Williams**

*Biochemistry Department, Dalhousie University, Halifax
 Nova Scotia, B3H 4H7, Canada.
**Department of Pharmacological Sciences, Health Sciences
 Center, State University of New York at Stony Brook
 Stony Brook, New York, 11794, U.S.A.

INTRODUCTION

The study of the acquisition of hormonal responsiveness
during development has the potential of identifying critical
factors involved in the establishment of hormonal regulation of
gene expression. In particular, choosing a developmental system
in which multiple distinctive genomic responses to the hormone
can be quantitated may lead to clearer understanding of common and
unique aspects in the differential programming of the activity of
the separate genes.

The chicken embryo has traditionally received considerable
attention as a practical and rewarding model for studying verte-
brate differentiation (1). Recently there has been particular
progress in delineating the development of the urogenital system
and of its responsiveness to estrogen. In a series of papers over
the past 5 years Teng & Teng have elegantly detailed studies on
the development of the embryonic Müllerian duct, the response of
the organ to estrogen, the ontogeny of the estrogen receptor
system, the composition and activity of chromatin and on ovalbumin gene expression and tubular gland cell differentiation (2)-
(11). These studies identify the 12th-16th days of embryonic
development as those in which a dramatic increase in hormonal
responsiveness takes place, followed by a further, but less pronounced, phase of maturation.

19

Our work has centered on the development of estrogen responsiveness in the embryonic chick liver (12)-(15). The rationale,
in part, is that the eventual comparison of development of distinctive responses in different target tissues such as liver and
Müllerian duct may give useful insights into the basic molecular
mechanisms involved. Furthermore, the liver appears to be a particularly advantageous target tissue for study because of the
relatively restricted and reversible nature of the responses
evoked (16). As part of the process of vitellogenesis estrogen
stimulates the hepatic production of specific proteins and lipids
which are eventually incorporated into the developing oocyte.
The proteins include vitellogenin, the large phospholipoglycopro-
tein precursor of yolk phosvitin and lipovitellin (16), the apoproteins B and II of very low density lipoprotein (VLDL) (17) (18),
and vitamin and mineral-binding proteins (19) (20). Estrogenic
regulation of the synthesis of these proteins appears to fall into
several classes, based on the presence or absence of a basal level
of synthesis in the absence of the hormone, and on the relative
kinetics of induction of the protein (21).

Liver cytosol from cockerels and embryonic chicks contains a
high-affinity specific estradiol-binding protein which is likely
a receptor (22) (23). Estrogen treatment in vivo results in
depletion of the cytosol sites along with elevation of receptor
activity in several different nuclear fractions. The relative
importance of these different receptor forms has not yet been
established (22)-(27). The salt-soluble form of nuclear receptor
accounts for about 70% of nuclear estrogen-binding sites in liver
from estrogen-treated 15-day chick embryos (28).

In this paper we document the development of the responsiveness to estrogen of the VLDL apoproteins (apo VLDL-B and apo VLDL-
II). These are the major apoproteins in VLDL particles in plasma
of estrogen-treated roosters, and have molecular weights of
350,000 and 9444 respectively (17) (29). The results are discussed in relation to earlier work on the ontogeny of the capacity
to produce vitellogenin (12) and to work on the embryonic cytosol
and soluble nuclear estrogen receptors (13).

METHODS

Animals and Injections

White leghorn chick embryos were used throughout these
studies (12) (13). This is an important point since some
different strains of domestic chickens exhibit significantly
different incubation periods (1). The procedures used for egg
incubation, injection and dissection of embryos are detailed
elsewhere (12) (14) (15). Relatively high doses of estradiol in
propylene glycol (0.5-2.5 mg/egg) were injected into the egg

white (14) (15) or yolk sac (12), and these doses were found to
be optimal. The amount of estrogen reaching the embryonic liver
is not known. The necessity of large doses of estrogen for substantial induction of egg yolk proteins in chick liver is widely
recognized (28) (30) (31). Tamoxifen citrate was dissolved in
propylene glycol (50 mg/ml).

Assay of Specific Estradiol Binding Activity

Embryonic liver cytosol receptor was assayed essentially as
reported by Lazier & Haggarty for the cockerel liver cytosol
receptor (22). Briefly, the tissue was homogenized in sucrose-
containing buffer in the presence of protease inhibitors. After
centrifugation at 100,000 x g the supernatant was treated with
ammonium sulfate (33% saturation) and the resulting precipitate
was dissolved in buffer containing 0.5 M KCl. Specific estradiol
binding activity was assayed by incubation of various concentrations of [^{3}H]-estradiol in the presence or absence of a 100 x
excess of diethylstilbestrol at 0° for 18 hr or by exchange at 25°,
followed by treatment with charcoal-dextran suspension at 0°.

Gel filtration on Sephacryl S-200 and trypsin-treatment of
embryonic cytosol receptor was as described earlier (22).

The salt-soluble nuclear receptor was prepared by 0.5 M KCl
extraction of crude nuclei and was assayed by the charcoal-dextran
technique (12).

Incubation of Liver and Supernatant Preparation

The vitellogenin ontogeny studies were carried out using
liver incubation and supernatant preparation techniques originally
reported by Luskey et al. (32). 1 gm of liver mince was incubated
for 4 hr at 38° in 5 ml of a modification of minimal essential
Eagles' medium and 50 µCi[^{3}H]-leucine (12). After incubation, 1 M
NaCl and 50 µg/ml phenylmethane sulfonyl fluoride (PMSF) and 1 mM
benzamidine were added. The medium and tissue were homogenized
together and the homogenate was dialysed and centrifuged at
100,000 x g for 1 hr. Supernatant was stored at -20°.

The liver incubations for the VLDL apoproteins differed from
the above method in that much lower quantities of tissue and
higher concentrations of isotope were used (33). In addition,
incubation was for 1 hr only, thus eliminating the necessity to
analyse the medium since no labeled apoprotein would be secreted
by that time. The incubated tissue was washed briefly with
phosphate-buffered saline (PBS) containing 1 mM leucine, and was
homogenized in PBS containing 1% Triton X-100 and 200 µg/ml PMSF.
The supernatant obtained after centrifugation at 100,000 x g was
stored at -20°. With both the vitellogenin and VLDL apoprotein

methods, the incorporation of [³H]-leucine into total supernatant
protein was linear over the time period studied.

Antibodies and Specific Immunoprecipitation Techniques

The techniques used for antigen purification and antibody
induction and characterization have been published for both
vitellogenin (12) and apo VLDL-B (33). In each case, direct
immunoprecipitation techniques were developed and optimized for
maximal precipitation.

Apo VLDL-II was purified from VLDL particles by gel filtration (17) and the antibody raised in rabbits by standard techniques
was further purified by chromatography on Sepharose-apo VLDL-B.
Indirect immunoprecipitation of apo VLDL-II was carried out by
incubation of the antibody (10 μl) with liver supernatant (10 μl)
for 1 hr at 0° followed by addition of goat anti-rabbit antiserum
(20 μl) for 20 min. at 0°. 1 ml of PBS containing 1% Triton X-100
and 200 μg/ml PMSF was added and the precipitate was sedimented in
a microfuge, washed twice with the PBS-Triton-PMSF solution and
once with PBS. The final pellet was dissolved in Protosol and
counted as described for apo VLDL-B (33). Non-specific immunoprecipitation was assessed by incubation of an equivalent amount
of pre-immune serum instead of the primary antibody. Both the
apo VLDL-II antibody and pre-immune serum were stored in the
presence of 1% Triton X-100 and 1% deoxycholate. Of a wide range
of incubation conditions tested, these were found to give optimal
precipitation of labeled apo VLDL-II (Blue & Williams, unpublished
data).

Gel Electrophoresis and Limited Proteolytic Mapping of Apo VLDL-B

Vitellogenin and apo VLDL-B immunoprecipitates were electrophoresed in 5% acrylamide gels in the presence of sodium dodecyl
sulfate (SDS) as described in reference (12) for the former protein and in references (14) (17) and (33) in the latter case.
Electrophoresis of apo VLDL-II was carried out in SDS/20% acrylamide gels (17).

The limited proteolytic cleavage technique of Cleveland et al.
(34) was used to examine embryonic basal and estrogen-induced apo
VLDL-B immunoprecipitates from [³⁵S]-methionine-labeled liver
supernatants. Following incubation with V-8 protease as indicated
in the text, the digests were boiled, electrophoresed on SDS/10%
acrylamide slab gels, fixed, stained, and subjected to fluorography (35) (36).

MATERIALS

All chemicals were of reagent grade and their sources have been identified previously (12) (17) (22) (33).

RESULTS

The Hepatic Estrogen Receptor System in Chick Embryo Liver

Liver nuclei from chicken embryos in the latter half of the incubation period contain small, but measurable, amounts of salt-soluble high-affinity estrogen binding sites (100-200 fmol/mg DNA) (12) (28). Injection of the egg with estradiol results in a dose-dependent several-fold increase in the concentration of the nuclear sites, up to about 600-800 fmol/mg DNA after 24-48 hr. The kinetics of the response are similar to those found for accumulation of the soluble estrogen nuclear receptor after depot injection of estrogen into hatched chickens (22) (31). In addition, the properties of the embryonic nuclear estrogen-binding sites (sedimentation, binding specificity and affinity) are indistinguishable from those in hatched birds (12).

We have examined the ontogeny of the soluble nuclear estrogen receptor and the acquisition of its responsiveness to exogenous estradiol (12). Injection of estradiol on the 8th day of embryonic development has little effect on the soluble nuclear receptor levels measured on day 10. Injection of the hormone on day 10 however does give a significant increase in receptor concentration on day 12 (Fig. 1), and on day 11 (data not shown). The extent of the increase in nuclear receptor at days 11-12 is only slightly less than that found at later stages. This suggests that the mechanism which gives rise to the accumulation of the soluble nuclear receptor is established on days 10-11. In line with observations with hatched chickens such a mechanism might involve translocation of cytoplasmic receptor, followed by a phase of nuclear receptor synthesis and/or stabilization (22) (37).

The ontogeny of cytoplasmic estrogen receptor in embryonic liver has been reported for two different strains of chicken (13) (23). While there are quantitative differences in the results of the two studies, the qualitative developmental patterns observed are closely similar. In the first report, Gschwendt found that the concentration of high-affinity estrogen-specific sites in an ammonium sulfate fraction from liver cytosol of a broiler strain of chicken increased from 344 fmol/gm liver (57 fmol/mg protein) at day 14 to 1850 fmol/gm (170 fmol/mg protein) at day 19 and thereafter fell within days to a level of about 300 fmol/gm (25 fmol/mg protein) which persisted for several weeks after hatch. Using white leghorn embryos, we examined some earlier stages, and found receptor concentrations of 124 ± 4 fmol/gm liver at day 10,

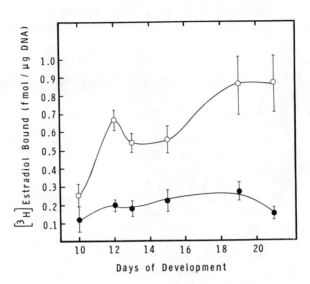

Fig. 1:   The effect of estradiol on the soluble nuclear estrogen
          receptor in embryonic chick liver.

          Embryonated eggs at different stages were injected with
          1.25 mg estradiol and after 48 hr the concentration of
          salt-soluble nuclear receptor sites in liver was deter-
          mined as described in the Methods section. o—o,
          estradiol-treated embryos; •—•, propylene-glycol-treated
          control embryos. Reproduced from (12).

which rose to give 846 ± 18 fmol/gm at day 19 followed by a decline
to the same level observed by Gschwendt (23).   Fig. 2 illustrates
these data in terms of fmol bound/mg protein.

          Comparison of the ontogenic patterns in Figs. 1 and 2 does
not reveal any apparent relationship between the cytosol receptor
concentration and that of the soluble nuclear receptor after 48 hr
of exposure to estrogen. With the dose used the nuclear receptor
response should still be maximal at this time (12). However the
nuclear receptor levels at day 21 do not reflect the peak in cytoplasmic binding at day 19. The nuclear response is just as large
in young cockerels, where the cytosol receptor concentration is

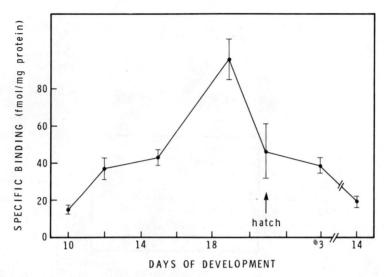

Fig. 2:   Ontogeny of the high-affinity estradiol-binding sites in
          embryonic liver cytosol.

          The cytosol ammonium sulfate fraction was prepared and
          assayed as described in the Methods section. Binding
          site concentration was determined by Scatchard analysis.
          The results are the mean ± range of 2 preparations of
          pooled livers except for day 14 after hatch which is the
          mean ± SEM for 16 preparations.

only 20% of that at day 19 (22). Similarly, the low cytosol
receptor concentration at day 10 does not seem to significantly
limit the nuclear receptor response when estrogen is given at that
stage.

     Gschwendt (23) investigated the possibility that the decline
in cytosol receptor levels after day 19 was due to diffusible
inhibitory or degradative activities present in the liver homogenate of the hatched chicken. Mixing experiments showed a small
effect, but it was insufficient to account for the difference in
the binding site concentrations. These experiments do not rule
out the possibility that the 19-day binding sites are stabilized
by some non-diffusible factor, or that there is a transient
development of a different class of binding site at this stage.

     We examined 19-day cytosol ammonium sulfate fractions for
evidence of binding-site heterogeneity. Fig. 3 shows a single

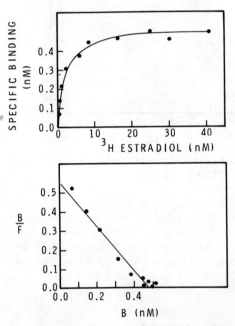

Fig. 3: High-affinity binding of [^{3}H]-estradiol by the 19 day embryonic cytosol ammonium sulfate fraction.

Pooled cytosol from 24 embryos was processed and assayed by incubation at 0° with a wide range of [^{3}H]-estradiol concentrations as described in the Methods section. Upper panel: Specific binding curve. Lower panel: Scatchard analysis of the same data.

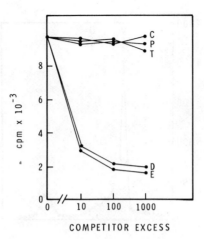

COMPETITOR EXCESS

Fig. 4: Binding specificity of the 19 day embryonic cytosol
receptor.

Binding of 2 nM [^{3}H]-estradiol in the presence or absence
of potential competitors was determined at 0° as described
in the Methods section. C, cortisol; T, testosterone;
P, progesterone; D, diethylstilbestrol; E, 17β-estradiol.

class of estradiol-binding sites over a wide range of ligand concentrations (which should be sufficient to distinguish type I and
type II estrogen-binding sites in rat uterus for example (38)).
The binding specificity is typical of the receptor in cockerel
liver (22)(Fig. 4). The behavior of the embryonic preparation on
gel filtration on Sephacryl S-200 is identical to cockerel receptor
(22)(Fig. 5). These studies suggest, although they do not of
course prove, that the 19-day cytosol estrogen-binding sites
represent a single receptor class, similar qualitatively to that
in hatched chickens.

The studies of the ontogeny of the cytoplasmic estrogen
receptor raise two immediate questions. First, what is the minimum concentration of cytoplasmic receptor at the early stages of
development which is consistent with estrogen-regulated expression
of specific genes? It is possible that different loci will exhibit
different requirements for receptor input. Second, does the
apparent transient elevation of cytoplasmic receptor at day 19 have
any consequences in terms of specific gene expression?

Ontogeny of Estrogenic Responses

Vitellogenin
The development of the capacity of embryonic liver to

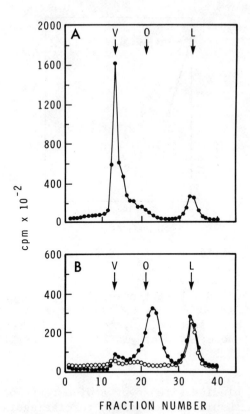

FRACTION NUMBER

Fig. 5:   Gel filtration of embryonic cytosol ammonium sulfate
          preparation and the effect of limited trypsin treatment.

          A: 19 day embryonic cytosol ammonium sulfate preparation
          was incubated with 10 nM [³H]-estradiol, charcoal-treated
          and subjected to gel filtration as described in reference
          22.   V, void volume; O, ovalbumin marker; L, elution
          position of [¹⁴C]-leucine.

          B: ●—●, Gel filtration of a preparation treated with
          trypsin prior to incubation with 10 nM [³H]-estradiol;
          o—o, Trypsinized preparation incubated with 10 nM [³H]-
          estradiol + 1 µM diethylstilbestrol.

respond to exogenous estradiol with vitellogenin synthesis was
reported in 1978 (12).   Embryonated eggs were injected with
estradiol at various stages of development and after 48 hr the
livers were cultured for 4 hr with [³H]-leucine and incorporation
into vitellogenin in the supernatant of the homogenized tissue and
medium was measured by specific immunoprecipitation followed

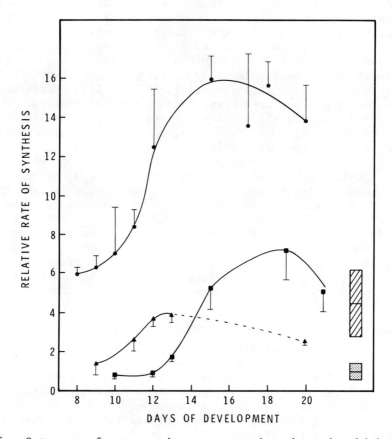

Fig. 6:   Ontogeny of estrogenic responses in embryonic chick liver

■, Vitellogenin synthesis by liver from estrogen-treated
embryos (redrawn from reference 12) (48 hr treatment).
●, Apo VLDL-B synthesis by liver from estrogen-treated
embryos (redrawn from reference 14) (18 hr treatment).
▲, Apo VLDL-II synthesis by liver from estrogen-treated
embryos (48 hr treatment).

The development stage on the abscissa refers to the time
of liver preparation. The hatched bar gives the mean
basal synthesis of apo VLDL-B at all stages (mean ± SD,
n = 27). The stippled bar gives the mean control value
for apo VLDL-II synthesis (mean ± SD, n = 18). The control value for vitellogenin synthesis is uniformly less
than 1% and is omitted from the graph (12).

by SDS/polyacrylamide gel electrophoresis of the immunoprecipitate.
The direct immunoprecipitation technique used gave relatively high
non-specific precipitation but the electrophoresis step permitted
positive identification of labeled vitellogenin. Synthesis of
vitellogenin by control (vehicle-treated) embryo livers was not
observed at any stage. This is consistent with observations in
roosters and cockerels (12) (39) (40). Fig. 6 illustrates the
results for livers cultured from estrogen-treated embryos. The
capacity for vitellogenin synthesis appears to be established by
days 13-15 of egg incubation. Traces of specific synthesis are
apparent in the 13-day livers (from embryos treated with estrogen
on day 11), but no vitellogenin synthesis is apparent before that
stage. Schjeide et al. (41) have recently reported that traces of
vitellogenin can be detected in the serum of 13-day embryos treated
with estrogen 4 days earlier, but that a substantial response
(measured as Ca^{++}-binding activity) could not be detected until
day 16-18 (after 4 days of hormone exposure). Our results suggest
that the level of synthesis of vitellogenin in the 15-21 day
embryos is roughly the same as that achieved in a primary response
to estrogen in cockerels (12), suggesting that the low cytosol receptor concentration in the cockerels does not limit estrogen
responsiveness.

Apo VLDL-B
        Following the analysis of rooster plasma apo VLDL-B and
characterization of specific antibody (17) we initiated a study on
the ontogeny of the response of this apoprotein to estrogen in the
embryo. Two features of this estrogen-regulated system made it
distinctive from the vitellogenin response. First, there is a
significant basal level of synthesis of apo VLDL-B in liver of
roostersunexposed to estrogen (33). Second, the induction kinetics
for the estrogen-regulated increment of apo VLDL-B synthesis were
notably faster than for vitellogenin (21). Following dose-response
and time course experiments (14) (15), we chose to examine the
ontogeny of the apo VLDL-B response 18 hr after estrogen treatment,
instead of after 48 hr as in the vitellogenin study. Another
difference in the experimental design was in the liver culture
technique (discussed in the Methods section). Data from (14) and
(15) are summarized in Fig. 6. Estrogen stimulation of apo VLDL-B
synthesis appears to be established at an earlier stage than does
the vitellogenin response. The relative induction kinetics for
the two loci mentioned above could provide a partial explanation
for the dissociation of the two responses, but the inductions at
day 12 (for apo VLDL-B) and day 13 (for vitellogenin) suggest that
additional factors are involved. It is interesting that Schjeide
et al. (41) also find that estrogen has a more pronounced effect
on apo VLDL-B accumulation in serum than on vitellogenin at the
earlier embryonic stages.

The basal level of synthesis of apo VLDL-B in propylene
glycol (vehicle) or untreated embryos averages about 5% of total
protein synthesis as judged by the immunoprecipitation technique.
We have further characterized the immunoprecipitates by electrophoresis in SDS/polyacrylamide gels and confirm that at least 80%
of the immunoprecipitated radioactivity in the control preparations
is associated with a protein with electrophoretic mobility identical to apo VLDL-B (14) (15). Furthermore, the basal level of
synthesis of apo VLDL-B is established in the liver tissue well
before estrogen-responsiveness is evident (14) (15). In 6-day
embryonic livers from untreated embryos, apo VLDL-B synthesis
accounts for 3.0 ± 0.3% of total protein synthesis; in 7-day livers
it is 3.9 ± 0.4%; at 8 days 5.4 ± 1.3%, and at 10 days 4.1 ± 0.7%.
The function and mechanism of regulation of this "constitutive"
synthesis in the normal embryos is unknown.

Tamoxifen, a widely studied antiestrogen, exhibits both
agonistic and antagonistic activities to estrogen in rodent uterus
(42). In the chicken however the compound appears to be a pure
antagonist, both in oviduct (43) and in liver (44) (45). Capony &
Williams (33) have shown that tamoxifen completely abolishes the
estrogen-induced increment in apo VLDL-B synthesis in rooster liver,
but has no effect on the basal level of synthesis. We therefore
examined the effect of tamoxifen on apo VLDL-B synthesis in the
embryo at estrogen-responsive and "pre-responsive" stages of development. The data in Table 1 confirm that tamoxifen is a pure
antagonist in the embryo with about the same dose-effectiveness
seen in roosters. The basal level of apo VLDL-B synthesis appears
to be tamoxifen-resistant and thus estrogen independent.

Table 1:   Effect of Tamoxifen on Apo VLDL-B Synthesis

Stage of Development	Treatment (18 hr)	Relative Rate of Apo VLDL-B Synthesis $\overline{X}$ % ± SD
18 days	E_2 (0.5 mg)	13.0 ± 2.9
	E_2 + Tam (0.5 mg)	3.7 ± 0.6
	E_2 + Tam (1.0 mg)	3.1 ± 0.4
	Vehicle	3.8 ± 0.2
	Tam (0.5 mg)	4.3 ± 0.8
	Tam (1.0 mg)	3.5 ± 0.6
10 days	Vehicle	5.6 ± 0.4
	Tam (0.5 mg)	5.3 ± 0.7
	Tam (1.0 mg)	5.2 ± 0.6
	Tam (1.5 mg)	6.3 ± 1.0

The existence of the estrogen-independent basal level of synthesis of apo VLDL-B raised the possibility that the basal synthesis
might reflect expression of a separate structural gene from that
regulated by estrogen. The electrophoretic similarity and immunochemical cross-reactivity do not favor such a model, but do not
rule it out since gene duplication could result in proteins of
similar gross characteristics. However, recent analysis of apo
VLDL-B immunoprecipitates by the sensitive limited proteolysis
mapping technique of Cleveland et al. (34) makes this possibility
unlikely. Fig. 7 shows that apo VLDL-B synthesized by liver from
a tamoxifen-treated 17-day embryo has a very similar cleavage
pattern to that from an estrogen-treated embryo. At least 18
bands of identical mobility can be seen.

In hatched chicks the basal rate of apo VLDL-B synthesis falls
from about 5% at the time of hatch to about 2-3% in 3 weeks. This
rate is found in roosters (33). In one set of experiments we observed a small decline in the estrogen-induced increment of apo
VLDL-B synthesis after hatch (A. Elbrecht & C. Lazier, unpublished
results). The increment in 12-20 day embryos is usually about 9%,
whereas it was 7-8% in the chicks up to 3 weeks post-hatch. Such
a decline however does not parallel the 80% loss in cytosol
receptor concentration which occurs between embryonic day 19 and
shortly after hatch.

The tissue specificity of basal and estrogen-induced apo VLDL-
B synthesis has been investigated in the 15-day and 9-day embryos
(14) (15). Although some tissues other than liver gave a degree
of [^{3}H]-leucine incorporation into the immunoprecipitates, electrophoretic analysis revealed this to be non-specific. Small intestine in particular showed no detectable apo VLDL-B synthesis.
This is interesting since Blue & Williams (46) have recently found
that rooster small intestine does support a significant degree of
estrogen-independent apo VLDL-B synthesis. The ontogeny of basal
apo VLDL-B gene expression in different organs thus appears to be
quite distinctive.

Apo VLDL-II
The kinetics of induction of apo VLDL-II are very similar to
those for vitellogenin (47) (Blue & Williams, unpublished results).
The ontogenic studies reported in Fig. 6 are thus based on 48 hr
treatment of embryos with estrogen. Although as presented in
terms of % protein synthesis the increment of induction of apo
VLDL-II does not seem to be as great as for vitellogenin or apo
VLDL-B, correction for leucine content and the molecular weight of
the protein reveals a considerable amount of synthesis evident
from days 11-12 of embryonic development. This pattern of estrogen
responsiveness is close to that observed for apo VLDL-B and quite
distinctive from that found earlier for vitellogenin.

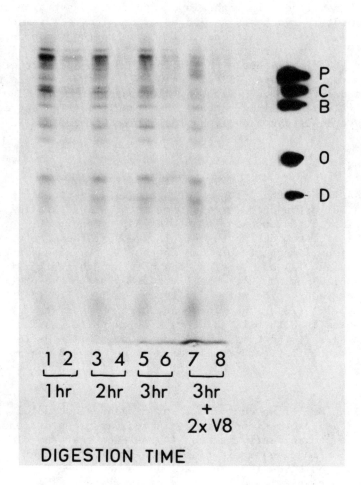

Fig. 7: Analysis of apo VLDL-B immunoprecipitates by the limited
proteolytic cleavage

Apo VLDL-B immunoprecipitates from liver supernatants of
tamoxifen or estradiol-treated embryos were subjected to
V-8 proteolytic cleavage by the method of Cleveland et al.
(34) and analysed by SDS/10% acrylamide slab gel electrophoresis and fluorography. Lanes 1,3,5,7, estrogen-
treated; Lanes 2,4,6,8, tamoxifen-treated 17-day embryos.
Marker proteins: P, phosphorylase; C, conalbumin; B,
bovine serum albumin; O, ovalbumin and D, DNase.

The basal level of synthesis of apo VLDL-II averages about 1% of total protein synthesis as judged by our indirect immunoprecipitation technique. Although this is corrected for non-specific precipitation using pre-immune serum, we feel that a considerable component of this synthesis is still due to non-specific effects. In the untreated rooster, less than 0.25% of hepatic protein synthesis is due to apo VLDL-II using electrophoretic and fluorographic analysis (Blue & Williams, unpublished results). The estrogen-induced synthesis can clearly be identified as apo VLDL-II by these techniques.

DISCUSSION

Comparison of the ontogeny of estrogenic responses in chick liver and Müllerian duct reveals some interesting parallels, and some distinct differences. In both cases, cytosol estrogen receptor is present from early stages. In the duct the cytosol receptor concentration is much higher than in the liver, reaches a peak earlier (at day 12) and remains constant through the remainder of the incubation period (2). The liver receptor on the other hand exhibits a gradual rise until day 19 and declines to 15-30% of the peak value (13) (23). This low concentration persists for at least 4 weeks in both male and female chickens (C. Lazier, unpublished results). There is however no proportionate decrease in estrogen inducibility of vitellogenin or apo VLDL-B accompanying the receptor loss (12) (A. Elbrecht & C. Lazier, unpublished results).

In both Müllerian duct and liver exogenous estradiol given at days 10-12 can provoke an increase in nuclear receptor concentrations. The stoichiometry is such in the duct that the classical translocation model entirely fits (4). In liver however nuclear accumulation of sites is more than can be accounted for by translocation alone, particularly at the early stages. The duct nuclear receptor responses are maximal by day 15, as is the proportion of nuclear receptor sites which are chromatin-bound (4) (5). This development of the duct receptor system corresponds closely to some, but not all, of the estrogenic responses in the organ. Responses of the first sort include estrogenic stimulation of ornithine decarboxylase activity and of development of epithelial tubular gland cells (6)-(9). Responses which lag behind the apparent maturation of the receptor mechanism include ductal growth, the concentration of ovalbumin mRNA/tubular gland cell and the relative rate of ovalbumin synthesis (10) (11). There is some indication of a limitation in translational capacity of the embryonic organ. The concentration of $mRNA_{ovalbumin}$ molecules/tubular gland cell is about the same on days 15 and 21 after 5 days of estrogen treatment, and the proportion of tubular gland cells in the magnum increases from 11 to 51%, but the relative rate of ovalbumin in synthesis increases from less than 1% to 10% in the same

period.   After hatching, the relative rate of ovalbumin synthesis
increases to over 30% (10).

A fundamental difference in the Müllerian duct and liver responses is the necessity for long term (5 day) primary hormone
treatment of the duct in order to give tubular gland cell differentiation and ovalbumin gene expression.   In liver there is no
evidence that differentiation of specialized cells is necessary
for specific genomic responses (16) and estrogen treatment for 5
hr is sufficient to detect increased apo VLDL-B synthesis (14).
In the hatched chicken, all parenchymal cells appear to be estrogen
responsive (48).   The embryonic liver contains a very high proportion of parenchymal cells (49), although the exact fraction at each
stage has not apparently been systematically studied.   The liver
grows prodigiously through embryogenesis – from 1 mg at day 5, to
100 mg at day 12 and 1g upon hatching (50).   Little is known about
the regulation of avian liver differentiation although it has been
observed that normal in ovo ultrastructural changes over days 5-11
can be obtained in organ culture in the presence of insulin (51).
The ultrastructure at this stage resembles that of the hatched
chicken (50).   It is impossible to say whether receptor development is an autonomous feature programmed in the organ or whether
extrinsic factors, possibly of endocrine origin, are important.

Our observations that the estrogen receptor system is present
in chick liver at days 10-12 and that the VLDL apoproteins are
estrogen-inducible at this time suggests that the receptor and
other components of the regulatory mechanisms are sufficiently
developed to give significant hormonal responses at this time.
This does not appear to be the case for vitellogenin induction,
as measured by the relative rate of synthesis of the protein.   As
discussed earlier, the difference in induction kinetics of apo
VLDL-B on one hand and vitellogenin and apo VLDL-II on the other
is not a sufficient basis for the apparent dissociation.
The possibility exists that there is a trivial explanation based
on the different methods used to incubate liver and prepare the
supernatants in the vitellogenin and VLDL apoprotein experiments.
This seems unlikely, but in view of the recent discovery that
there are 2 distinctive vitellogenins in avian liver (35), we are
examining inducibility of apo VLDL-B and of the 2 vitellogenins
over the critical 10-14 day stages using a highly sensitive direct
electrophoretic analysis of the supernatants.

Temporal dissociation of genomic responses to estrogen in
development raises some interesting possible explanations.
Postulates of receptor heterogeneity and differential development
of specific essential forms of receptor seem unlikely, but await
definitive proof of receptor singularity in target cells.   A more
conventional explanation would lie at the level of chromosome
structure and organization.   Vitellogenin gene regulatory sites may

be inaccessible to receptor or the protein components of the sites
may be underdeveloped at the unresponsive "receptor-positive"
stages. Another possibility is that all of the estrogen responsive
genes are transcribed at days 11-12, but that only the VLDL apoprotein transcripts are properly processed and translated. Such an
explanation could have important implications with regard to the
specificity of these processes. It is not clear whether the translational lag for ovalbumin mRNA in Müllerian duct (referred to
above) is specific to that mRNA, or whether it also applies to
other estrogen-induced proteins such as ovomucoid and conalbumin.

An obvious experimental approach to deal with these considerations would be to investigate inducibility of the estrogen-
responsive genes at the level of the specific mRNA. Recent suc-
cesses in cloning cDNA sequences corresponding to specific hepatic
estrogen-induced mRNAs make this a feasible approach (52) (53).

SUMMARY

We have examined the development of responsiveness to estrogen
by embryonic chick liver with a view to determining common and
unique factors involved in the establishment of different genomic
responses to the hormone. The major apoproteins of chick VLDL,
apo VLDL-B and apo VLDL-II, both appear to be estrogen inducible at
an earlier stage of embryonic development than is vitellogenin.
Apo VLDL-B, but not vitellogenin, exhibits a significant level of
hepatic synthesis in the absence of estrogen treatment. This
basal synthesis is tamoxifen-resistant and is detectable at very
early stages of hepatic development, well before estrogen responsiveness is seen. Immunological cross-reactivity, electrophoretic
behavior and the results of limited proteolysis mapping suggest
that the apo VLDL-B synthesized under basal and estrogen-stimulated
conditions is the same (or a very similar) protein.

Inducibility of the VLDL apoproteins appears to parallel the
appearance of the hepatic estrogen receptor system at days 10-12
while vitellogenin induction is delayed by several days. Cytosol
receptor concentration undergoes a gradual increase up to the 19th
day of development and thereafter declines. The properties of the
19-day receptor are very similar to those of cytosol receptor in
hatched chicks, but the fall in concentration does not appear to be
proportionately related to inducibility of estrogenic responses, as
measured by the relative rates of synthesis in vitro.

ACKNOWELDGEMENTS

These studies were supported by grants from the Medical
Research Council of Canada (MA 4880) to C.B.L., and from the
National Institutes of Health, U.S.A. (AM 18171) to D.L.W. Tamox-
ifen citrate was a gift to D.L.W. from Imperial Chemical Industries
Ltd.

REFERENCES

1. Hamburger, V. & Hamilton, H.L. (1951) J. Morphol. 88, 49-92.
2. Teng, C.S. & Teng, C.T. (1975) Biochem. J. 150, 183-190.
3. Teng, C.S. & Teng, C.T. (1975) Biochem. J. 150, 191-194.
4. Teng, C.S. & Teng, C.T. (1976) Biochem. J. 154, 1-9.
5. Teng, C.S. & Teng, C.T. (1978) Biochem. J. 172, 361-370.
6. Teng, C.S. & Teng, C.T. (1979) in "The Ontogeny of Receptor and Reproductive Hormone Action" (Hamilton, T.H., Clark, J.H. & Sadler, W.H., eds), Raven Press, New York, pp. 421-440.
7. Teng, C.T. & Teng, C.S. (1980) Biochem. J. 185, 169-175.
8. Teng, C.S. & Teng, C.T. (1978) Biochem. J. 176, 143-149.
9. Andrews, G.K. & Teng, C.S. (1979) Biochem. J. 182, 257-269.
10. Andrews, G.K. & Teng, C.S. (1979) Biochem. J. 182, 271-286.
11. Teng, C.S. (1980) Adv. Biosci. 25, 77-94.
12. Lazier, C.B. (1978) Biochem. J. 174, 143-152.
13. Lazier, C.B. (1980) Adv. Biosci. 25, 125-139.
14. Nadin-Davis, S.A., Lazier, C.B., Capony, F. & Williams, D.L. (1980) Submitted for publication.
15. Nadin-Davis, S.A. (1979) M.Sc. Thesis, Dalhousie University.
16. Tata, J.R. & Smith, D.F. (1979) Rec. Prog. Hor. Res. 35, 47-95.
17. Williams, D.L. (1979) Biochemistry 18, 1056-1063.
18. Chan, L., Jackson, R.L., O'Malley, B.W. & Means, A.R. (1976) J. Clin. Invest. 58, 368-379.
19. Murthy, U.S. & Adiga, P.R. (1978) Biochem. J. 170, 331-335.
20. Lee, D.C., McKnight, G.S. & Palmiter, R.D. (1978) J. Biol. Chem. 253, 3494-3503.
21. Williams, D.L., Wang, S.Y. & Capony, F. (1979) J. Steroid Biochem. 11, 231-236.
22. Lazier, C.B. & Haggarty, A.J. (1979) Biochem. J. 180, 347-353.
23. Gschwendt, M. (1977) Eur. J. Biochem. 80, 461-468.
24. Gschwendt, M. & Kittstein, W. (1974) Biochim. Biophys. Acta 361, 84-96.
25. Lebeau, M.C., Massol, N., Lemonnier, M., Schmelck, P.-H., Mester, J. & Baulieu, E.-E. (1977) in "Hormonal Receptors in Digestive Tract Physiology" (Bonfils, S., Fromageot, P. & Rosselin, G., eds), North Holland Publishers, Amsterdam, pp. 183-195.
26. Alberga, A., Tran, A. & Baulieu, E.-E. (1979) Nucleic Acids Res. 7, 2031-2044.
27. Barrack, E.R., Hawkins, E.F. & Coffey, D.S. (1979) in "Steroid Hormone Receptor Systems" (Leavitt, W.W. & Clark, J.A., eds), Plenum Press, New York, pp. 47-70.
28. Gschwendt, M. (1977) FEBS Lett. 75, 272-276.
29. Jackson, R.L., Lin, M.Y., Chan, L. & Means, A.R. (1977) J. Biol. Chem. 252, 250-253.
30. Burns, A.T.H., Deeley, R.G., Gordon, J.I., Udell, D.S., Mullinix, K.P. & Goldberger, R.F. (1978) Proc. Nat. Acad. Sci. (U.S.A.) 75, 1815-1819.

31. Joss, U., Bassand, C. & Dierks-Ventling, C. (1976) FEBS
     Lett. 66, 293-298.
32. Luskey, K.L., Brown, M.S. & Goldstein, J.L. (1974) J. Biol.
     Chem. 249, 5939-5947.
33. Capony, F. & Williams, D.L. (1980) Biochemistry, in press.
34. Cleveland, D.W., Fischer, S.G., Kirschner, N.W. & Laemmli,
     U.K. (1977) J.Biol. Chem. 252, 1102-1113.
35. Wang, S.-Y. & Williams, D.L. (1980) Biochemistry, in press.
36. Bonner, W.M. & Laskey, R.A. (1974) Eur. J. Biochem. 46,
     83-88.
37. Schneider, W. & Gschwendt, M. (1977) Hoppe-Seyler's Z.
     Physiol. Chem. 358, 1583-1590.
38. Clark, J.H., Markaverich, B., Upchurch, S., Eriksson, H. &
     Hardin, J.W. (1979) in "Steroid Hormone Receptor Systems"
     (Leavitt, W.W. & Clark, J.H., eds), Plenum Press, New York,
     pp. 17-46.
39. Deeley, R.G., Gordon, J.J., Burns, A.T., Mullinix, K.P.,
     Binastein, M. & Goldberger, R.F. (1977) J. Biol. Chem. 252,
     8310-8319.
40. Jost, J.-P., Ohno, T., Panyim, S. & Schuerch, A.P. (1978)
     Eur. J. Biochem. 84, 355-364.
41. Schjeide, O.A., Kelley, J.L., Schjeide, S., Milius, R. &
     Alaupovic, P. (1980) Comp. Biochem. Physiol. 65B, 231-237.
42. Jordan, V.C., Clark, E.R. & Allen, K.E. (1980) in "Non-
     Steroidal Antioestrogens: Subcellular Pharmacology and
     Antitumour Activity" (Sutherland, R.L. & Jordan, V.C., eds),
     Academic Press, London, in press.
43. Sutherland, R.L., Mester, J. & Baulieu, E.-E. (1977) Nature
     267, 434-435.
44. Lazier, C.B. & Alford, W.S. (1977) Biochem. J. 164, 659-667.
45. Lazier, C.B., Capony, F. & Williams, D.L. (1980) in "Non-
     Steroidal Antioestrogens: Subcellular Pharmacology and Anti-
     tumour Activity" (Sutherland, R.L. & Jordan, V.C., eds),
     Academic Press, London, in press.
46. Blue, M.-L. & Williams, D.L. (1980) manuscript submitted.
47. Chan, L., Jackson, R.L. & Means, A.R. (1978) Circulation
     Res. 43, 209-217.
48. Wachsmuth, E.D. & Jost, J.-P. (1976) Biochim. Biophys. Acta
     437, 454-461.
49. Skea, B.R. & Nemeth, A.M. (1969) Proc. Nat. Acad. Sci.
     (U.S.A.) 64, 795-802.
50. Benzo, C.A. & Nemeth, A.M. (1971). J. Cell Biol. 48, 235-247.
51. Benzo, C.A. & De La Haba, G. (1972) J. Cell Physiol. 79, 53-
     64.
52. King, C.R., Udell, D.S. & Deeley, R.G. (1979) J. Biol. Chem.
     254, 6781-6786.
53. Ohno, T., Cozens, P.J., Cato, A.C.B. & Jost, J.-P. (1980)
     Biochim. Biophys. Acta 606, 34-46.

BIOCHEMICAL AND ESTROGENIC ACTIVITY OF SOME DIETHYLSTILBESTROL METABOLITES AND ANALOGS IN THE MOUSE UTERUS

Kenneth S. Korach

Laboratory of Reproductive and Developmental Toxicology
National Institute of Environmental Health Sciences
P.O. Box 12233, Research Triangle Park, NC   27709

INTRODUCTION

Diethylstilbestrol (DES) is a potent non-steroidal estrogen first synthesized and described by Dodds in 1938 (1). The compound has been used extensively as a medicinal estrogen due to its oral potency which is comparable to the natural estrogen 17β-estradiol. In recent years, several reports from studies with humans have indicated an association between in utero exposure to DES and the development of reproductive tract cancers (2,3). Vaginal adeno-carcinoma has been reported in exposed female offspring (4). Male human subjects have not shown any indication of cancers but reproductive tract lesions are present (5). In addition to these lesions, the offspring in both sexes suffer from a variety of fertility problems (6).

Prenatal DES exposure in laboratory animals such as mice (7), rats (8), and hamsters (9) has indicated some of the same findings as those reported in humans. The exact mechanism of the DES effects is not yet known, which leads to a great deal of speculation concerning the site of the effect. Secondly, the role of DES itself in this problem is still unresolved. The question of whether DES produces toxic effects by itself or through some metabolic product is of continuing interest. Metzler has shown that DES can be oxidatively metabolized to a number of reactive products. These products have been shown to interact with cellular macromolecules (10) and supports earlier work suggesting covalent binding of DES to DNA as a possible mechanism of its carcinogenesis (11).

A second question involves whether the toxic action of DES is manifested through its potent estrogenic activity or through its above-mentioned chemical metabolism. Recently, the concept of persistent estrogen stimulation or hyperestrogenicity has been suggested in a cause/effect relationship to the induction of reproductive tract lesions (12). Therefore, we became interested in the estrogenicity of DES and some of its metabolites and analogs. Prior to this report, we have indicated the various activities of these DES compounds as falling into two classes: those which retain their estrogenic properties and those which become inactive (13). In addition, we found a divergent activity of these compounds when comparing their in vivo and in vitro activity (14). In this report a further description is made of the estrogenic activity and intracellular mechanism of some DES compounds as it relates to their action in the mouse uterus.

MATERIALS AND METHODS

General Procedures. Protein concentrations of all cytosol preparations were determined in duplicate by the method of Lowry et al. (15). DNA was quantified by the ethidium bromide procedure as outlined by LePecq and Paoletti (16) or by the Burton procedure (17) using calf thymus DNA (Sigma Chemical Co.) as the standard. DNA synthesis was measured by the method of Harris and Gorski as previously described (18). All other chemicals were reagent grade and obtained from commercial sources. Proton NMR was performed on a Varian XL-100 by Dr. Richard Cox of the Chemistry Section, NIEHS. Stability of the various compounds was checked by thin-layer chromatography (TLC) in previously described systems (19). Separation and isolation of pseudo-DES was accomplished by Dr. J. Kepler using high pressure liquid chromatography (HPLC) (Waters Associates).

Steroids and DES Compounds. [2,4,6,7-^{3}H] Estradiol-17β (110 Ci/mmol) and ^{3}H-R-5020 (87 Ci/mmol) were purchased from New England Nuclear (Boston, MA) and brought to greater than 98% radiochemical purity by TLC (benzene/ethyl ether 1:1). A Varian radiochromatogram scanner (LB-2723) was used for analysis; steroids were also identified by reference to simultaneously chromatographed unlabeled standards. Unlabeled compounds were obtained from Steraloids, Inc. (Wilton, NH) and used without further purification. The three indanyl ring compounds, indenestrol A (IA), indenestrol B (IB), and indanestrol (I) were synthesized by Dr. Manfred Metzler (University of Wurzburg) by the method described by Adler and Hagglund (20). Pseudo-DES (PD) was synthesized by Dr. Jack Kepler (Research Triangle Institute). The other compounds were previous gifts of Dr. Manfred Metzler and were synthesized and characterized as described elsewhere (13,19).

Binding Assays. Nuclear estrogen receptor levels were quantified by the exchange assay of Anderson et al. (21) as recently modified (22). Cytoplasmic estrogen receptors were determined by the protamine sulfate procedure (23). The equilibrium competition assay of Korenman (24) and cytosol receptor association rates were determined as previously described (25). Cytosolic progesterone receptor levels were determined by the method outlined by Leavitt et al. (26) using labeled R-5020 as the assay ligand.

Uterotropic Assays. Bioassay experiments were performed identical to previous reports (13,14). The dynamic uterotropic assay of Katzenellenbogen et al. (27) was utilized as indicated earlier (14). Immature (21 day) and ovariectomized adult CD-1 mice were used throughout these experiments.

RESULTS

A study of the estrogenicity of DES and its metabolites and analogs should certainly involve a description of the compound's metabolism. Although that is not the purpose of this paper, a diagrammatic representation of various metabolic routes for DES is given in Fig. 1. The reader is directed toward a recent review (28) and the work of various investigators who have studied DES metabolism in detail and whose papers present the chemical evidence and structural identification of the various compounds (29,30,31). A new nomenclature recently described by Metzler and McLachlan will be used throughout the text to describe the various compounds (32). Pathways A and F involving ring hydroxylation of DES were described by Engel and associates using an in vitro system of rat liver microsomes (33,34). Work from in vivo metabolism studies using Syrian hamsters and rats has supported those findings (35,38). In addition, there are a number of possible combinations of metabolic routes. An example is the identification of an ortho quinone dienestrol compound which presumably would arise from pathways A or F and E. PD has been identified as a product of bacterial metabolism of DES. This is relevant to in vivo studies when you consider the enterohepatic circulation of DES. Therefore, pathway B is suggested and illustrates ψ-DES as both a possible metabolic product and precursor to 1-hydroxy-ψ-DES. This compound is a significant urinary metabolite in the mouse (36). Identification of urinary metabolites has also demonstrated the formation of 1-hydroxy-DES (28). Since significant amounts of these compounds are found in rodent urine, it is possible that pathway C results in their formation as an end product with no further metabolic activity to form indenestrol. Z,Z-Dienestrol is the major urinary metabolite of DES in all species studied so far (28). The description and mechanism of its formation has been studied primarily by Metzler (38). Pathways D and E involving different intermediates have been suggested

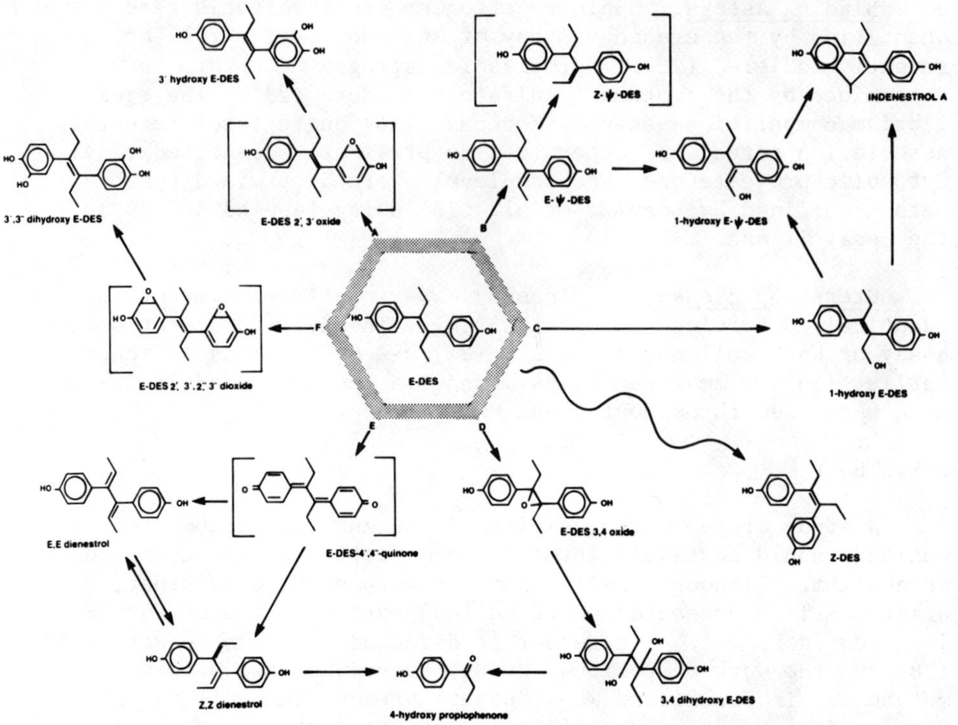

Figure 1. Proposed Pathway of DES Metabolism

in the past to be responsible for its formation (10,38). It should
be evident from Fig. 1 and the above-mentioned text that the
hormonal, toxic and/or fetotoxic nature of DES may reside in one
or a number of the above-mentioned compounds.

Considering the extensive metabolism of DES, it is interesting
to determine whether the established hormonal activity resides in
the parent compound or one of the various metabolites. Estrogenicity of these compounds was analyzed in the mouse uterus
because of the marked sensitivity of this tissue to estrogens (39)
and because of its possible correlation with previous studies
involving metabolism (19) and toxicity (7) of DES in the mouse.
We know the binding of the hormone with the soluble cytoplasmic
receptor molecule is the primary interaction leading to subsequent
hormonal responses (see Rev. 40). This binding can be studied
directly using labeled compounds or can be determined by using a
comparative binding analysis (22). The data can then be analyzed
according to the method of Korenman (24). In Fig. 2 we illustrate
the binding affinity of various DES metabolites under equilibrium

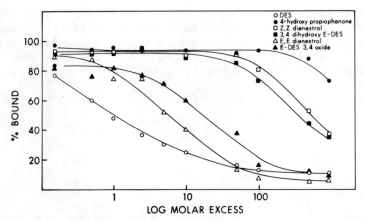

<u>Figure 2.</u> Competitive equilibrium binding plot of mouse
uterine cytosol and DES metabolites. A 100 µl aliquot of mouse
uterine cytosol was incubated with 5 nM labeled estradiol and one
of the following concentrations (1 nM to 2.5 µM) of unlabeled
competitors. The compounds are denoted in the figure. Incubations
were allowed to achieve equilibrium at 4°C for 18 hr and the bound
receptor was assayed by protamine precipitation as described in the
Methods section.

binding conditions. DES is included as a comparative standard to
illustrate the high affinity binding of the parent compound. A
previous study has shown that DES interacts with mouse uterine
cytosol in a similar manner as the natural ligand 17β-estradiol
(13). In these experiments the only two compounds which demonstrated reasonable binding affinity were E,E-dienestrol and E-DES
3,4-oxide. The other three compounds which are possible components
of metabolic pathways D and E did not show strong interaction
with the receptor. Preliminary binding experiments (data not
presented) with the dicatechol-DES (3',4',3",4"-tetrahydroxy E-DES)
proposed in pathway F have indicated an affinity for the mouse
cytosol receptor which is in the range of E,E-dienestrol.

Bouton and Raynaud (41) have pointed out the use of multiple
assay conditions for determining the interaction of various
steroid derivatives with soluble receptor molecules. Figure 3
illustrates the binding patterns of additional DES metabolites
and analogs under a variety of experimental conditions. In
Fig. 3A are the competitive binding patterns produced under the
same equilibrium conditions as Fig. 2 (e.g., 18 hr, 4°C). DES is
again used as a standard. Both indenestrol isomers, indenestrol
A (IA) and indenestrol B (IB), possess strong binding affinity
which is slightly better than DES. Pseudo-DES (PD) and DES gave
identical patterns, whereas the unsaturated indane derivative,

indanestrol (I), showed poor affinity. When assay conditions
were changed to a shorter time to indicate association, the
compounds with the stronger binding affinity again demonstrated
similar interaction (Fig. 3B). There was a slight parallel shift
to the right for IA and IB but it is unclear how significant this

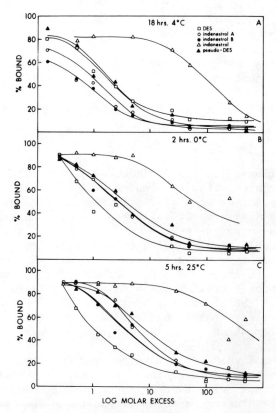

Figure 3. Competitive binding analyses under different
incubation conditions. Amounts of cytosol, labeled estradiol and
competitors were the same as Fig. 2. The compounds are listed in
the figure (□) DES, (○) indenestrol A, (●) indenestrol B,
(△) indanestrol and (▲) pseudo-DES. Incubation conditions were
(A) 18 hr, 4°C; (B) 2 hr, 0°C; and (C) 5 hr, 25°C. Bound receptor
was assayed by protamine precipitation as described in Fig. 2.

Table 1. Binding Affinities and Uterotropic
Activities of Various DES Compounds.

Compound	Structure	C_{50}[a]	K_a[b]	K_a[c]	Doubling[d] dose	Metabolic[e] pathway
ESTRADIOL-17β		1.6±0.5	15.0±0.3	12.5	5.0±1.0	—
INDENESTROL A		0.7±0.1	22.0±3.0	14.0	107±14	B,C
INDENESTROL B		0.7+−0.1	22.0±6.0	15.0	111±8	B,C
E-DES		1.0±0.1	15.0±2.0	14.0	7.0±2	—
E-Pseudo-DES		1.1±0.2	15.0±3.0	14.5	600±20	B
E,E-Dienestrol		5.0±0.8	4.2±0.6	6.2	14.2±6	E
E-DES 3,4 oxide		17±2	1.0±0.2	—	14.1±2	D
INDANESTROL		60±5	0.3±0.03	48.0	1,120±50	B,C
Z-DES		130±10	0.12±0.05	—	—	—
3,4 dihydroxy E-DES		334 = 92	0.07±0.03	—	3,374±760	D
Z,Z Dienestrol		367±72	0.05±0.01	—	15,000	D,E
4-hydroxy propiophenone		1000±50	—	—	—	D,E

a) Nanomolar concentration of competitor required for 50% inhibition of specific binding of [³H]-estradiol. Results are expressed as the mean + S.E. for a minimum of four determinations.
b) Calculated values of K_a in nM⁻¹ units using the C_{50} value by the method of Korenman (24).
c) Calculated value of K_a in nM⁻¹ units from data generated in Fig. 4 using a competitive inhibitor model (44).
d) Values are expressed as the dose (μg/kg) of compound required to produce a two-fold increase above the control values of the uterine wet weight/body weight ratio in 21-day year-old CD-1 mice treated for 3 days.
e) Designation of the metabolic pathway of which the compound is a component as illustrated in Fig. 1.

was. I showed poor binding affinity under these conditions
similar to that seen in Fig. 3A but appeared to show a slight
parallel shift to the left. This might suggest a better association
of this ligand with the receptor than determined from Fig. 3A.
Conditions that demonstrate differences in dissociation (Fig. 3C)
indicated a similar interaction for DES as in Fig. 2 or 3A, but
the IA, IB and PD compounds showed slight parallel shifting to the
right. The I compound was also shifted significantly to the right
of the curve. According to Bouton and Raynaud (41) this would
indicate a faster dissociation of the compounds from the receptor
as compared to DES.

The determination of whether a compound may be interacting
with the receptor in a competitive or noncompetitive manner (see
Rev. 42) is difficult to ascertain from semi-logarithmic plots
as used in Fig. 2 and 3. Although the shapes of the curves were
similar and parallel shifting did occur, which was suggestive of
a competitive interaction differing only in binding affinity, a
further analysis was performed. Uterine cytosol was incubated
with a variety of competitor concentrations (e.g., DES metabolites)
in the form of a saturation analysis (22). The concentrations of
metabolites used were judged as being below, equal, or above the
proposed competitor concentration from the binding curve (Fig. 2
and 3, Table 1). This wide range of competitor concentrations
gave a complete analysis which helped to eliminate a number of
possible noncompetitive types of interactions (43).

The data in Fig. 4 were obtained using PD as the competitor
and are representative of curves generated for most of the
metabolites studied. In all cases, the curves gave a pattern
which was interpreted as being indicative of a competitive
interaction. There was no indication of irreversible binding
which could have been detected from these analyses (44).

Recent work has suggested multiple estrogen binding components
in uterine cytosol (15). This raised the question of whether the
metabolites were interacting with the receptor or some other
binder. Mouse uterine cytosol was incubated with increasing concentrations of unlabeled metabolites and a saturating concentration
of labeled estradiol and then analyzed for component binding on
sucrose gradients (14). Results of such an analysis are illustrated
in Fig. 5 and demonstrate a definite dose inhibition of the
estradiol binding to mouse cytosol receptor. Approximately 50 nM
or 10-fold excess of compound was required to inhibit 50% of the
estradiol binding. Under these experimental conditions, using
glycerol in the buffer, the mouse uterine cytosol sediments at
approximately 6 s (22). This is clearly evident in the figure and
illustrates a receptor specific interaction. Secondly, the data
suggest there is no shifting of binding forms due to the binding
of the metabolites since all interactions were detected in the 6 s

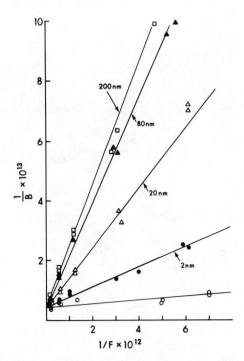

Figure 4.   Lineweaver-Burke analysis of competitive interactions
with mouse cytosol receptor.   Cytosol samples (100 μl) were
incubated with labeled estradiol (0.2 to 5.0 nM) (○) above or in
the presence of (●) 2 nM, (△) 20 nM, (▲) 80 nM or (□) 200 nM
of unlabeled pseudo-DES.   Incubations were performed at 4°C for 18
hr.   Bound and unbound fractions were determined as previously
described (22).   Unweighed linear regression analysis of the lines
gave correlation coefficients > 0.9.

region of the gradient.   Figure 5 shows the results of studies
using IA, but additional experiments with a number of the other
compounds gave similar findings (data not presented).

    To demonstrate whether the compounds could react rapidly with
the cytosol receptor to either interfere or block the binding of
estradiol, a study was performed on the association rate reaction
of the receptor.   These studies are designed to measure and
investigate the early initial rates of association of the ligand
and the receptor (23,25).   Data from these studies are presented
in Fig. 6 using IA as the ligand.   There is a clear diminution of
the association rate when the receptor is pre-incubated with the
metabolite.   A dose-related inhibition is seen with between one-
and five-fold excess of compound required to block 50% of the
reaction.   Similar studies using some of the other metabolites
have demonstrated comparable results.

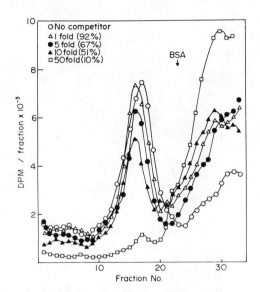

Figure 5. Sucrose density gradient analysis of mouse uterine cytosol binding of indenestrol A. A 500 µl aliquot of mouse uterine cytosol was incubated for 4 hr at 4°C with 5 nM of labeled estradiol and the following concentrations of unlabeled IA. None (◯) , 5 nM (△), 25 nM (●), 50 nM (▲) or 250 nM (□). After the incubation, 400 µl aliquots were layered on chilled, preformed 5-20% sucrose gradients and processed as previously described (14). A bovine serum albumin (BSA) standard was processed simultaneously and its position is given in the figure.

        A composite of the in vitro receptor binding data from studies with the mouse uterine cytosol receptor and the various compounds is given in Table 1. Some of these data are tabulated from previous studies (13,14). The table lists the C_{50} value for each compound studied, which was obtained from the equilibrium binding curves in Fig. 1 and 3A. This C_{50} was used to calculate an apparent K_a for the metabolite cytosol receptor interaction using the method of Korenman (24) and is also listed in Table 1. Lineweaver-Burke plots were constructed from the data generated in Fig. 4 and an approximate K_a' was calculated according to a competitive inhibitor model (44). These values are listed in Table 1 for the compounds studied. Since the amount of compound was limited, not all of the compounds were investigated in this manner.

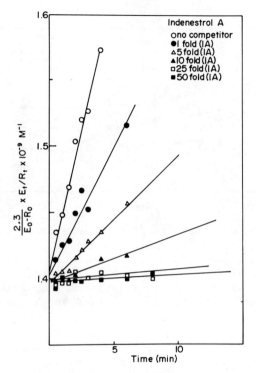

Figure 6. A series of association rate reactions (24) were performed on a group of samples preincubated for 2 hr with unlabeled competitor as described in Fig. 5. Results are single aliquot determinations and rate calculations are based on lines having a correlation coefficient > 0.9.

The in vivo estrogenicity of these compounds was tested in a bioassay using stimulation of the immature mouse uterus. Table 1 gives the dose of compound required to produce twice the uterine weight increase relative to control values. The response curves generated from such studies gave the classical sigmoid shape (data not shown). The metabolites gave similar curves as DES, but differed by parallel shifting to the right, indicating greater dose requirements to elicit the response. It is apparent from the table that the in vivo response of the compounds is not directly related to its cytosol receptor affinity. The IA and IB which possessed similar high affinity for the receptor showed rather poor estrogenicity, requiring a 20-fold difference for stimulation. PD was even a poorer estrogen and showed a requirement of approximately 100-fold the DES or estradiol doses. I, which is a saturated isomer of IA or IB possessed poor binding and estrogenic activity. Two compounds studied, E,E-dienestrol and E-DES 3,4-oxide, showed rather good estrogenic activity and binding affinity.

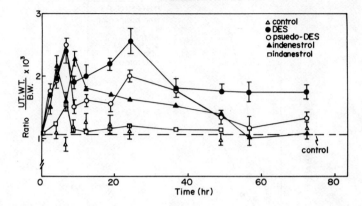

<u>Figure 7</u>. Temporal pattern of uterine stimulation produced
by some DES metabolites. Sexually immature (21 day old) CD-1 mice
were injected with either 100 µl of saline/ethanol (△), 20 µg/kg
doses of DES (●), PD (○), IA (▲) or I (□). At the specified
time, animals were killed and uteri were removed, trimmed of fat,
blotted and weighed. Results are expressed as the uterine weight
(mg) to body weight (g) ratio.

The last three compounds listed, which are components in the D
and E metabolic schemes illustrated in Fig. 1, showed very poor
binding affinity for the cytosol receptor with C_{50} and K_a values
which were 300-fold that of DES. This correlated with the <u>in vivo</u>
estrogenicity of these compounds which was 600 to 3000-fold less
than DES.

    In order to further study the variant relationship between
receptor binding of DES metabolites and their biological activity,
the uterotropic response of these particular compounds was investigated as a temporal event similar to the experiments of
Katzenellenbogen et al. (27). In Fig. 7, the uterine wet weight
increase is followed after a single injection of compound. DES
(20 µg/kg) gives a biphasic result with early stimulation at 4 to
6 hr and a second stimulation which peaks at 24 hr. Values then
decline slightly but stayed significantly elevated above control.
IA or IB (not shown) gave comparable early increases to those of
DES, but the response never peaked again and continually decreased
until it was similar to control by 56 hr. PD gave both an early
and a late increase in uterine weight, but the response started to
decline, similar to IA, and approached control values by 56 hr.
A 20 µg/kg dose of I gave a very transient response with minimal
stimulation by 6 hr which returned to control values by 8 hr and
did not increase again.

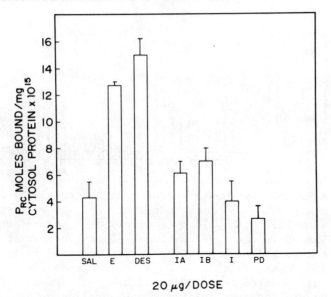

Figure 8.   Induction of uterine cytosol progesterone receptor.
Groups of 4 castrate (7 day) mice were injected with either 100
µl of saline/ethanol or a 20 µg/kg dose of one of the DES compounds
listed.   Animals were sacrificed 24 hr later and the uteri were
removed and progesterone receptor determined by the technique
outlined in the Methods section.   Data is expressed as the femtamoles
of specific progesterone binding per mg cytosol protein.

Estrogen stimulation and response in the uterus has been
linked to the induction of cytosolic progesterone receptor (P-
receptor) (26).   This experimental end point was investigated in
the castrate mouse uterus 24 hr after a single injection of the
various metabolites.   Figure 8 illustrates the levels of cytosol
P-receptor induced by the compounds.   Estradiol and DES stimulate
receptor levels by three- to four-fold at a dose of 20 µg/kg,
which is comparable to the dose used in the uterotropic assays of
Fig. 7.   Both I and PD produced levels which were equivalent or
slightly below control values.   IA and IB produced levels which
were only slightly above control with the level of IB consistently
higher than IA.

Growth and stimulation of cell division in the uterus have
been used as major end points of estrogen action (46).   Since all
compounds except I showed significant net weight increases above
control at 24 hr (Fig. 7), we investigated whether or not these
compounds could stimulate DNA synthesis in the uterus at 24 hr
after a single injection.   The dose response of this effect is
shown in Fig. 9.   The data are expressed as the percent increase

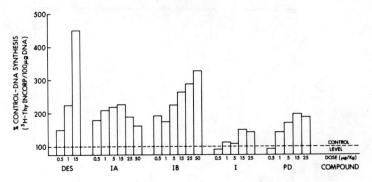

Figure 9. DNA synthesis in the mouse uterus 24 hr after exposure to some DES compounds. Castrate animals were injected in groups of 4 animals with saline (control) or a dose of one of the compounds listed in the figure. Twenty-four hours after injection the animals were killed and DNA synthesis measured by the method of Harris and Gorski (18). The data are expressed as the labeled thymidine incorporated into 100 µg of DNA. The results are then expressed as the response relative to the saline control. Each compound group has a saline control and the respective values are based on that control.

above the saline control which is given as 100%. DES gave a significant stimulation with a dose of 0.5 µg/kg and the response continued to increase over four-fold at 15 µg/kg dose. PD gave a weaker effect than DES at the doses used in these experiments and never matched the response of the 1 µg/kg DES even at a 25-fold higher dose.

I showed the poorest response of all the compounds studied with doses of 5 µg/kg not stimulating DNA synthesis above the control levels. A 15 or 24 µg/kg dose of I gave a partial response which did not appear to show a further increase. The unsaturated indenestrol isomers gave responses which were somewhat better than I and PD. At lower doses of IA or IB (0.5-1.0 µg/kg) the response was comparable to DES; at the higher doses (15-50 µg/kg) the overall response was significantly lower. DNA synthesis patterns with IA showed a progressive rise in activity which then declined from doses of 15-50 µg/kg whereas IB showed a pattern which progressively increased from 5-50 µg/kg.

The varying uterotropic responses observed in our studies such as the bioassay response (Table 1), uterotropic stimulation (Fig. 7), progesterone receptor synthesis (Fig. 8) and DNA synthesis (Fig. 9) may be due to variation in receptor translocation and distribution. These patterns for cytosol and nuclear estrogen receptors are illustrated in Fig. 10. Saline controls did not

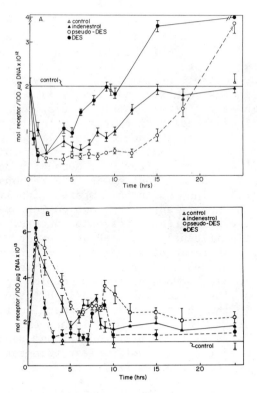

Figure 10. Mouse uterine receptor distribution pattern after treatment with DES compounds. Adult castrate (5 day) mice were injected with either saline ($\triangle$), unlabeled DES (10 µg/kg) ($\bullet$) or 20 µg/kg doses of PD ($\bigcirc$) or IA ($\blacktriangle$). At appropriate times, a group of three animals were killed and the tissue processed for cytosol (A) or nuclear (B) receptor levels. Specifics of the receptor assay techniques are described in the Methods section. Results are the mean $\pm$ S.D. of triplicate samples.

vary greater than 2% over the 24-hr time course of the experiment. DES (10 µg/kg dose) shows a characteristic pattern of depletion and replenishment of cytosol receptor (Fig. 10A). Replenishment equals the zero time control levels by 10 hrs and exceeds these levels for up to 24 hrs. IA depletes the receptor in a similar manner, but does not replenish the receptor at a comparable rate. In the experiments performed thus far, we have not noticed any excessive replenishment with this analog similar to DES. In experiments performed with PD, there was a consistent pattern of depletion with delayed replenishment. Although, contrary to the indenestrol data, there is some excess replenishment with PD similar to DES.

Nuclear receptor patterns varied between the three compounds (Fig. 10B). DES gave a pattern similar to that recently reported for estradiol (22,47). There is an initial translocation event at 1 hr which then declines to control values by 3 hrs. The nuclear levels remain near control for up to 7 hrs, at which time there is a second nuclear increase in receptor levels (7.5-9 hrs). The values then remain near control from 10-24 hrs. Indenestrol shows an identical level of translocation at 1 hr, but appears to cause retention of the complex in the nuclei for a longer period of time. There is a minimal nuclear level reached at 5 hrs which then increases from 6.5 to 8 hrs. After this second increase, which appears to be similar in magnitude to the DES response, there is a fall to near control values which then stays slightly elevated for the remainder of the experiment. PD shows nuclear receptor pattern similar to IA, but even a greater retention occurs. The minimum level (~6 hr) is significantly elevated above that in the control or the DES group. Clearance of receptor IA or PD complex from the nuclear compartment showed similar rates, which were slower than those of the DES complex. More of the PD complex appeared to stay in the nucleus than the other two compounds, but the amounts of receptor present in the nucleus at 7-8 hrs were equivalent. The PD levels then increased again around 9-10 hrs and stayed significantly elevated up to 24 hrs. Additional results indicate that there were no further peaks of nuclear receptor for any of the compounds after the increases at 7-9 hrs.

DISCUSSION

It appears from recent metabolism work (28) that the metabolic fate of DES is simply not conjugation and excretion (48). Instead, as diagrammed in Figure 1, there is a considerable amount of oxidative metabolism (28). The question of the effectiveness of DES as a hormone and/or toxic agent has to also consider the hormonal activity of the metabolic products. It should again be pointed out that the pathways in Figure 1 are from reported pathways (28) or are the authors' own interpretation of pathways suggested in other reports (28,34). It should also be pointed out, that in some cases only some of the possible isomers of the compounds are illustrated, but this is mainly because these are the structures suggested from the metabolic studies. Secondly, various compounds are unstable and have not as yet been isolated such as the ring epoxide compounds in pathways A and F. Although the synthesis and isolation of the catechol DES compounds has been made (33,34), Z,Z-dienestrol is the major urinary metabolite of DES in all species studied (28). The compound had been suggested to arise through a stilbene epoxide (38) but recent studies indicate that it may occur through some peroxidase mediated reactions (10). The compound is weakly estrogenic, so its formation would result in a decreased or inactivity of the DES dose. Its isomeric form

E,E-dienestrol, on the other hand, possess good in vitro and in vivo activity, although this isomer has not been isolated and apparently is not formed metabolically in the body (38).

Pathway D shows a metabolic pattern which progressively decreases in estrogenic potency, since the E-DES 3,4-oxide remains fairly active. The dihydroxy compound shows a significant difference in activity of some 20-fold with the receptor and 200-fold in vivo. This large decrease in uterotropic activity may be due to the compounds further breakdown in vivo to either Z,Z-dienestrol or the cleavage product 4-hydroxy propiophenone which are both hormonally inactive. The Z-DES isomer was reported by Winkler et al. (49) to be poorly estrogenic in vivo, our receptor binding data (Table 1) would support those findings. How effective this isomerization of E-DES to Z-DES is in reducing the activity of DES in the body is unknown, mainly because of the lack of knowledge concerning how much of the isomer is formed in vivo. The chemical reactivity of the possible ring oxide compounds in pathways A and F has been discussed previously (10,33). Their hormonal activity on the other hand has never been determined, primarily due to their chemical instability in the assays. Although, as mentioned above, preliminary results using a dicatechol DES compound have indicated good cytosol receptor interactions with an affinity similar to E,E-dienestrol. Additional and more complete studies with the ring oxide compounds must await better synthetic procedures.

The final pathways B and C involve metabolites in which isomerization of the stilbene double bond (B) or allylic hydroxylation (C) are the main metabolic activities. Compounds in these pathways show the greatest variance in receptor binding activity and uterotropic response. It is difficult, because of this variation in activity, to state whether these compounds should be considered estrogenic or even possibly antiestrogenic. Although, it is obvious from the studies we have performed thus far, the hormonal activity is somewhat less than E-DES. Gottschlich and Metzler (35) have reported an alternative pathway for IA formation, which is not in Figure 1. In their pathway IA is formed from Z,Z-dienestrol. If this were the mechanism and would occur to a significant extent, then the estrogenicity of E-DES would be decreased as it was metabolized to Z,Z-dienestrol, but then hormonal activity would reoccur as IA was formed from Z,Z-dienestrol. Further studies on both the hormonal activity and metabolic pathways of these compounds will be required to more clearly answer these questions.

Our original studies were conducted when IA, IB and PD were considered DES analogs (14). Recently, Metzler's work has indicated these compounds may be actual metabolic products of DES (28).

Therefore, we further investigated their action in the mouse uterus. The data in our study clearly indicates that these compounds interact in vitro in varying degrees with the mouse cytosol estrogen receptor. Data from both the competitive binding curves (Figure 2 and 3) and the Lineweaver-Burke analysis (Figure 4) indicate a competitive interaction. This type of multiple analysis is necessary since we have indicated earlier that a fluorinated derivative of DES does not show competitive binding (50), but may possibly be a metaffinoid inhibitor (43). An attempt was made to establish the association/dissociation rate of the metabolite receptor complex by the methods outlined by Bouton and Raynaud (41). Comparison of Figures 3A, B and C indicates a slight parallel shift of the IA and IB binding curves to the right. The significance of this is unclear, but may suggest a slower association of these ligands with the receptor as compared to DES. Dissociation of the metabolites from the receptor appeared to be significant (Fig. 3C) since the pattern with I shifted from a C_{50} of ~60 nM to ~200 nM. The IA, IB and PD compounds also produced shifts which would be indicative of a faster dissociation rate than DES, but the effect was less dramatic.

Sucrose density gradients (Figure 5) and rate inhibition reactions (Fig. 6) indicate that these compounds act directly with the cytosol receptor. This interaction is specific enough to illustrate a dose effect. Recent studies have suggested multiple binding components in rat uterine cytosol (45). These binders show different steroid binding characteristics than the classical receptor and have different sedimentation properties. Our data indicate that in these studies the compounds are binding to the 6 s high affinity cytosol receptor of the mouse uterus (22). There is no indication from the gradient patterns that competition was occurring with other cytosol binding proteins, since no other regions (e.g., particularly 4 s) showed an inhibition. Actually, the levels increased in the free steroid region of the gradient as expected, since the labeled ligand was being displaced from the receptor. In an earlier study (13), we demonstrated that binding of the various DES compounds did not change the sedimentation properties of the receptor. Although, Jordan and Prestwich (51) have demonstrated that Tamoxifen interacts with both an 8s and 4s binder in the rat uterine cytosol. These findings were only possible when using labeled Tamoxifen which allowed demonstration of the 4s binding. It is possible when labeled DES metabolites are available, that we can investigate whether a similar interaction is occurring in the mouse cytosol with a 4s binder. Until then, we must rely on the competitive inhibition and displacement techniques. Results of the rate inhibition experiments show specificity for the interaction of the DES compounds. We have previously shown the specificity and sensitivity of the technique (25). When IA was used as the competing ligand (Fig. 6) the association rate was inhibited by 50% using a 5-fold excess. This agreed with the concentration required in Fig. 3B (5-fold) after the parallel shifting of the binding curve under the association type analysis. Therefore, IA and some of the other DES compounds could act quite effectively to block the binding of estradiol to the receptor. Such an interaction could possibly alter or hamper the normal estrogenic response in these tissues.

A major point in our studies has involved the determination of the discrepancy between the in vitro and in vivo activities. As shown in Fig. 7, a single injection of the same dose of DES compounds produced similar early responses (0 to 10 hr). DES and PD were the only compounds to give the biphasic uterine response pattern (14,52). This effect was quantitatively greater for DES than PD. IA showed an early response but no later effect. DES, PD and IA appeared to translocate comparable amounts of receptor at 1 hr (Fig. 10) and showed similar early uterotropic responses. This same correlation has been demonstrated earlier with estriol (53). I, on the other hand, gave a very poor response at this dose, which was not surprising considering its binding affinity for the receptor and probably indicates its inability to translocate an effective amount of receptor, possibly because of its rapid dissociation from the receptor (Fig. 3C).

A number of studies have indicated the induction of progesterone cytosol receptor as a correlate to estrogen action (26,54). The DES metabolites used in these studies showed a poorer response than DES in inducing this activity. Although, previous studies (54) with the mouse uterus have indicated 40 hr as the maximum time of progesterone receptor induction after a single injection. We chose 24 hr in order to relate this response to other parameters being investigated (Fig. 7, 9 and 10). The poor response by I is not surprising and probably relates to its poor uterotropic activity (Fig. 7). PD on the other hand, shows P-receptor levels lower than control which is not consistent with its uterotropic response. IA and IB did not show the biphasic or extended uterine stimulation, but did produce a partial P-receptor induction. DES or E_2 produced almost a 4-fold increase which is consistent with a previous report (26). A couple of points should be considered at this time. Since only one time point (e.g., 24 hr) was chosen for these studies, the possibility exists that the compounds may produce varying rates of induction. For example, IA or IB may be starting to stimulate P-receptor synthesis at 24 hr and will give a similar response as DES at some later time. Although, such a weak response with PD at 24 hr would not suggest this mechanism is occurring with this compound. The second point involves specificity and characteristics of the P-receptor induced. Studies are presently in progress to determine what differences, if any, may exist in the induced P-receptor such as sedimentation value

and ligand binding specificity. Since estrogenic substances act
on the liver to increase the concentration of plasma binding
proteins (55), it is important to determine if all the DES compounds
are inducing (i.e., to whatever degree) the same protein. Although,
the assay utilized R-5020 as the binding ligand and this should
have eliminated any interference with the results due to plasma
progesterone binding. Additionally, no experiments have as yet
been performed to determine if these DES compounds could react
with the progesterone receptor.

In an earlier study (14), we indicated that histological
examination of bioassay uteri showed tissue hyperplasia from
treatment with DES, IA and IB. Samples from the PD treatment gave
evidence of cellular hypertrophy. This uterine tissue response
was further investigated in this study by measuring the ability of
these compounds to stimulate DNA synthesis. DES again showed a
significant dose response. Responses by the indenestrol compounds
were effective at the lower doses, but showed a significant diver-
gence in activity at higher doses. As the dose increases IA
produces a decrease in DNA synthesis, while IB continues to produce
an increase. The nuclear receptor distribution from studies with
IA indicated a pattern similar to DES (Fig. 10), but quantitatively
the receptor levels were slightly higher. At present, we have not
performed a complete analysis of receptor distribution using IB to
determine whether the nuclear receptor pattern could explain the
differences in DNA synthesis between the two isomers. This difference in IA and IB activities is indeed an intriguing one, since
the only structural difference in the compounds is the position of
the double bond. Consequently, the structure of I produced by
the indene ring saturation results in a reorientation of the
phenolic rings and weak uterine responses and binding affinity.
DNA synthesis (Fig. 9) and receptor translocation (Fig. 10) studies
with PD were not consistent with the P-receptor induction experiments (Fig. 8). DNA synthesis was only partially stimulated with
PD compared to the results with DES but this may be related to the
earlier observation of hypertrophy rather than hyperplasia in the
stimulated uteri (14). The activity appears to increase and plateau
after a dose of 15 µg/kg PD and there was no indication of the
activity decreasing at higher doses. The poor P-receptor induction
and partial DNA synthesis would suggest that these two hormone
responsive processes may not be interrelated. Similar findings
have been reported in the hamster uterus indicating a variation in
binding affinity and uterine response and P-receptor induction (26).
Those results involved CI-628 and were not quantitatively on the
same order as ours and DNA synthesis was not one of the parameters
determined.

One of the easiest explanations for this difference in activity would involve some type of hormone difference in the receptor

genomic interaction. Certainly, this can not be discounted at the present time, but properly labeled metabolites will be required before such studies can be considered. The idea of altered inter-action had been proposed as an explanation of antiestrogen action (56). It is plausible to consider that some of these DES compounds, particularly those showing this variance in activities, could be acting in only one uterine cell type. Recent work suggesting preferential action of Nafoxidine in one cell type of the uterus has been reported (57). Experimentally, the data would show partial stimulation, when actually only part of the tissue is responding. We are presently involved in determining which cell types are responding to the DES metabolites.

The role of the estrogen receptor in this variant activity is unclear, although, it has been shown in vivo that the hormone nuclear receptor complex is related to the uterotropic response (52,53). Presently, it is inconclusive whether the receptor is the "answer" or simply an unrelated "bystander." Previously, we indicated that the mouse uterus produces two increases in nuclear receptor at different times (47). Further, we have demonstrated that this second increase was required to elicit a full uterine response (52). Receptor patterns determined during the course of those and earlier studies (22) suggested that the mouse uterus exhibits a rapid and efficient clearance of nuclear receptor, even when doses of 166 µg/kg of estriol were used. In addition the cytosol receptor pattern demonstrates a replenishment of assayable complex after 2 hr which becomes equivalent to pretreatment levels by 10-12 hr. In the case of the DES compounds, particularly PD, there are both nuclear events, but also significantly high nuclear receptor levels during the 3-6 hr time period between the two increases. We have suggested that this differential level of complex at this time is altering or muting the estrogenic response (14), since it is not allowing proper processing of the nuclear receptor complex. This concept is in agreement with previously published work concerning the mechanism of antiestrogen action (58). On the other hand, PD also shows retarded replenishment of cytosol complex which may also be involved in the mechanism. Therefore, it is clear that the compounds produce some estrogenic activity, though their mechanism may be different than those presently con-ceived for the natural estrogen hormone. Further studies requiring properly labeled ligands will be needed in order to more fully investigate these mechanisms.

SUMMARY

DES is metabolized to a number of compounds through a minimum of three main metabolic routes. These routes result in some inactivity of DES as an estrogen, but the majority appear to produce estrogenic by-products, which in some cases produce divergent in vivo and in vitro hormone activities. Therefore, if DES undergoes this type of metabolism, then large doses or repeated ingestion could produce a body burden of compounds with a wide range of hormonal activities possessing some possibly toxic or carcinogenic nature. It is apparent that these types of findings must also be considered when DES is used as an estrogenic test substance. The studies in this report have only attempted to ascertain the hormonal activity of these compounds and do not address the questions of their toxic or carcinogenic nature.

ACKNOWLEDGEMENT

      The author is indebted to Ms. Christine Fox-Davies and Mr. Mark Swaisgood for their invaluable technical aid during the course of these studies. The author is grateful to Manfred Metzler for supplying the majority of the DES compounds and for his and John McLachlan's collaboration in the earlier studies.

REFERENCES

1.   Dodds, E. C. (1938) Acta Med. Scand. Suppl. 90: 141-145.
2.   Herbst, A. L., Ulfelder, H. and Poskanzer, D. C. (1971) N. Engl. J. Med. 284: 878-881.
3.   Gunning, J. E. (1976) Obstet. Gynecol. Surv. (Suppl) 31: 827-833.
4.   Herbst, A. L., Poskanzer, D. C., Robboy, S. J., Friedlander, L. and Scully, R. E. (1975) N. Engl. J. Med. 292: 334-339.
5.   Gill, W. B., Schumacher, G. F. B. and Bibbo, M. (1977) J. Urology 117: 477-480.
6.   Sieghler, A. M., Wang, C. and Friberg, J. (1979) Fert. Steril. 31: 601-607.
7.   McLachlan, J. A. (1977) J. Toxicol. Environ. Hlth. 2: 527-537.
8.   Boylan, E. S. (1978) Biol. Reprod. 19: 854-863.
9.   Rustia, M. and Shubik, P. (1979) Cancer Res. 39: 4636-4644.
10.   Metzler, M. and McLachlan, J. A. (1978) Biochem. Biophys. Res. Comm. 85: 874-884.
11.   Blackburn, G. M., Thompson, M. H. and King, H. W. S. (1976) Biochem. J. 158: 643-646.
12.   McCormack, S. and Clark, J. H. (1979) Science 204: 629-631.
13.   Korach, K. S., Metzler, M. and McLachlan, J. A. (1978) Proc. Natl. Acad. Sci. 75: 468-471.
14.   Korach, K. S., Metzler, M. and McLachlan, J. A. (1979) J. Biol. Chem. 254: 8963-8968.
15.   Lowry, D. H., Rosebrough, N. J., Farr, A. L., and Randall, R. J. (1951) J. Biol. Chem. 193: 265-275.
16.   LePecq, J-B and Paoletti, C. (1966) Anal. Biochem. 17: 100-107.
17.   Burton, K. A. (1956) Biochem. J. 62: 315-323.

18. Harris, J. and Gorski, J. (1978) Endocrinology 103: 240-245.
19. Metzler, M. (1976) J. Toxicol. Environ. Hlth (Suppl.) 1: 21-35.
20. Adler, E. and Hagglund, B. (1945) Arkiv Kemi Mineral Geol. 19: 1-15.
21. Anderson, J. W., Clark, J. H. and Peck, E. J. (1972) Biochem. J. 126: 561-567.
22. Korach, K. S. (1979) Endocrinology 104: 1324-1332.
23. Korach, K. S. and Muldoon, T. G. (1974) Endocrinology 94: 785-793.
24. Korenman, S. G. (1969) Steroids 13: 163-177.
25. Korach, K. S. and Muldoon, T. G. (1974) Biochemistry 13: 1932-1938.
26. Leavitt, W. W., Chen, T. J. and Allen, T. C. (1977) Ann. N. Y. Acad. Sci. 286: 210-225.
27. Katzenellenbogen, B. S., Iwamoto, H. S., Heiman, D. F., Lan, H. C. and Katzenellenbogen, J. A. (1978) Mol. Cell Endocrinol 10: 103-113.
28. Metzler, M. (1980) C. R. C. Rev. In press.
29. Metzler, M. (1978) Tetrahedron 34: 3113-3117.
30. Gottschlich, R. and Metzler, M. (1979) Anal. Biochem. 92: 199-202.
31. Engel, L. L., Marshall, P. J., Orr, J. C., Reinhold, V. N. and Carter, P. (1978) Biomed. Mass Spec. 5: 582-586.
32. Metzler, M. and McLachlan, J. A. (1978) J. Environ. Pathol. Toxciol. 2: 579-581.
33. Engel, L. L., Weidenfeld, J. and Merriam, G. R. (1976) J. Toxicol. Environ. Hlth. (Suppl.) 1: 37-54.
34. Weidenfeld, J., Carter, P., Reinhold, V. N., Tanner, S. B., and Engel, L. L. (1978) Biomed. Mass Spec. 5: 587-590.
35. Gottschlich, R. and Metzler, M. (1980) Xenobiotica (In press).
36. Metzler, M. and McLachlan, J. A. (1978) Biochem. Pharmacol. 27: 1087-1094.
37. Gottschlich, R. and Metzler, M. (1980) J. Environ. Pathol. Toxicol. In press.
38. Metzler, M. (1975) Biochem. Pharmacol. 24: 1449-1453.
39. Rulin, B. L., Dorfman, A. S., Black, L. and Dorfman, R. I. (1951) Endocrinology 49: 429-438.
40. O'Malley, B. W. and Means, A. R. (1974) Science 183: 610-620.
41. Bouton, M. M. and Raynaud, J. P. (1978) J. Steroid Biochem. 9: 9-15.
42. Clark, J. H. and Peck, E. J. (1977) in Receptors and Hormone Action I (O'Malley, B. W. and Birnbaumer, L., eds.) Academic Press, New York, 383-410.
43. Van Den Brink, F. G. (1977) in Kinetics of Drug Action (Van Rossum, J. M., ed.) Springer-Verlag, New York, 169-254.
44. Webb, J. L. (1965) Enzyme and Metabolic Inhibitors. Vol. 1, p. 149-191, Academic Press, New York.
45. Clark, J. H., Hardin, J. W., Upchurch, S. and Eriksson, H. (1978) J. Biol. Chem. 253: 7630-7636.

46. Martin, L. and Finn, C. A. (1968) J. Endocrinol. 41: 363–368.
47. Korach, K. S. and Ford, E. B. (1978) Biochem. Biophys. Res. Commun. 83: 327–333.
48. Gawienowski, A. M., Knoche, H. W. and Moser, H. C. (1962) Biochim. Biophys. Acta 65: 150–159.
49. Winkler, V. W., Nyman, M. A. and Egan, R. S. (1971) Steroids 17: 197–203.
50. McLachlan, J. A., Baucom, K., Korach, K. S., Levy, L. and Metzler, M. (1979) Steroids 33: 543–547.
51. Jordon, V. C. and Prestwich, G. (1977) Mol. Cell Endocrinol. 8: 179–188.
52. Korach, K. S., Fox-Davies, C. and Baker, V. (1980) Endocrinology (In press).
53. Clark, J. H., Anderson, J. N. and Peck, E. J. (1972) Biochem. Biophys. Res. Commun. 48: 1460–1468.
54. Philibert, D. and Raynaud, J. P. (1977) in Progesterone Receptors in Normal Neoplastic Tissues (McGuire, W. L., Raynaud, J. P. and Baulieu, E-E., eds.) Raven Press, New York, 227–243.
55. Westphal, U. (1971) Steroid-Protein Interactions. p. 237–290. Springer-Verlag, New York.
56. Ruh, T. S. and Baudendistel, L. J. (1978) Endocrinology 102: 1838–1846.
57. Clark, J. H., Hardin, J. W., Padykula, H. A. and Cardasis, C. A. (1978) Proc. Natl. Acad. Sci. 75: 2781–2787.
58. Koseki, Y., Zava, D., Chamness, G. C. and McGuire, W. L., (1977) Endocrinology 101: 1104–1110.

ETIOLOGY OF DES-INDUCED UTERINE TUMORS IN THE SYRIAN HAMSTER

Wendell W. Leavitt, Rawden W. Evans and William J. Hendry, III

Worcester Foundation for Experimental Biology

Shrewsbury, Massachusetts 01545

SUMMARY

This paper describes a new experimental model system for the induction of endometrial adenocarcinoma in hamster uterus following diethylstilbestrol (DES) treatment of the newborn female. We propose that DES acts as an initiator during early development and that other estrogens act as promoters to stimulate tumor development in the adult uterus. DES directly affects the uterus as was shown by the failure of neonatal ovariectomy to prevent early DES-induced uterine growth. Subsequently, ovarian estrogen secretion from anovulatory, polyfollicular ovaries modifies the DES-altered uterus starting between 20 and 30 days of age and continuing into adult life. Early DES effects on the uterus include stimulation of endometrial cellular differentiation and progesterone receptor production. Permanent changes in uterine collagen, DNA and progesterone receptor content were noted, but the responsiveness of the DES-altered uterus to estrogen and progestin action was not impaired. Morphogenetic changes included an increase in extracellular connective tissue elements and striking alterations in endometrial cell composition such as hyperplasia of luminal and glandular epithelia and a massive inflammatory response in the stroma. Endometrial adenocarcinomas occurred in DES-treated animals in association with exposure to either endogenous estrogen from anovulatory ovaries or exogenous estrogen treatment of the ovariectomized animal. Endometrial tumors had relatively high concentrations of estrogen and progesterone receptors, suggesting a sensitivity to hormone action. Thus, these studies (a) demonstrate the utility of this animal model for the preparation of experimental endometrial tumors, and (b) suggest that DES acts as an initiator to transform uterine cells during early development, and estrogen exposure later in life acts as a promoter to stimulate growth and proliferation of DES-transformed cells.

63

INTRODUCTION

Estrogens have been implicated as important etiologic agents in cancer of the reproductive system (1-3). However, the exact role played by estrogens in the carcinogenic transformation of target cells is not known (4). The synthetic estrogen, diethylstilbestrol (DES), has been widely used for estrogen replacement therapy (5), as a "morning after" contraceptive (6), as a growth-promoting agent in livestock (7), and for the treatment of threatened abortion in women (8). The use of DES during pregnancy was found to induce congenital abnormalities and neoplasia of the female reproductive tract when administered during critical stages of development (9). The DES syndrome occurs in the female progeny of mothers who took DES for threatened abortion, and such women characteristically have a high incidence of vaginal adenosis, dysplasia and a possible predisposition to clear-cell carcinoma of the vagina and cervix (10). Newborn rodents exposed to DES develop symptoms akin to those observed in women with the DES-syndrome (11,12). These include alteration of Müllerian duct development with the Müllerian epithelium growing down beyond the cervix into the upper vagina. In addition to this teratogenic action of DES on Müllerian duct development, it is possible that DES itself has carcinogenic potential. However, it is not clear whether DES acts as an initiator or promoter of carcinogenesis nor is it certain whether DES is carcinogenic by virtue of its estrogenic activity (1).

There is need for experimental model systems for the study of hormone-dependent tumors of the reproductive system. While there are several systems available for work on breast cancer, an experimental paradigm of endometrial cancer is lacking. It came to our attention while studying DES-induced developmental changes in female hamster reproductive organs that there was a high incidence of endometrial hyperplasia and endometrial adenocarcinoma in animals that had been treated on the day of birth with DES (13). We report here on our studies of DES-induced changes in uterine growth, morphology and steroid receptor levels. We found that alteration of uterine target cells occurs by direct action of DES during the neonatal period, and endometrial tumors result from chronic exposure of the DES-modified uterus to estrogen action in adult life.

MATERIALS AND METHODS

Animals

Female hamster pups were each injected subcutaneously with 100 µg DES (40 mg/kg body weight) in 50 µl corn oil vehicle on the day of birth (day 1). Controls received the vehicle. In order to determine whether endogenous ovarian steroids contribute to the alteration of the reproductive system, animals were either ovariectomized or subjected to sham surgery on day 3 of life and then were studied at vari-

ous intervals thereafter. To test the hypothesis that ovarian estrogen may act later in life as a promoter of DES-induced lesions in the
uterus, the following groups of control and DES animals were compared:
(a) ovaries intact, (b) ovariectomized and (c) ovariectomized with
estrogen replacement given by means of a subcutaneous pellet of estradiol sealed in Silastic tubing (14).

Cytological preparations

Tissues were fixed in formalin, paraffin embedded, sectioned at
6 μm and stained with hematoxylin and eosin for routine light microscopic study. Other tissues were fixed for 24 h in 2% glutaraldehyde
and 2% formaldehyde in 67 mM cacodylate buffer, pH 7.35, embedded in
methacrylate, and thin (2 μm) sections stained with acid fuchsin and
methylene blue for light microscopy. Transmission electron microscopy
(TEM) was carried out on material fixed in 2% glutaraldehyde, 2.5%
formaldehyde, 0.001% $CaCl_2$ in 67 mM cacodylate buffer for 1 h. Specimens were postfixed in 1% OsO_4 for 2 h, dehydrated and embedded in
Epon. TEM was done using a JEOL 100S electron microscope.

Receptor assays

Cytosol and nuclear estrogen and progesterone receptors were
measured by equilibrium binding assays as previously developed and
validated in our laboratory (15,16). Specific [^{3}H]-steroid binding
data were analyzed by the Scatchard plot method (17) to provide total
progesterone receptor (Rp) and estrogen receptor (Re) levels.
Receptor sedimentation studies were performed with linear 5-20%
sucrose gradients as detailed elsewhere (18).

Other assays

Protein was measured according to Sedmak and Grossberg (19). DNA
was assayed by the Burton (20) method. Collagen was determined by the
hydroxyproline method of Bergman and Loxley (21). Steroid radioimmunoassays were performed as before (14) using specific antibodies for
estradiol (E_2) and progesterone (P).

RESULTS

Uterine growth in the neonatal hamster

To determine whether endogenous ovarian steroid secretion contributes to DES-induced uterine growth during postnatal development, 3-
day-old control and DES-treated hamsters were ovariectomized (ovex) or

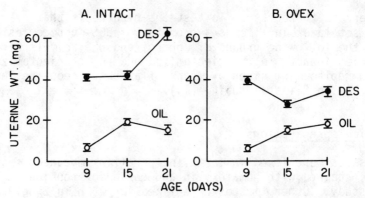

Fig. 1. Uterine development in hamsters treated on the day of birth
(day 1) with DES or oil vehicle. At day 3, animals were either subjected to a sham surgical procedure (intact, panel A) or ovariectomized (ovex, panel B). Each point represents the mean ± SEM (n = 8 or
more). DES = 100 µg DES/animal (40 mg/kg) administered in 50 µl oil.
OIL = corn oil vehicle (control).

Table 1. Comparison of Serum Steroid Levels in Intact and
          Neonatally Ovariectomized Animals

Steroid	Age (days)	INTACT OIL	INTACT DES	OVARIECTOMIZED OIL	OVARIECTOMIZED DES
Estradiol (pg/ml)	9	21 ± 3.1	23 ± 2.5	29 ± 5.2	26 ± 3.1
	15	29 ± 4.9	19 ± 4.2	16 ± 1.0	20 ± 1.5
	21	10 ± 1.9	16 ± 3.2	13 ± 2.3	10 ± 3.1
	30	40	150	-	-
Progesterone (ng/ml)	9	< 0.3	< 0.3	< 0.3	< 0.3
	15	< 0.3	< 0.3	< 0.3	< 0.3
	21	1.4 ± 0.2	< 0.3	0.4 ± .02	0.3 ± .02
	30	6.5	0.3	-	-

Assay sensitivity was: estradiol (6 pg/ml) and progesterone (0.3
ng/ml). Animals were given 100 µg DES or 50 µl oil vehicle at birth
(day 1) and, on day 3, either were ovariectomized or subjected to a
sham surgical procedure (Intact). Each value represents the mean ±
SEM. Results for 30 days are from a serum pool.

subjected to sham surgery (intact) and studied at 9, 15 and 21 days of age. Neonatal DES treatment produced a 6-fold increase in uterine weight at day 9 and a 2-fold elevation in uterine mass at day 15 in both the intact and ovex groups of animals (Fig. 1). Since the same increment of uterine growth was observed in ovariectomized and intact animals, it can be concluded that DES-induced uterine growth up to day 15 was the result of direct action of DES as opposed to an indirect effect mediated by stimulation of ovarian steroid secretion.

Measurement of serum estradiol (E_2) and progesterone (P) confirmed that E_2 levels were low (10-30 pg/ml) and P was nondetectable (<0.3 ng/ml) from 9 to 15 days (Table 1). No differences in serum E_2 were observed comparing intact and ovariectomized animals, further demonstrating that ovarian estrogen production was minimal during the first 2 weeks of life. However, ovarian-dependent uterine growth became apparent by day 21, indicating that ovarian estrogen secretion may begin to modify DES-induced uterine changes at this age and beyond. In intact animals, serum steroid levels increase between day 21 and day 30 (Table 1). Control animals reach puberty during this interval with E_2 and P levels rising in association with the onset of ovulatory cycles (22). In contrast, DES animals do not have ovulatory cycles as evidenced by the relative absence of serum P (<1 ng/ml) and the sustained E_2 levels of 100-150 pg/ml. Thus, in the intact DES animal, uterine growth commences during the neonatal period in response to DES action, and the DES-modified uterus is subsequently exposed to endogenous estrogen action at puberty and beyond from anovulatory ovaries which secrete high levels of E_2 and lower-than-normal levels of P.

Ontogeny of estrogen and progesterone receptors

The ontogeny of cytosol Re and Rp in uterus and vagina of DES-treated and control hamsters was studied at 10, 20 and 30 days of age (13). In the control animal, cytosol Rp remained low in uterus and vagina until day 20, and then Rp levels rose between day 20 and day 30 in response to the prepubertal increase in ovarian estrogen secretion. In the DES-treated animal, cytosol Rp was increased at day 10 in both uterus and vagina, and uterine Rp, but not vaginal Rp remained elevated on days 20 and 30 (Fig. 2). Cytosol Re was increased in uterus but not vagina at day 10 after DES exposure on day 1, and thereafter uterine Re levels dropped to control values between day 10 and day 30. The ratio of cytosol Rp to cytosol Re was higher in the uterus and vagina of the DES animal at all times studied, perhaps suggesting that neonatal DES treatment permanently increases Rp numbers relative to Re in estrogen target cells (Fig. 3).

To determine whether neonatal DES treatment induced permanent changes in receptor numbers, control and DES-treated hamsters were ovariectomized beginning on day 21 and studied at various intervals thereafter (13). At 9-15 days after ovariectomy, uterine weight, but

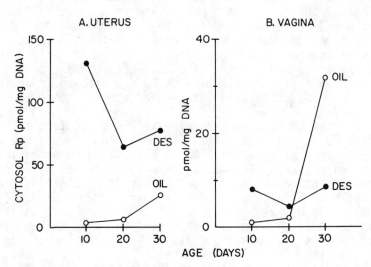

Fig. 2. Cytosol progesterone receptor (Rp) concentration in uterus and vagina of hamsters treated on day 1 of postnatal life with DES or oil vehicle. Rp was measured as described in Materials and Methods. Each point represents the mean of duplicate assays performed on a pool of cytosol.

not vaginal weight, was significantly higher in the DES animal as compared to control. There was a significant increase in uterine Rp content (pmol/uterus) and concentration (pmol/g tissue and pmol/mg DNA) in the DES animal. Nuclear Re levels in vagina and uterus of the ovariectomized DES animal were significantly elevated when expressed either per organ (pmol/uterus) or on a tissue weight basis (pmol/g tissue). However, when nuclear Re was expressed on a cellular basis (pmol/mg DNA), there was no difference between DES and control animals (13). These results demonstrate permanent, ovarian-independent changes in uterine Rp numbers up to day 30 following DES treatment on day 1 of life. Although nuclear Re concentration is higher in the DES uterus when expressed on a tissue weight basis, this difference cannot be attributed to differences in the numbers of receptors per cell. Rather, these results support the conclusion that the cellular composition of the uterus is modified by neonatal DES treatment with an attendant permanent change in the cellular Rp content. It follows, therefore, that the primary effect of DES is on cell differentiation rather than alteration of receptor systems.

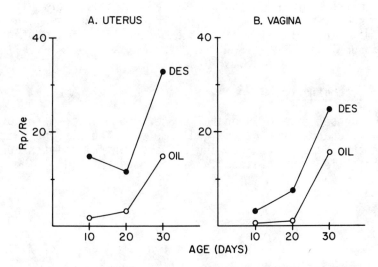

Fig. 3.   Ratio of progesterone receptor (Rp) to estrogen receptor
(Re) in uterine and vaginal cytosol following neonatal treatment
with DES or oil vehicle. The Rp and Re values used to calculate the
Rp/Re ratio were measured by equilibrium binding assays as in Fig. 2.

Responsiveness to estrogen action

Uterine weight, DNA and cytosol Rp responses to estrogen action
were measured using ovariectomized control (oil vehicle) and DES
animals (Fig. 4). After 3 days of E_2 treatment (0, 0.1, 1, and 10 µg/
animal/day), similar patterns of uterine weight response were observed
in DES and control animals (Fig. 4). However, DES uteri weighed more
than controls at each dose of E_2, resulting in an upward shift in the
dose-response curve of DES uteri. The uterine DNA content (mg DNA/
uterus) was higher in DES animals than in oil controls at each dose of
E_2, but uterine DNA concentration (mg DNA/g tissue) was not different
in oil and DES animals. These results show that the DES uterus contains significantly more cells, and this difference in cellularity is
maintained during estrogen stimulation. Cytosol Rp content (pmol/
uterus) was higher in the DES uterus as compared to control, and
estrogen priming increased Rp levels in both preparations. However,
it should be noted that the cellular Rp concentration of unprimed
uteri was higher for DES (7 pmol/mg DNA) than control (2 pmol/mg DNA)
groups, and that estrogen priming raised the cellular Rp concentration

to the same maximum value (20 pmol/mg DNA). Since the difference observed in cellular Rp content of DES and control uteri disappeared upon estrogen stimulation, the higher baseline Rp level in the DES uterus may represent a persistent estrogen-like effect of neonatal DES exposure.

Uterine cytopathology

The consequence of neonatal DES exposure in terms of uterine structural change is striking and complex. The uterine weight difference that is observed between DES and control animals during early postnatal life is maintained into adulthood (Fig. 4). The DES-induced

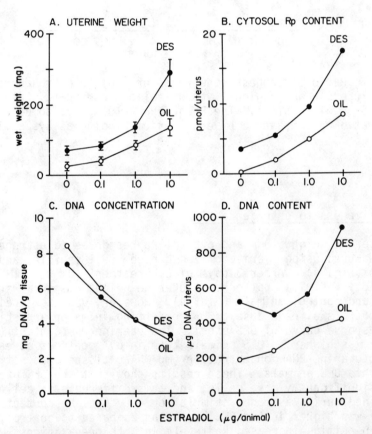

Fig. 4. Uterine response to estrogen action. DES-treated and control (OIL) animals were ovariectomized at day 25 and treated with 0, 0.1, 1, and 10 μg E_2/animal/day for 3 days beginning on day 35. Animals were autopsied 24 h after the last injection and uterine weight, DNA and cytosol Rp determined.

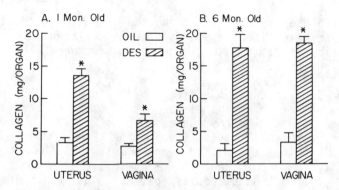

Fig. 5. Uterine collagen content in intact animals at 1 and 6 months of age. Intact animals were treated with DES (hatched bars) or oil vehicle (open bars) on day 1. Collagen was determined by hydroxyproline assay (21). * = P<0.01.

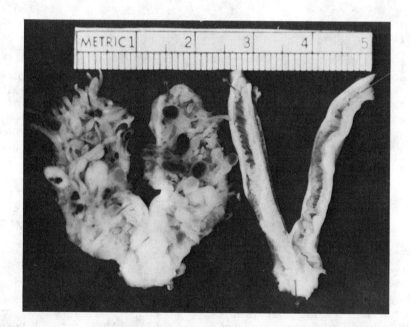

Fig. 6. Endometrial abnormalities induced by neonatal DES exposure (left) as compared to control (right). Uteri were obtained at 120 days of age from intact animals, and each uterine horn was opened longitudinally to expose the endometrial lining. The control animal was taken on day 4 (proestrus) of the estrous cycle. Polyps, cysts and hyperplastic endometrium are routinely found in the DES uterus at this stage of development.

increase in uterine mass is accounted for by an increase in extracellular connective tissue elements such as collagen (Fig. 5) in addition
to dramatic alterations in endometrial structure (Fig. 6) and cell
composition (Figs. 7-9).

The DES-altered endometrium appears to be in part an exaggeration
of the normal cellular and tissue differentiation that is observed in
control animals during the estrous cycle (23,24). The mucosa becomes
heavily convoluted into ridges or polyps (Fig. 6). The invaginated
regions of luminal epithelium reach almost into the myometrium.
Mitotic figures are evident in the luminal epithelium and, to some
extent, appear in the glandular epithelium as well. The hyperplastic
luminal epithelium is widely pseudostratified (Fig. 7). The glandular epithelial cells are cytologically distinct from the luminal epithelial cells, and the glands vary considerably in the degree of distension by heterogenous secretion with some becoming greatly enlarged
and cystic (Fig. 7b).

Fig. 7.   Photomicrographs a-d are 2 μm methacrylate sections, stained
with acid fuchsin and methylene blue. Fixation was 2% glutaraldehyde
and 2% formaldehyde in 0.067M cacodylate buffer, pH 7.35 for 24 h.

    a.   A partial cross-section through the uterus of a control
hamster, 120 days of age, on the third day of the estrous cycle.
Note the lumen (L) surrounded by the columnar luminal epithelium.
Glands (g) occur within the cellular stroma. Note the high cellularity of the stroma. Note the thickness of the myometrium (M) in
this control animal. X 250.

    b.   A partial cross-section through the uterus of a hamster
treated on day 1 with 100 μg DES and fixed on day 122. Note that the
lumen (L) is divided by large outgrowths of the uterine wall. The
luminal epithelium is pseudostratified. Glands (g) in the stroma
frequently contain a large lumen and have irregular epithelial
borders. The myometrium is distinctly reduced in thickness when
compared to the control animal (Fig. 7a). X 250.

    c.   A higher magnification photomicrograph through a portion of
the uterine wall of an animal treated with DES as in Fig. 7b. Note
that the tall luminal epithelium is definitely pseudostratified and
contains empty spaces surrounded by circularly arranged cells. The
adjacent stroma contains spindle-shaped and ovoid cells. A portion of
a gland within the stroma shows an epithelium that resembles somewhat
the appearance of the luminal epithelium. X 2,000.

    d.   A higher magnification photomicrograph of a control uterus
similar to Fig. 7a. Note that the luminal epithelium is simple
columnar and approximately one-half the height of the epithelium in
the DES-treated animal (Fig. 7c). The stroma in the control uterus
contains closely packed cells. The glandular epithelium is simple
low columnar in section and borders a small lumen. X 2,000.
(Prepared by Dr. J.M. Price, University Massachusetts Medical School).

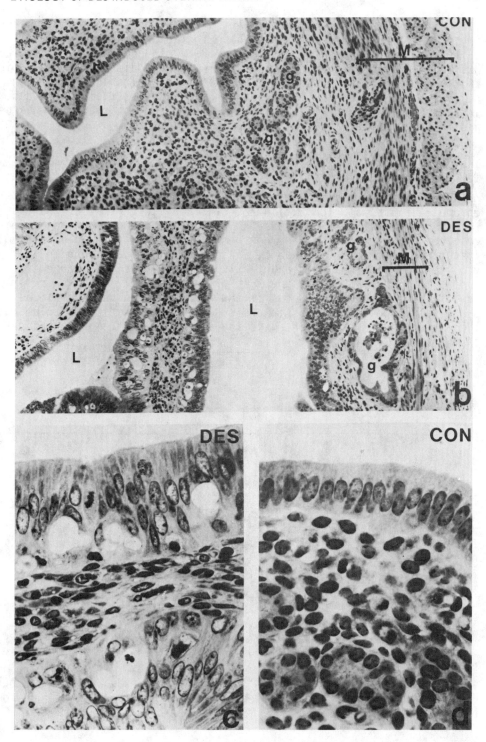

An interesting ultrastructural feature of the DES-exposed uterus is the prevalence of nuclear bodies in the epithelial and stromal cells (Figs. 8 and 9). Recent work by Padykula and associates (25,26) has demonstrated that the incidence of nuclear bodies in uterine epithelium is correlated with the degree of estrogenization. Although nuclear bodies occur in many types of normal cells, their prevalence in tumor cells and in virally-infected cells suggest that they may be associated with cell growth and/or replication (27).

Marked changes were noted in the stromal compartment of the DES-altered uterus (Fig. 9). There is an abundance of cells and extracellular matrix. The high cellularity originates from a massive expression of a local immune and/or inflammatory response throughout the endometrial stroma. In particular, plasma cells in various phases of secretory activity are numerous throughout the stroma, but most are concentrated beneath the basement membrane of the luminal epithelium. Tissue eosinophils are abundant, and heterophils occur both in the uterine lumen and in the glandular lumena. Lymphocytes, monocytes, macrophages and mast cells are also present in the stroma. A conspicuous feature of the DES uterus is the presence of a well-developed system of lymphatic vessels in the superficial stroma. This elaborate lymphatic system may be linked to the strong cellular manifestations of mucosal immunologic activity.

Fig. 8.   Electron micrographs a-c are of the luminal epithelium of a DES-treated animal similar to Fig. 7b. The uterus was fixed in 2% glutaraldehyde and 2.5% formaldehyde, 0.001% calcium chloride in 0.067M cacodylate buffer, pH 7.35 for one hour. Following postfixation in 1% OsO_4 in 0.1M cacodylate for 2 h, the tissue was dehydrated and embedded in Epon.

a.   The nuclei of these cells are euchromatic and often irregular in profile. The cytoplasm contains a variety of organelles, particularly in the supranuclear cytoplasm. The large dense granules in the supranuclear cytoplasm may represent the lysosomal system whereas the small granules immediately below the free surface may be secretory material. A nuclear body (arrow) is seen in the nucleus of one epithelial cell. X 8,000.

b. and c. Sections of two nuclear bodies are shown. Each nuclear body has a central core of small electron-opaque granules surrounded by a fibrous capsule. X 30,000 (Prepared by Dr. J.M. Price, Univ. Massachusetts Medical School).

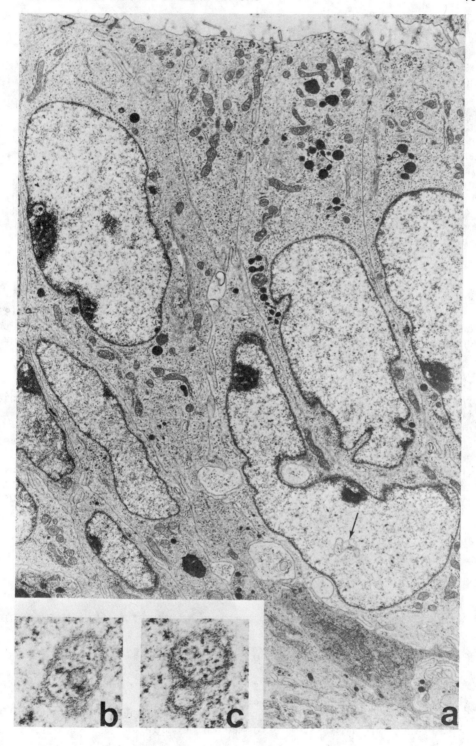

Tumorigenesis

Rustia (28) found a high (28-50%) percentage of reproductive
tract neoplasms in the female progeny of hamster mothers given 20 or
40 mg DES/kg during late pregnancy. Similar reproductive abnormalities are produced in mice after DES exposure during the neonatal
period (12,29). We found that when female hamsters were treated on
the day of birth with 100 µg DES (40 mg/kg), there was a high incidence of endometrial hyperplasia and endometrial adenocarcinoma in DES
animals as compared to no such problems in controls (13) (Fig. 10).
Other DES-induced abnormalities included anovulatory ovaries with
cystic follicles; metaplasia and inflammation of oviducts; squamous
cell metaplasia and fibromuscular development of the cervix; and hyperplasia of the vaginal epithelium. In an earlier study (13), endometrial hyperplasia occurred in 28/28 DES animals at 4-7 months of
age, whereas endometrial tumors were found in animals with intact
ovaries or in ovariectomized animals bearing E_2 implants but were not
present in chronically ovariectomized DES animals. We have completed
a second larger series (Table 2) which shows essentially the same results as the first. Endometrial adenocarcinomas occur in the DES
animal in the presence of either endogenous estrogen (intact ovaries)
or exogenous estrogen (ovariectomized with E_2 implant) but not in the
absence of estrogen (ovariectomized). These results support the hypothesis that exposure of the DES-altered uterus to estrogen in adult
life increases the growth and/or the incidence of endometrial tumors.
This hypothesis is further supported by the finding of a positive
relationship between serum E_2 levels and the incidence of endometrial
tumors in the groups studied (Fig. 11). DES animals with intact
ovaries have chronically reduced serum P and elevated serum E_2 as
compared to control hamsters undergoing normal estrous cycles. Ovariectomy reduced E_2 and P to nondetectable levels, and replacement
therapy with an E_2 implant raised serum E_2 in the ovariectomized
animal to around 100 pg/ml which approximated the value observed in
the intact DES animal (Fig. 11). These results support the conclusion
that chronic exposure to elevated E_2 ($\sim$100 pg/ml serum) is responsible
for promoting endometrial tumor development in the DES animal.

Fig. 9.   Electron micrograph of the superficial uterine stroma of a
DES-treated animal similar to the one shown in Fig. 8. The close
packing of the stromal cells is evident. Sections through five plasma
(PC) cells occur among fibroblasts. Note the nuclear body (arrow)
within the nucleus of uterine fibroblast. X 8,000. (Prepared by Dr.
J.M. Price, Univ. Massachusetts Medical School).

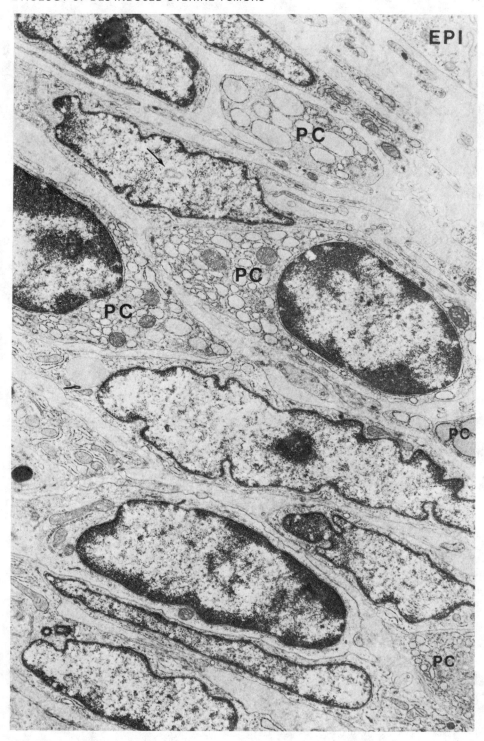

Receptor levels in endometrial tumors

Steroid receptors were measured in the uterus and endometrial tumors obtained from adult E_2-treated animals (Fig. 12). The uterus of the DES animal had levels of cytosol Re and Rp that were equivalent to those observed in the control. In addition, the concentration of Re and Rp in endometrial tumor tissue was the same as that observed in nontumorous uterine tissue. The presence of Re and Rp support the idea that the endometrial tumors in the DES animal are hormone sensitive.

Response to progestin action

Studies done recently in our laboratory (14,16,30,31) have revealed that P has a rapid specific effect on nuclear Re levels in the estrogen-primed uterus. P does not interrupt Re translocation nor does it compromise cytosol Re levels. Rather P appears to act by way of RNA and protein synthesis to reduce the retention of nuclear Re and thus modulate estrogen action. We were interested to determine whether P had a similar effect in the DES uterus. Young adult hamsters were ovariectomized and implanted with Silastic E_2 pellets.

Table 2. Incidence of Endometrial Tumors in Adult Hamsters
          Exposed to DES during Neonatal Life

	Control	DES
Intact ovaries	0/35 (0%)	11/29 (38%)
Ovariectomized	0/34 (0%)	0/18 (0%)
Ovariectomized + E_2 Implant	0/28 (0%)	30/35 (86%)

Animals were treated on the day of birth with either 50 μl corn oil vehicle or 100 μg DES in 50 μl oil. Animals were autopsied between 3 and 10 months of age. E_2 implant = Silastic tube filled with crystalline estradiol and placed subcutaneously. Ovariectomies were performed on day 3 of life. E_2 implants were introduced after 3 weeks of age.

Fig. 10. Endometrial adenocarcinoma in DES-altered uterus of an adult hamster at 7 months of age after placement of subcutaneous estradiol implant for 4 months. Tissue was fixed in formalin, embedded in paraffin, sectioned at 6 μm and stained with H and E. Upper figure is low power view and lower figure is higher magnification of endometrial tumor cells. This represents a typical finding at this age for DES-treated hamsters with intact ovaries or after ovariectomy and chronic exposure to exogenous estrogen.

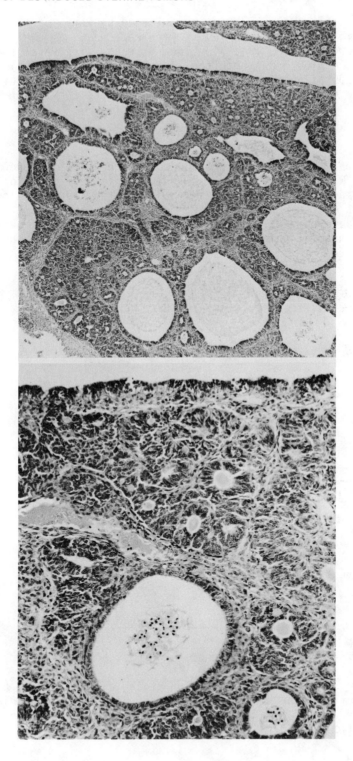

Estrogen withdrawal (-E) was accomplished by removing the E_2 implant, and within 4 h nuclear Re levels were reduced by about 20% in DES and control groups (Fig. 13). Combined estrogen withdrawal and P treatment (2.5 mg/100 g BW) resulted in a 50% decrease in nuclear Re in both groups of animals. Thus, the nuclear Re responses of the DES uterus to estrogen withdrawal and progestin action appear to be normal.

DISCUSSION

Animal model systems are needed for the study of endometrial cancer. We have developed a new experimental paradigm for the induction of endometrial adenocarcinoma in hamster uterus following DES treatment of the newborn female. Our results indicate that DES-induced developmental changes in uterine target cells are associated with endometrial tumor development during estrogen exposure in later

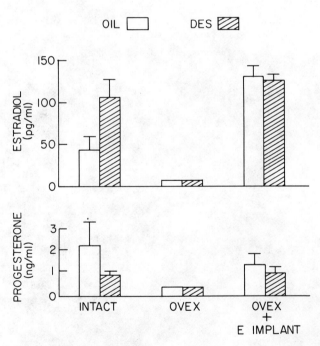

Fig. 11. Serum steroid levels in intact, ovariectomized (ovex) and ovariectomized plus E implant groups studied for endometrial tumor incidence (Table 2). Serum estradiol and progesterone were measured by specific RIA.

life. We propose that DES acts as an initiator to transform uterine
cells during early development, and that ovarian estrogen acts subsequently as a promoter to stimulate growth and proliferation of the
DES-transformed cells in the adult uterus.

Our observation in hamsters of DES-induced endometrial lesions
may be pertinent to the human population exposed to DES in utero. In
both DES-exposed women and experimental animals, vaginal lesions are
confined to the cranial aspect of the organ (10,32-36). The upper
portion of the vagina develops from the Müllerian ducts while the
lower part is derived from the urogenital sinus (37). Thus, DES-
induced lesions of the female genital tract occur in tissues derived
from the embryonic Müllerian ducts. Clinical and experimental manifestations of perinatal DES exposure appear to be common in the vagina
and cervix. The apparent lower frequency of uterine problems in DES
women may be related to the lack of appropriate study rather than an
absence of uterine lesions since examination of the uterus is not a
routine gynecological procedure. Our experimental results suggest
that pathological changes in the endometrium of women exposed to DES
in utero are possible, and that these changes may advance to neoplasia
with advancing age and extended periods of estrogen exposure.

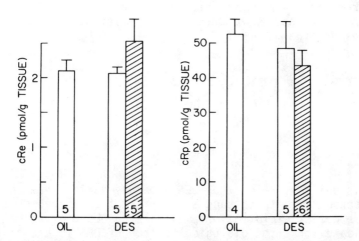

Fig. 12. Cytosol (c) receptor levels in endometrial tumor and nontumorous portion of uterus. Control = oil treatment at birth and
sacrifice on day 4 of estrous cycle at 200 days of age. DES treatment
was at day 1 and autopsy was at 200 days old. Tumor tissue (hatched
bars) was separated from the nontumorous portion of the uterus (open
bars), and each was assayed separately for cRe and cRp content. Each
bar represents the mean ± SEM with n shown at the base of each bar.

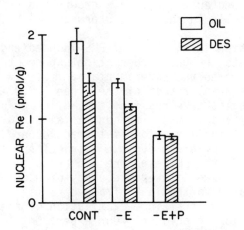

Fig. 13.   Uterine nuclear Re response to estrogen withdrawal (-E) and estrogen withdrawal plus progesterone treatment (-E +P).   Animals were treated with DES or oil vehicle on the day of birth and ovariectomized at day 25.   Silastic tubes containing crystalline E_2 (E implants) were placed subcutaneously at the time of ovariectomy.   Ten days later (day 35), the animals were given the following treatments: control (CONT) = E implant left in place; -E = E implant removed for 4 h; -E +P = E implant removed and progesterone (2.5 mg/animal) treatment for 4 h. Nuclear Re was measured as described in Materials and Methods.   Each bar represents the mean ± SEM (n = 4).

        It is our contention that DES exposure during development of the female reproductive tract causes transformation of one or more types of uterine cells.   Information available on DES and vaginal cancer (38) indicates that the biological effect of DES is one of teratogenesis, rather than carcinogenesis.   This view contends that DES induces congenital alterations in the vaginal epithelium where the possibility of neoplastic transformation can occur at a later age through a mutagenic agent other than DES (38).   The stroma induces and specifies the morphogenesis and cytodifferentiation of the epithelia of the Müllerian ducts and urogenital sinus during development of the uterus and vagina in mice, and this process is age dependent (39).   These age-dependent tissue interactions also appear to be involved in the induction and perpetuation of ovary-independent vaginal hyperplasia in neonatally estrogenized mice (40). Recent studies of morphogenesis in other organs have yielded results which may be pertinent to the situation in both the normal and DES-altered uterus. Mesenchymal tissues produce growth-stimulating substances that induce mitotic activity in the adjacent epithelial cells (41). Of further interest are studies on the involvement of extracellular materials associated with tissue surfaces in epithelial morphogenesis (41).

Our view is that DES acts as an initiator during development to cause permanent changes in uterine cells which are recruited during estrogen stimulation in later life. Support for the idea that DES exposure during embryonic development increases the sensitivity of hamster target organs to carcinogen action later in life was provided recently (42). Furthermore, evidence from studies with the DES-treated neonatal mouse indicate there is an alteration of antigenic determinants in the affected reproductive organs (43). However, the nature of the DES-induced permanent cellular changes is an intriguing question. While our studies indicate differences in uterine steroid receptor concentrations in both prepubertal and adult animals after neonatal DES exposure, we have uncovered no evidence of changes in either the physicochemical or functional properties of these receptor systems. Therefore, we interpret the change in uterine steroid receptor levels to be a consequence of alteration in the cellular composition of the organ due to early DES action. Apparently, exposure of the neonatal hamster to DES affects the pattern of cell differentiation in the uterus and ultimately results in a permanent change in the course of organ development.

Normal development is a dynamic process involving both the formation and breakdown of cell-cell associations and tissue structures. This concept is particularly relevant to the mammalian uterus, an organ which undergoes constant cyclic remodeling during adult life. As is the case for early events of uterine and vaginal development, the adult cyclic pattern of reproductive tract differentiation is also dependent on stromal-epithelial interactions. The evidence for this has been reviewed recently by Cunha et al. (44). There is compelling evidence that remodeling of the stromal extracellular matrix plays an important role in certain normal and abnormal developmental processes in the urogenital tract.

The morphological sequelae to neonatal DES exposure which we observe in the hamster uterus take on added significance in light of these developmental concepts. The inflammatory response in the uterine stroma is a very striking and consistent finding in the neonatal DES-exposed hamster. In the postpartum rat and opossum uterus, Padykula and associates have demonstrated extensive infiltration by heterophils, eosinophils, monocyte-macrophages, lymphocytes and plasma cells at the same time that rapid collagen degradation is occurring (45,46). Based upon cytological observations and existing information on uterine collagenase activity, Padykula suggested that this inflammatory response is a result of the release of new antigenic sites by the action of collagenase and other extracellular proteases (47). Relevant to this hypothesis is the possibility that lysosomal function and estrogen action are linked in target organs (48). Furthermore, recent studies have shown elevated activity of the lysosomal enzyme cathepsin B1 associated with vaginal pathology after prenatal DES exposure in women (49), and that leupeptin-sensitive protease activity may contribute to cell membrane and growth modifications elicited by E_2 treatment in endometrial cells in vitro (50). It is possible that enzyme-induced modification of cell membranes could play an important role in mediating the changes in cellular function often associated with tumorigenic transformation. Indeed, various membrane proteins are known to play a role in such functions as cell-cell recognition, immune response, proliferative activity and substrate adherence. Such considerations are consistent with the view that tumorigenesis is simply a problem of anomalous cellular differentiation where the underlying heritable cellular change is epigenetic in nature; as evidenced by observations that the cancerous state is not irreversibly fixed in a cell and may revert to the normal state (51). Thus, the cancerous state may result from the persistent activation of biosynthetic regulatory systems found in normal cells. According to this view, neonatal DES exposure could induce a heritable change in certain sensitive cell types during early stages of uterine organogenesis. Phenotypic expression of this change might then occur in later life in response to subsequent estrogen action.

It is well documented that exposure of neonatal rodents to estrogen (or androgen) causes a permanent alteration in the hypothalamo-pituitary-ovarian axis resulting in persistent vaginal cornification and polyfollicular, anovulatory ovaries at maturity. The midcycle ovulatory LH surge fails to occur in such persistent estrous animals, and the ovaries continue to produce follicles and estrogen for a prolonged period. Thus, the persistent estrous syndrome induced by neonatal DES exposure in the hamster is in marked contrast to the presence of cyclic ovarian function and menstrual cycles in DES women (52). It is perhaps pertinent that progestin may reverse some DES-induced abnormalities in the human (53), and that periodic exposure of DES-induced lesions to progestin during the luteal phase of the menstrual cycle may play a protective role in suppressing their development. In contrast, the DES-treated hamster exhibits constant estrogen production from anovulatory ovaries, and chronic estrogen exposure promotes the proliferation of DES-induced lesions. Therefore, it will be important to determine whether progestin treatment can reverse or prevent the growth of DES-induced lesions, and whether the neonatal rodent model is really appropriate for understanding the DES syndrome in the human.

ACKNOWLEDGMENT

This work was supported by NSF grant PCM77-25630; NIH grants CA 23362, CA 23693, and HD 15132; and a grant from the UpJohn Co. We appreciate the excellent technical assistance of Jacqueline Tetrault, Michael Muto and William Robidoux. We are especially grateful to Drs. Helen A. Padykula and J. Michael Price, Anatomy Department, University of Massachusetts Medical School, Worcester, MA for the preparation and interpretation of histological material. Dr. Norval W. King, Jr., New England Regional Primate Center, Southborough, MA collaborated on the cytopathological work.

REFERENCES

1. Lipsett, M.B. (1979) Cancer 43: 1967-1981.
2. Gurpide, E. (1976) Cancer 38: 503-508.
3. Siiteri, P.K. (1978) Cancer Res 38: 4360-4366.
4. Hertz, R. (1979) J Steroid Biochem 11: 435-442.
5. Noller, K.L., and C.R. Fish (1974) Med Clin N Amer 58: 793-810.
6. Kuchera, L.K. (1974) Contraception 10: 47-54.
7. McMartin, K.E. (1978) J Environ Pathol Toxicol 1: 279-313.
8. Smith, O.W. (1948) Am J Obstet Gynecol 56: 821-834.
9. Herbst, A.L., H. Ulfelder, and D.C. Poskanzer (1971) N Engl J Med 284: 878-881.
10. Herbst, A.L., R.E. Scully, and S.J. Robboy (1979). In: J.M. Rice, ed. "Perinatal Carcinogenesis", Natl Cancer Inst Monograph 51: 25-35.
11. Forsberg, J.-G. (1973) Am J Obstet Gynecol 115: 1025-1043.
12. McLachlan, J.A. (1979). In: J.M. Rice, ed. "Perinatal Carcinogenesis", Natl Cancer Inst Monograph 51: 67-72.
13. Leavitt, W.W., R.W. Evans, W.J. Hendry III, and K.I.H. Williams (1980). In: R.L. Sutherland and V.C. Jordan, eds. "Non-steroidal Antiestrogens. Subcellular Pharmacology and Antitumor Activity", Academic Press, Sydney (in press).
14. Evans, R.W., T.J. Chen, W.J. Hendry III, and W.W. Leavitt (1980) Endocrinology 107: 383-390.
15. Leavitt, W.W., T.J. Chen, Y.S. Do, B.D. Carlton, and T.C. Allen (1978). In: B.W. O'Malley and L. Birnbaumer, eds. "Receptors and Hormone Action", vol 2, Academic Press, New York, pp 157-188.
16. Leavitt, W.W., T.J. Chen, and R.W. Evans (1979). In: W.W. Leavitt and J.H. Clark, eds. "Steroid Hormone Receptor Systems", Plenum Pub Corp, New York, pp 179-222.
17. Scatchard, G. (1949) Ann NY Acad Sci 51: 660-672.
18. Leavitt, W.W., D.O. Toft, C.A. Strott, and B.W. O'Malley (1974) Endocrinology 94: 1041-1053
19. Sedmak, J.J., and S.E. Grossberg (1977) Ann Biochem 97: 544-552
20. Burton, K. (1956) J Biochem 62: 315-323.
21. Bergman, I., and R. Loxley (1969) Analyst 94: 575-584.
22. Vomachka, A.J., and G.S. Greenwald (1979) Endocrinology 105: 960-966.

23. Brenner, R.M., N.B. West, R.L. Norman, B.A. Sandow, and H.G. Verhage (1979). In: W.W. Leavitt and J.H. Clark, eds. "Steroid Hormone Receptor Systems", Plenum Pub Corp, New York, pp 173-196.
24. Sandow, B.A., N.B. West, R.L. Norman, and R.M. Brenner (1979) Am J Anat 156: 15-36.
25. Clark, J.H., J.W. Hardin, H.A. Padykula, and C.A. Cardasis (1978) Proc Natl Acad Sci USA 75: 2781-2784.
26. Padykula, H.A., and J.H. Clark (1980). In: H. Busch, ed. "The Cell Nucleus", vol 9, Academic Press, New York (in press).
27. Krishnan, A., B.G. Uzman, and E.T. Hedley-Whyte (1967) J Ultrastruct Res 19: 563-582.
28. Rustia, M., and P. Shubik (1976) Cancer Lett 1: 139-146.
29. McLachlan, J.A. (1977) J Toxicol Environ Health 2: 527-537.
30. Evans, R.W., and W.W. Leavitt (1980) Endocrinology 107: 1261-1263.
31. Evans, R.W., and W.W. Leavitt (1980) Proc Natl Acad Sci USA 77: 5856-5860.
32. Robboy, S.J., R.E. Scully, and A.L. Herbst (1975) J Reprod Med 15: 13-18.
33. Ulfelder, J (1976) Cancer 38: 426-431.
34. Herbst, A.L., S.J. Robboy, R.E. Scully, and D.C. Poskanzer (1974) Am J Obstet Gynecol 119: 713-724.
35. Forsberg, J.G. (1975) Am J Obstet Gynecol 121: 101-104.
36. Kalland, T., T.M. Forsberg, and J.G. Forsberg (1978) Obstet Gynecol 51: 464-467.
37. Cunha, G.R. (1975) Am J Anat 143: 387-392.
38. Edgren, R.A. (1976). In: K.M. Menon, and J.R. Reel, eds. "Steroid Hormone Action and Cancer", Plenum Pub Corp, New York, pp 95-106.
39. Cunha, G.R. (1976) J Exp Zool 196: 361-370.
40. Cunha, G.R., G. Lung, and K. Kato (1977) Dev Biol 56: 52-67.
41. Goldin, G.V. (1980) Quart Rev Biol 55: 251-265.
42. Rustia, M., and P. Shubik (1979) Cancer Res 39: 4636-4644.
43. Forsberg, J.G. (1979). In: J.M. Rice, ed. "Perinatal Carcinogenesis", Natl Cancer Inst Monograph 51: 41-56.
44. Cunha, G.R., L.W.K. Chung, J.M. Shannon, and B.A. Reese (1980) Biol Reprod 22: 19-42.
45. Padykula, H.A., and J.M. Taylor (1976) Anat Rec 184: 5-26.
46. Padykula, H.A., and A.G. Campbell (1976) Anat Rec 184: 27-48.
47. Padykula, H.A. (1976) Anat Rec 184: 49-72.
48. Hirsch, P.C., and C.M. Szego (1974) J Steroid Biochem 5: 533-542.
49. Pietras, R.J., C.M. Szego, C.E. Mangan, B.J. Seeler, M.M. Burtnett, and M. Orevi (1978) Obstet Gynecol 52: 321-327.
50. Pietras, R.J., and C.M. Szego (1979) J Cell Biol 81: 649-663.
51. Braun, A.C. (1977) "The Story of Cancer; On Its Nature, Causes and Control", Addison-Wesley Publ Co., Reading, MA, 308 pp.
52. Barnes, A.B. (1979) Fertil Steril 32: 148-153.
53. Herbst, A.L., S.J. Robboy, and R.W. Scully (1974) Am J Obstet Gynecol 118: 607-615.

NEONATAL STIMULATION OF THE UTERUS BY CLOMIPHENE, TAMOXIFEN AND NAFOXIDINE: RELATIONSHIP TO THE DEVELOPMENT OF REPRODUCTIVE TRACT ABNORMALITIES

James H. Clark, Sylvia C. Guthrie and
Shirley A. McCormack
Department of Cell Biology
Baylor College of Medicine
Houston, TX 77030

INTRODUCTION

Triphenylethylene derivatives, such as Clomid and Tamoxifen, are drugs that are in common use for the induction of ovulation and treatment of breast cancer, respectively. They are generally considered to be estrogen antagonists; however, it is well known that they may also act as agonists (15). While most investigators have been primarily interested in their antagonistic properties, we have concentrated on their estrogenic capacities. Triphenylethylene drugs cause long-term retention of the estrogen receptor in the nuclei of uterine cells and this is accompanied by a sustained stimulatio. of uterotropic activity (6-8, 10, 12, 17, 20, 29). This stimulation is primarily due to the ability of these drugs to stimulate the epithelium of the uterine lumen, whereas estradiol, a physiological estrogen, causes all tissues of the uterus to grow (9, 10, 17, 34). Therefore, even though these drugs are decidedly anti-estrogenic in some tissues, they are long acting estrogens in others. Since chronic exposure to estrogens is known to result in preneoplastic and neoplastic changes in the reproductive tract (22), we considered the possibility that triphenylethylene derivatives might cause such changes in the fetal and neonatal rat (5,30).

NEONATAL EXPOSURE AND ABNORMALITIES OF THE REPRODUCTIVE TRACT

Neonatal female rats were injected on day 1 of life with either Nafoxidine (1 to 100 μg per rat) or Clomid (10 to 500 μg per rat). Each compound was dissolved in absolute ethanol stirred into warmed (45°C) sesame oil until the ethanol had evaporated, and injected subcutaneously in the nape of the neck. Clomid is a mixture of cis and trans isomers and was used as such because this is the form which is administered to women. The animals were weaned at 21 days of age and the time of vaginal opening was noted. Vaginal smears were examined for 3 to 4 weeks before autopsy. The ovaries, oviducts, and uteri were removed between days 60 and 100 of life and were prepared for routine histological analysis.

Vaginal opening occurred in 86 percent of the rats injected with 100 µg of Nafoxidine or 50 µg of Clomid between days 26 and 34. Control rats have vaginal opening between days 35 and 50. The vaginal smears of treated rats did not show normal cyclic changes, and a high incidence of estrus smears was noted. Therefore, these animals are probably acyclic and in a state which outwardly resembles persistent estrus. These responses are typical of masculinized female rats; however, a more extensive evaluation of these animals is required before this can be stated with certainty.

Abnormalities of the reproductive tract involved a complicated array of anomalies. These included atrophic ovaries with accompanying atrophic uteri in some animals, while others showed cystic ovaries and enlarged uteri. Hypertrophy of the oviducts was a common observation. An examination of the histology of the uterine tissue revealed various stages of uterine hyperplasia and squamous metaplasia. Tumors of the uterus were also observed in rats that received Clomid or Nafoxidine. Uterine tumors were observed in only a few animals; however, no animals older than 100 days were used in this study. The incidence of uterine tumors may increase considerably in older rats. Other abnormalities include hypertrophied and hyperplastic oviducts; ovarian, oviductual, and uterine inflammation accompanied by pyometra; atrophic ovaries which contained few follicles, a condition that was usually accompanied by atrophic uteri; liquid filled periovarian sacs with small atrophic ovaries; and hilus cell tumors of the ovary. Control animals that received oil injections did not manifest any reproductive tract abnormalities and were cyclic. The types and frequency of abnormalities varied widely among the various treatment groups. The high dose of either Clomid (500 µg) or Nafoxidine (100 µg) produced some form of abnormality in 80 to 100 percent of the animals. Although intermediate and lower doses have not been completely evaluated, our results indicate that 10 to 50 percent of the animals will be adversely affected. For a more detailed report of these findings see Clark and McCormack (5).

FETAL EXPOSURE AND REPRODUCTIVE TRACT ABNORMALITIES

Rats were mated and the morning that copulatory plugs were

found was designated as day zero of pregnancy. Clomid (2.0 mg/kg
body weight) was injected on days 0, 5 and 12 of pregnancy in
either water or oil. Both methods were equally effective. At
birth the number of pups were adjusted to 8 per mother rat. The
pups remained with the mother rat until the day of weaning (day
21) without further handling except for weekly determinations of
body weight. At weaning males and females were separated and
caged in groups of four and checked daily for preputial separation
or vaginal opening. Once this was determined, rats were kept
undisturbed until the termination of the experiment at 15 weeks.
The rat mothers were also sacrificed at this time. Vaginal smears
were obtained on the day of sacrifice and the ovaries, oviducts,
uterus and vagina were removed. These were placed in Bouin's fixative for subsequent sectioning and staining by routine hematoxylyn
and eosin procedures.

     Rats which were injected on day 0 did not become pregnant.
This is in agreement with the observations of others (12, 32,
36); however, when the rats were autopsied 6, 8 and 15 weeks later,
the uteri showed extreme stromal and glandular development with
hyalinization and small angular nuclei, an almost obliterated
lumen and severely metaplastic and disorganized luminal epithelium.
Two of the 5 animals had follicular cysts while 3 had many very
large corpora lutea showing a peculiar fatty degeneration or vacuolization. Oviducts of these rats showed fluid distension with
destruction of the epithelium in some areas. The incidence of
atypical or abnormal epithelial tissues in these animals is shown
in Table 1.

     Three of the rats treated on day 5 became pregnant and deli-
vered normal pups on day 21. When the rats were killed 15 weeks
later, the reproductive tract of both offspring and mothers showed
a remarkable array of abnormal or atypical conditions (Table 1).
The incidence of disorganization and vacuolated epithelium in the
vagina and cervix of the offspring is reminiscent of the vaginal
adenosis which has been observed in young girls whose mothers had
received diethylstilbestrol during pregnancy. These abnormalities
of the epithelium were also observed in the uterus and oviduct of
both offspring and rat mothers. Disorganized hyperplastic epithelium which appeared to be invasive was observed in the uterus and
vagina of offspring and mothers. The high incidence of sloughing
of non-cornified cells, cysts (both uterine and ovarian), degenerating epithelium, extensive metaplasia and hyperplastic vacuolated
epithelium indicate the extent of the abnormalities which can be
produced by Clomid. In addition, leucocytic infiltration of the
intercellular spaces and glands of the stroma and epithelium of
the uterus was observed. This was occasionally seen in the follicles and corpora lutea of the ovaries of both offspring and mothers.

In addition to the abnormalities shown in Table 1, the uteri of the two rats that did not have litters contained extremely wide glandular stroma with a few glandular cysts and low atrophic luminal epithelium.

Of the 6 females injected on day 12, only 4 had litters successfully. One mother bore only 3 pups, two of which were stillborn and one which died 2 days later. A second female went 9 days beyond normal delivery date at which time a laparotomy revealed one uterine horn, ovary and oviduct grossly normal and containing no conceptuses while the other side had a very large ovarian tumor with adhesions to the oviduct, uterus, intestine and body wall. This tumor measured 7 x 10 x 6 cm and contained the necrotic remains of at least 3 pups. Histological examination of the other uterine horn revealed disorganized and possibly invasive epithelium with nests of degenerating stromal cells. The uterine epithelium was metaplastic and cornified throughout the lower half of the uterus. The female pups of these mothers appeared normal at 3 weeks of age, but by 7 weeks areas of luminal epithelial metaplasia had appeared in the uterus. At 15 weeks, the epithelial metaplasia and general extensive stromal development with glandular hyperplasia was marked. In 2 females the cervical epithelium showed proliferation, downgrowth and glandular invasion of the stroma. The ovaries seemed normal but the oviducts were distended with fluid and contained cysts without epithelium. One of 9 male pups had testicular tubules in which spermatogenesis did not proceed beyond secondary spermatocytes. Interstitial cells were abundant. The epididymis was filled only with fluid and cell fragments and showed local cysts with inflammatory reaction. The remaining male offspring appeared normal. For a more detailed account of these findings see McCormack and Clark (30).

ESTROGENIC STIMULATION DURING NEONATAL EXPOSURE

The reproductive tract abnormalities described above are similar to those which have been observed in rats and mice treated during the neonatal period with estrogens (35). Since triphenylethylenes also possess estrogenic properties and are able to stimulate epithelial cell growth (9, 10, 11, 25) we examined their capacity to stimulate uterotropic responses during this period.

Female rat pups of the Sprague-Dawley strain were injected subcutaneously in the nape of the neck on day 5 of life with 100 μg of the following hormones or drugs dissolved in 0.1 ml of oil: testosterone, dihydrotestosterone, corticosterone, progesterone, estradiol, estriol, Nafoxidine, Tamoxifen, Enclomiphene and Zuclomiphene. The animals were killed on day 9, the uteri were removed, trimmed to remove fat and mesentery and weighed. They were immediately placed in Bouin's Fixative for histological

Table 1: Incidence of Epithelial Abnormalities in Rats Treated with Clomid During Pregnancy

Rats were injected with Clomid (2.0 mg/kg body weight) on day 1, 5, or 12 of pregnancy. Rat mothers (n=12) and offspring (n=28) were autopsied 100 days post-partum. Control females either received no treatment or 0.1 ml of oil. Results are expressed as percent of total no. of rats per group.

Abnormality Organ	Experimental Group	Highly Dis-Organized Epithelium	Extensive Hyperplastic Vacuolated Atypical Epithelium	Extensive Metaplastic Epithelium	Cysts
vagina	control	-	-	-	-
	mothers	0	10	0	24
	offspring	0	0	0	8
cervix	control	0	0	0	4
	mothers	12	35	35	0
	offspring	14	21	18	0
uterus	control	0	0	0	8
	mothers	12	47	47	12
	offspring	14	46	68	25
oviduct	control	0	0	0	0
	mother	0	6	0	18
	offspring	0	11	0	0

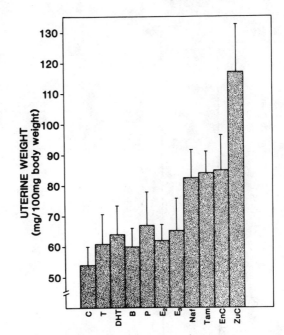

Figure 1. The effect of various steroids and triphenylethylene
derivatives on uterine growth in neonatal rats. Female rats were
injected on day 5 of life with saline (C), testosterone (T), dihydrotestosterone (DHT), corticosterone (B), progesterone (P),
estradiol (E_2), estriol (E_3), Nafoxidine (Naf), Tamoxifen (Tam),
Enclomiphene (EnC) or Zuclomiphene (ZuC). Each compound was injected in oil, 100 μg/0.1 ml, and the uterine weights were determined on day 9.

preparation after weighing.

   None of the steroid hormones caused a significant elevation
in uterine weight 96 hours after injection (Fig 1). In contrast,
all of the triphenylethylene drugs were effective. The estrogenic
properties of these drugs are even more pronounced when the histology of the uterus is examined (Fig 2). The luminal epithelium
from control animals was low cuboidal with round nuclei and the
cell height was just adequate to accomodate the nuclei. All of
the triphenylethylene derivatives caused extensive epithelial
hypertrophy with cell heights 3-5 times that of the long axis of
the ovoid nuclei.

   Hypertrophy and hyperplasia were also present in the stromal
and myometrial layers in the uteri from animals treated with Zuclomiphene. In addition, luminal distension was also observed in

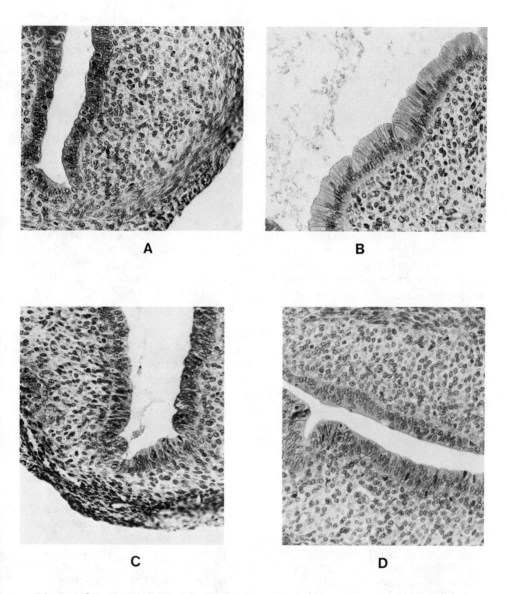

Figure 2. Representative uterine histology of rats treated with saline (A), Zuclomiphene (B), testosterone (C), and estradiol (D). Uterine histology from rats treated wtih Nafoxidine, Tamox- ifen or Enclomiphene does not differ from that shown for Zuclomi- phene. Likewise, treatment with dihydrotestosterone, corticos- terone, progesterone, estriol was similar to that shown for testosterone.

these uteri which resembles that seen in older animals treated
with estradiol. Slight stimulation of the stromal and myometrial
layers was also noted with the other triphenylethylene derivatives
and with estradiol. No stimulation of these tissue layers was
observed with estriol, corticosterone, progesterone, testosterone
or dihydrotestosterone.

DISCUSSION

These results indicate that a single injection of Clomid or
Nafoxidine during fetal or neonatal life of the rat will cause a
wide number of abnormalities of the reproductive tract. These abnormalities may arise from the intense and sustained estrogenic
stimulation of the epithelial lining of these organs (Fig. 1).
The ability of triphenylethelene derivatives to cause epithelial
cell stimulation appears to be a property common to these drugs. This
occurs even in the case of Enclomiphene which is widely considered
to be primarily an anti-estrogen (Fig. 1). Zuclomiphene is clearly
more uterotropic than the other triphenylethylene derivatives and
is capable of stimulating cell growth in all three tissue layers
of the neonatal uterus.

Continuous exposure to high levels of estrogen during fetal and/
or neonatal life is known to increase the incidence of preneoplastic
and neoplastic changes in the reproductive tract (18, 19, 21, 35).
The abnormalities that were observed in the maternal tissues may
also result from a similar hyperestrogenization. We have observed
extensive epithelial cell stimulation in adult cycling rats (unpublished results) and we assume that this takes place in the pregnant
rat.

These results also show that the sustained estrogenic stimulation of the neonatal rat uterus is specific for triphenylethylene
derivatives. The steroid hormones that were administered appear
to have little or no stimulatory effect when they are given as a
single injection. Multiple daily injections of estradiol are
required to cause uterotropic stimulation in the neonate and subsequent development of abnormalities in the adult rodent (35). Multiple injections probably cause continuous receptor occupancy and
continuous uterotropic stimulation over a period of several days
in a way similar to that seen in the animals treated with a single
dose of the triphenylethylene derivatives.

Although we have not ruled out the possibility of indirect
effects of triphenylethylene derivatives, it seems likely that
these drugs are acting directly on the various target tissues. We
have observed previously that Nafoxidine causes long-term retention
of the estrogen receptor by uterine nuclei by a sustained stimulation
of uterine growth up to 19 days after a single injection (6). This

effect also occurs in the neonatal rat (11), and therefore, it is likely that the abnormalities which we have observed are due to long-term estrogenic stimulation during critical periods of reproductive tract development.

We have also shown that Clomid is estrogenic in the uterine endometrium of the ovariectomized baboon (11). This estrogenicity was evident not only from the cellular hypertrophy but also from stimulation of nuclear bodies in epithelial and stromal cells. Nuclear bodies are of unknown function, however, they are associated with intense transcriptional activity and estrogen receptor binding in uterine nuclei (9, 10). Such nuclear bodies have often been identified in neoplastic cells (1, 14).

These observations in the baboon and rat imply that similar estrogenic responses to Clomid may occur in the human. A survey of the literature indicates that similar responses do occur in humans; however, they have been over-looked or deemphasized. This is understandable since these studies were designed to determine the effects of Clomid on ovulation. Ovulation was judged by endometrial biopsy and the desired endpoint was a secretory endometrium (31). Simple endometrial proliferation was taken as evidence that no ovulation had occurred and was assumed to be due to endogenous estrogens. The alternative explanation that endometrial proliferation was due to the inherent estrogenicity of Clomid was not considered. This too is understandable since the evidence in existence at that time for the anti-estrogenic function of Clomid was substantial. Clomid caused decreased vaginal cornification, as judged by decreased pyknotic index, increased the incidence of hot flashes in some women and decreased the fern pattern in cervical mucous (24, 31, 33). As discussed in the introduction, these divergent effects may result from the ability of Clomid to act as a cell specific agonist/antagonist. Therefore, it may function as a anti-estrogen in the vaginal mucosa while acting as an estrogen in the uterine endometrium, and thus, explain the results discussed above.

The effect of Clomid on epithelial cells of the uterus is similar to that which is observed by the unopposed action of estradiol (hyperestrogenization). Since hyperestrogenization is correlated with the development of endometrial carcinoma (22), the possibility that this may occur in women must be considered. However, it seems unlikely that Clomid would result in the development of cancer in women who exhibit ovulation and menstruation as a result of Clomid treatment. Indeed it has been shown that Clomid can be used to treat endometrial hyperplasia and presumably reduce the risk of cancer (27, 37). However, in women who do not develop a luteal phase, and hence do not benefit from the modifying influences of progesterone, caution should be used.

The endometrial epithelium in these women could become hyperestro-
genized and thus provide an environment favorable for the development of cancer.

The estrogenic effects of Clomid in cell types other than those
of the reproductive tract also bear consideration. Clomid is known
to bind estrogen receptors in the hypothalamus and pituitary where
it is generally considered to have an inhibitory effect on the
estrogenic control of gonadotropin secretion (15, 26). Boyer (2)
suggested that low doses of Clomid stimulated gonadotropin secretion
because it antagonized the negative feed-back of endogenous estrogens. He also suggested that high doses inhibit gonadotropin
secretion by virtue of their abiliity to act as estrogens. This
differential response may also be due to cell specific agonist/anta-
gonist effects, i.e., Clomid may have a positive effect on some
hypothalamic or pituitary cells while it may have negative (antagonistic) effects in others. Hsueh et al. (22) have shown that Clomid
increases the sensitivity of pituitary cells to LH-RH in a fashion
similar to that observed with estradiol.

Triphenylethylene derivatives, especially Tamoxifen, are used
in the treatment of estrogen dependent breast cancer. Here again
the rationale is based on the assumption that these drugs are
anti-estrogens and this appears to be the case most of the time.
However, it is predictable from our findings that some mammary
cancers will respond to Tamoxifen as though it were an estrogen.
We have observed a hormone dependent transplantable mammary tumor
line in the mouse which does have this positive response to Nafoxidine (a drug similar to Tamoxifen; unpublished observation, Watson,
Medina and Clark). In addition, Chamness et al. (3) have recently
shown that neonatal treatment with Tamoxifen causes reproductive
tract abnormalities similar to those reported in this and previous
studies (6, 28).

REFERENCES

1. Bouteille, M., Kalifat, S.R. and Delarue, J., 1967,
        J. Ultrastructure Res., 19:474.
2. Boyer, R.M., 1970, Endocrinology, 86:629
3. Chamness, G.C., Bannayan, G.A., Landry, L.A., Sheridan, P.J.,
        and McGuire, W.L., 1979, Biol. Reprod., 21:1087.
4. Clark, J.H. and Gorski, J., 1979, Science, 169:76.
5. Clark, J.H. and McCormack, S.A., 1977, Science, 197:164.
6. Clark, J.H., Anderson, J.N., and Peck, E.J., Jr., 1973, Ster-
        oids, 22:707.
7. Clark, J.H., Anderson, J.N., and Peck, E.J., Jr., 1974, Nature,
        251:446.
8. Clark, J.H., Paszko, Z., and Peck, E.J., Jr., 1977, Endocrin-
        ology, 100:91.

9.   Clark, J.H., Hardin, J.W., McCormack, S.A., and Padykula, H.A.,
        1978, in: "Hormones, Receptors and Breast Cancer," W.L.
        McGuire, ed., Raven Press, New York.
10. Clark, J.H., Hardin, J.W. Padykula, H.A., and Cardasis, C.A.
        1978, Proc. Natl. Acad. Sci. USA, 75:2781.
11. Clark, J.H., McCormack, S.A., Kling, R., Hodges, D., and
        Hardin, J.W., in press, in: "Control Mechanisms in Animal
        Cells," S. Iacobell, ed., Raven Press, New York.
12. Davis, P., Syne, J.S., and Nicholson, R.J., 1979, Endocrino-
        logy, 105:1336.
13. Davidson, O.W., Wada, K., and Schuchner, E.B., 1965, Fertil.
        Steril., 16:495.
14. Dupuy-Coin, A.M., Kalifat, S.R., and Bouteille, M., 1972,
        J. Ultrastruct. Res., 38:174.
15. Eisenfeld, A.J., 1970, Endocrinology, 86:1313.
16. Emmens, C.W., 1970, Ann. Rev. Pharmacol., 4:237.
17. Ferguson, E.R., and Katzenellenbogen, B.S., 1977, Endocrino-
        logy, 100:1242.
18. Forsberg, J.G., 1975, Am. J. Obstet. Gynecol., 121:101.
19. Furth, J., Ueda, G., and Clifton, K.H., 1973, in: "Methods
        in Cancer Research," H. Busch, ed., Academic Press,
        New York. Vol. X.
20. Hardin, J.W., Clark, J.H., Glasser, S.R. and Peck, E.J., Jr.,
        1976, Biochemistry, 15:1370.
21. Herbst, A.L., Ulfelder, H., and Poskanzer, D.C., 1971, N.
        Engl. J. Med., 284:878.
22. Hertz, R., 1974, Cancer, 38:534.
23. Hsueh, A.J.W., Erickson, G.F., and Yen, S.S.C., 1978, Nature,
        273:57.
24. Jones, G.S., and de Morales-Ruehsen, M., 1965, Fertil and
        Steril., 16:461.
25. Jordan, V.C., Dix, C.J. and Prestwich, G., 1979, in: "Steroid
        Hormone Receptor Systems," W. Leavitt, and J.H. Clark,
        eds., Plenum Press, New York.
26. Kistner, R.W., 1975, in: "Progress in Infertility," S.J.
        Berhman and R.W. Kistner, eds., Little, Brown, and Co.,
        Boston.
27. Kistner, R.W., Gore, H., and Hertig, A.T., 1966, Am. J. Obst.
        and Gynec., 95:1011.
28. Kling, O.R., and Westfahl, P.K., 1978, Biol. Reprod., 18:392.
29. Markaverich, B.M., Clark, J.H., and Hardin, J.W., 1978, Bio-
        chemistry, 17:3146.
30. McCormack, S.A. and Clark, J.H., 1979, Science, 204:629.
31. Pildes, R.B., 1965, Am. J. Obst. and Gynec., 91:466.
32. Prasad, M.R.N., Segal, S.J. and Kalra, S.P., 1965, Fertil.
        Steril., 16:101.
33. Riley, G.M. and Evans, T.M., 1964, Am. J. Obst. and Gynec.,
        89:97.
34. Ruh, T.S. and Baudensdistel, L.H., 1977, Endocrinology, 100:
        420.

35. Takasugi, N. and Bern, H.A., 1964, J. Natl. Cancer Inst., 33:
         855.
36. Staples, P.E., 1966, Endocrinology, 78:82.
37. Whitelaw, M.J., 1963, Fertil. and Steril., 14:540.

EFFECT OF ESTRADIOL AND PROGESTERONE ON THE SECRETORY IMMUNE

SYSTEM IN THE FEMALE GENITAL TRACT

Charles R. Wira and David A. Sullivan

Department of Physiology
Dartmouth Medical School
Hanover, N.H. 03755

INTRODUCTION

The presence of a local secretory immune system which both synthesizes and releases Immunoglobulin A (IgA) has been identified at mucosal surfaces of the body[1-3]. A number of investigators have found that while IgA is a minor fraction of total immunoglobulins in the blood, it is the predominant class of antibody in external secretions[4,5]. In secretory fluids, IgA exists as a dimer in combination with two polypeptides, the J (or joining) chain and secretory component[6]. Recent information suggests that secretory component, which is present in epithelial cells acts as a receptor for IgA and mediates dimeric IgA transport[7-10]. The female genital tract appears to be a part of the local immune system because (a) IgA is the principal immunoglobulin in genital tract secretions[11,12]; (b) IgA-positive cells are present in uterine and cervical tissues[13,14]; and (c) the presence of antigens on luminal surfaces leads to the appearance of IgA antibodies in the secretions and IgA-positive plasma cells in the tissues of the genital tract[15,16].

Immunoglobulins in the genital tract are under hormonal control. Previous studies from our laboratory indicated that IgA as well as IgG in rat uterine secretions change during the estrous cycle[12,17]. We observed that IgA was highest at proestrus, remained somewhat elevated at estrus and then declined at diestrus. IgG, in contrast, was highest at proestrus, dropped at estrus and remained low at diestrus. Our interest in the cyclic patterns of both immunoglobulins led to the observation that estradiol, when administered in vivo to ovariectomized or hypophysectomized rats,

increased the levels of IgA and IgG in the uterine lumen. This
increase, however, was abolished when progesterone was given
simultaneously with estradiol. We have also observed that this
response is specific for estradiol and is both dose and time
dependent[17,18]. The present study extends these observations in
an attempt to identify the underlying changes in the uterine
response to estradiol which give rise to the appearance of IgA and
IgG in uterine secretions.

MATERIALS AND METHODS

General Procedures

     Female Sprague-Dawley rats (Charles River Breeding Labs)
were kept in constant temperature rooms with 12 hr intervals of
light and dark. Animals at various stages of the estrous cycle
were chosen after daily vaginal smears indicated that each rat
had at least two normal four day estrous cycles. Ovariectomies
were performed 6-15 days before each experiment. Uterine content
was collected as described earlier[17]. Briefly, after decapitation,
the uterine vascular bed was perfused with saline through the
descending aorta. Following 2-3 washings of the intact uterus to
remove adherent debris, the lumena of both horns were perfused with
0.1 ml of sterile saline. Recovered fluid was centrifuged and the
supernatant was lyophilized and stored -20°C until assayed. Plasma
samples were obtained at the time of decapitation or by direct
cardiac puncture of rats that had been previously anesthetized
with ether. In order to measure circulating lymphocytes, blood
was immediately mixed with 10 μl sodium heparin (Calbiochem, B
grade, 1000 USP/ml). Duplicate aliquots (10 μl) of blood were
then diluted into 10 ml of 0.15 M NaCl. To measure nucleated
cells, all samples were lysed prior to counting by adding 2 drops
of Zap-oglbulin II (Coulter Diagnostics). Determinations were
made with a Model F Coulter Counter (Coulter Electronics, Inc.,
Hialeah, FL at Attenuation 1, Threshold 10, and Aperture at 4 or
8). Blood smears for differential counts were prepared at the
time of blood collection.

Analysis of IgA and IgG

     Immunoglobulin measurements were determined by radioimmuno-
assay using either the immunosorbent[17] or the double antibody
precipitation techniques described below. Rabbit anti-rat heavy
chain IgG antibody (Miles Labs, Elkhart, IN) and goat anti-rat
IgA prepared against IgA rich serum from rats with IR22 immuno-
cytomas (a gift from Dr. H. Bazin, Université Catholique de
Louvain, Belgium) were coupled to cyanogen-bromide activated

microcrystalline cellulose for the immunosorbent assay. Antigen
components of the radioimmunoassay (rat IgG and rat IgA immunocytoma serum) were radiolabeled with ^{125}I using lactoperoxidase
bound Sepharose 4B. Bound IgA and/or IgG was separated from unbound by centrifugation of the microcrystalline-coupled antibody
comples[17]. Lyophilized uterine samples were reconstituted with
50-100 μl of distilled water just prior to use. Tissue IgA levels
were determined by homogenizing uteri with a Polytron in TKM
buffer (50 mM Trizma-HCl, 25 mM KCl, 5 mM $MgCl_2$, pH 7.5) and centrifuging 2x at 10,000 x g for 4 min. Cytosols were analyzed by
double-antibody precipitation using anti-rat IgA (Bazin) and
rabbit anti-goat IgG (Miles-Yeda).

Immunofluorescence Analysis

Uteri were surgically removed and immediately frozen in
liquid nitrogen until used. Specimens were transferred to a
cryostat (-20° C) without thawing and cut into 8 μ sections.
Immunofluorescence staining was carried out with the IgG fraction
of goat anti-rat IgA which was conjugated with fluorescein iso-
thiocyanate (FITC, Sigma Chemical Co., St. Louis, MO). For details
of this procedure, see Wira et al.[19]. FITC-conjugates (initial
concentration, 10 mg/ml) were used at a 1:28 dilution. Sections
were evaluated with a Zeiss Photo III Microscope illuminated by a
HB-200 mercury vapor lamp. Zeiss excitation and barrier filters
for fluorescein were used.

Chromatographic Analysis of Uterine Fluid

Fractionation of uterine fluid, IgG and β-galactosidase were
carried out by Sepharose 6B (Pharmacia, Piscataway, NJ) chromatography. Uterine fluid was obtained from ovariectomized rats
treated with estradiol (1 μg/day for 2 or 3 days). Elution was
performed with TKM buffer with bovine plasma albumin (1 mg/ml,
Calbiochem, La Jolla, CA). Radioimmunoassays of IgA and IgG were
by double-antibody precipitation. IgG standard and β-galactosidase were purchased from Miles Labs, and Boehringer Mannheim,
Gmbh, West Germany, respectively. β-galactosidase was reacted
with O-nitrophenyl β-D-galactoside (Sigma) and monitored spectro-
photometrically at 405 nM.

Analysis of Secretory Component.

The presence of secretory component in uterine fluid was
determined by Ouchterlony analysis. The endpoint of this assay
was an immunoprecipitin band which formed when uterine fluid containing secretory component was placed in one well and reacted

with anti-rat secretory component that was a gift from Dr. B.
Underdown, University of Toronto, Canada. Assays were carried out
on Meloy plates (Springfield, VA) that contained 1.0% agarose in
barbital buffer (ionic strength 0.05, pH 8.6). Reacting products,
which consisted of 10 µl of anti-secretory component versus 5 µl
of uterine fluid, were incubated for 24 hrs at room temperature.

RESULTS

Estradiol and Progesterone Effects on IgA and IgG in Uterine Secretions of the Ovariectomized Rat.

Figure 1 shows the levels of IgA and IgG present in uterine
secretions of ovariectomized rats following treatment with estradiol for three days. Both immunoglobulins increased after 2 to 3
days of hormone treatment while controls which received only solvent showed no change. In other studies, we observed that prolonged daily treatment with estradiol for 7 to 14 days failed to maintain the uterine increase in IgA and IgG measured at 3 days[17,18].
No significant variations in serum levels of either IgA or IgG
were noted during the course of these experiments.

Figure 2 indicates that the stimulatory effect measured after
three days of estradiol treatment did not occur in ovariectomized
rats when progesterone (P) was administered along with estradiol
(E_2). This antagonism existed irrespective of whether progesterone
was given on all three days (E_2-3P), on the last 2 days (E_2-2P),
or on the last day (E_2-1P) of a 3 day estradiol treatment. In
contrast, progesterone by itself had no effect. The levels of IgA
and IgG in serum of hormonally treated ovariectomized rats were
essentially identical to those present in animals that received
only solvent.

Estradiol and Progesterone Effects on Lymphocytes in Blood and on the Movement of IgA-positive Cells into the Rat Uterus.

In light of the marked hormonal changes in IgA and IgG in
the uterine lumen, we were interested in the possible role of
estradiol and progesterone in cellular migration of lymphocytes to
the rat uterus. Figure 3 shows the effect of estradiol on the
number of lymphocytes in blood. When 1 µg of estradiol was administered daily to ovariectomized rats for three days, the number
of circulating lymphocytes gradually declined on days 2 and 3 by
20-35% of the control population. By doing differential smears on
each of the blood samples, we observed that 80-90% of the nucleated
cell population in both the control and hormonally treated groups
consisted of lymphocytes. In other studies, blood lymphocytes
were measured when progesterone (2 mg/day) was administered

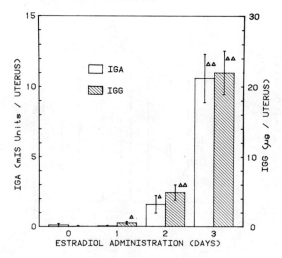

Figure 1. IgA and IgG in the uterine flushings of ovariectomized rats following the administration of estradiol (1.0 µg/0.1 ml) in ethyl laurate given daily for 1, 2 or 3 days. Controls received only ethyl laurate. The bars represent the mean of 5 animals per group and the vertical lines on the bars represent the standard error. Δ, significantly (P<0.005) greater than control; ΔΔ, significantly (P<.05) greater than control. From Wira and Sandoe[17].

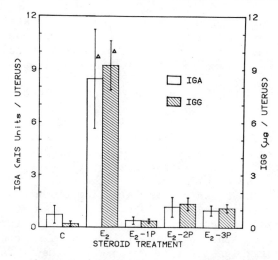

Figure 2. The effect of estradiol and progesterone on IgA and IgG in the uterine flushings of ovariectomized rats Animals were injected with estradiol (1.0 µg/day) and/or progesterone (2.0 mg/day) for 3 days. Progesterone was administered either along with estradiol on all 3 days (E_2-3P), on the last 2 days (E_2-2P) or on the last day (E_2-1P)of a 3 day estradiol treatment. Each bar is the mean±SE of 5 animals. Δ, significantly (P<.01) greater than other groups. From Wira and Sandoe[17].

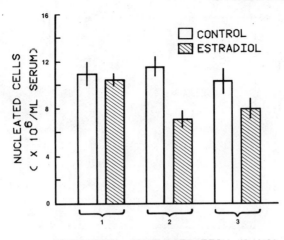

ESTRADIOL ADMINISTRATION (DAYS)

Figure 3.   The effect of estradiol on circulating nucleated cells
in the blood of ovariectomized rats.   Animals were injected with
estradiol (1.0 μg/day in saline for 1, 2 or 3 days.   Twenty-four
hours after the last injection, rats were anesthetized and blood
was collected by direct cardiac puncture.   Bars and brackets indicate the mean±SE of 4-5 animals/group.   From Wira et al.[19].

along with estradiol (1 μg/day) to ovariectomized rats[19].   As was
the case for IgA and IgG in the rat uterine secretions, administration of progesterone along with estradiol (E$_2$-3P) blocked the
estradiol-induced decrease in circulating blood lymphocytes.

The decrease in the number of circulating blood lymphocytes
by estradiol is paralleled by the infiltration of IgA-positive
cells into the uteri of ovariectomized rats.   Using fluoresceinated
anti-rat IgA (FITC-anti IgA), direct fluorescence examination
indicated that IgA-positive cells accumulate in the uteri of
ovariectomized rats treated with estradiol (1 μg/day) for 3 days.
The appearance of these cells appears to be related to the days of
hormone exposure.   As shown in Fig 4A in the absence of estradiol,
no IgA-positive cells were found in the uteri of ovariectomized
rats.   With estradiol treatment, IgA-positive cells appeared in
both the endometrium and myometrium (Fig 4B).   Time course studies
indicated that a few IgA-positive cells were present 24 hours after
a single injection of estradiol.   As judged by a representative
sampling of segments from a number of uteri, greater numbers of
IgA-positive cells were found in the uteri of rats treated with
estradiol for 2 and 3 days.   In other studies, we observed that
progesterone blocked the hormonally-induced accumulation of IgA-
positive cells in the uterus .   Antagonism was complete, however,
only when progesterone was administered for the last 2 days or
for all 3 days along with estradiol.

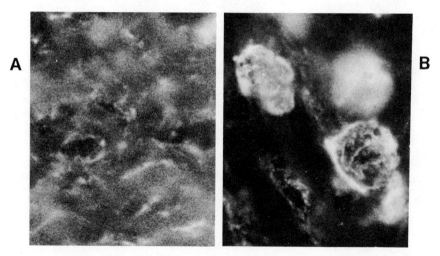

Figure 4. IgA-positive cells in the uteri of ovariectomized rats
treated with estradiol. Frozen sections (7-8 μ) were stained with
fluorceinated anti-rat IgA. A. Section from the uterus of an
animal that received saline for 3 days. B. Uterine section from
an animal that received daily injections of estradiol (1.0 μg/
0.1 ml saline) for 3 days.

While it is clear that the uterine IgA response involves the
infiltration of IgA-positive cells into the tissues, it is unlikely that IgG- positive cells are involved in the increase in
IgG in the uterine secretions. Immunofluorescent analysis with
FITC-anti IgG failed to demonstrate the presence of IgG-positive
cells in uteri from estradiol-treated rats (1 μg/day, for 1, 2 or
3 days). Since IgG-positive cells were present in control sections
of rat intestine, the absence of IgG-positive cells in the uterus
cannot be accounted for by antisera-related problems.

Estradiol Stimulation of IgA and IgG Movement from the Uterus
into the Uterine Lumen.

The movement of IgA but not IgG from the uterus into the
lumen is against a concentration gradient. As seen in Table I,
the concentration of IgA in the uterus following estradiol
treatment was significantly lower than that in the uterine lumen.
In contrast, the concentration of IgG in the uterus was greater
than that measured in the lumen. These results suggest that IgA
moves into the lumen by a mechanism that is distinct from that
which regulates the appearance of IgG.

Table 1.   The Concentration of IgA and IgG in the
Uterus and in the Uterine Secretions Following
the Treatment of Ovariectomized Rats with Estradiol[a]

Immunoglobulin	Uterus	Uterine Fluid
IgA	0.006 ± 0.0021[b] (4)[f]	0.130 ± 0.0150[c] (4)
IgG	0.36 ± 0.0210[d] (4)	0.016 ± 0.0054[e] (4)

[a]Rats were injected with estradiol (1 µg/day for 3 days) in saline; [b]IgA expressed as mIS units/mg tissue; [c]mIS units/µl uterine fluid; [d]IgG expressed as µg/mg tissue; [e]µg/µl uterine fluid; [f]number of rats in each group.

IgA movement is closely related to epithelial cells that line the uterine lumen[20]. In the absence of estradiol, very little IgA was found within these cells. Some however was identified in the basement membrane region adjacent to the epithelial cells. With estradiol (1 µg/day) for 3 days, we observed that IgA increased markedly in these cells at a time that coincided with the maximal accumulation of IgA in the uterine lumen.

Analysis of uterine fluid by Sepharose-6B chromatography indicated that IgA consisted of a single peak, which was of higher molecular weight than IgG (Figure 5). Uterine IgA had an elution profile that was analogous to the elution peak of β-galactosidase an enzyme of 540,000 M.W. Also shown is the elution profile of uterine IgG which was indistinguishable from rat IgG standard.

Secretory Component in the Rat Uterus

Both the stage of the estrous cycle and treatment of ovariectomized rats with estradiol influence the appearance of secretory component in uterine secretions. As seen in Table 2, secretory component was detected in the uterine secretions of intact female rats at the proestrus but not at the diestrous stage of the estrous cycle. Table 2 also shows that secretory component was present in the uterine secretions of ovariectomized rats treated with estradiol (1 µg/day for 3 days) but was unmeasurable in saline-injected controls. Secretory component was not detected in serum taken from either control or hormonally treated groups. In other studies using FITC-anti rat secretory component, secretory component increased in uterine epithelial cells in response to estradiol[20].

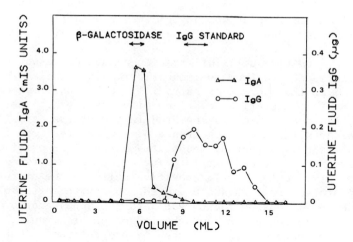

Figure 5. Fractionation by Sepharose 6B of IgA and IgG in the uterine fluid of ovariectomized rats treated with estradiol (1.0 µg in 0.1 ml saline) daily for 2 and 3 days.

Table 2. The Presence of Secretory Component in Uterine Flushings of Rats at Various Stages of the Estrous Cycle, Following Ovariectomy and After Estradiol Treatment

| | Stage of Estrous Cycle | | | | Ovariectomy + |
	Proestrus	Estrus	Diestrus	Ovariectomy	Estradiol[a]
Percentage of Positive Responses	100	20	0	0	100
Number in Group[b]	8	5	7	5	5

[a]Rats were injected with 0.1 ml of saline containing 1 µg of estradiol daily for 3 days. Ovariectomized control rats received only saline; [b]indicates the number of rats within each group.

DISCUSSION

These results show that IgA is under sex hormonal control and that estradiol affects at least two parameters of the uterine secretory immune system. Evidence to support this hypothesis comes from our observations that estradiol influences both the infiltration of IgA-positive cells into the uterus and the movement of high molecular weight IgA into the uterine secretions by a process that involves uterine epithelial cells.

That IgA-positive cell infiltration occurs in response to estradiol is indicated from our immunoflourescent studies which showed that, in the absence of estradiol, no IgA-positive cells were present in the uteri of ovariectomized rats. With estradiol treatment, IgA-positive cells appeared in the uterus at a time that coincided with the disappearance of lymphocytes from the blood. This suggests that at least some of the IgA-positive cells in the uterus are of blood origin. The correlation between circulating lymphocytes and IgA-positive cells in the uterus also holds when progesterone is administered along with estradiol. Under these conditions we found that both the appearance of IgA-positive cells in the uterus and the reduction of circulating lymphocytes in the blood were blocked by progesterone. Others have shown that lymphocytes accumulate in mucosal tissues in a hormonally dependent way and that Peyer's patches and mesenteric lymph nodes are a primary source of lymphocytes which migrate to the mucosal tissues of the mammary gland[22]. These studies further demonstrated that prolactin, progesterone and estrogen, when given either alone or in combination, resulted in an increase in IgA-containing plasma cells in the mammary tissues of virgin female mice. Selective migration of lymphocytes was demonstrated experimentally by the ability of injected in vitro labeled IgA-positive cells from the mesenteric lymph nodes and Peyer's patches to populate the mammary glands of hormonally treated mice in greater numbers than did cells from peripheral lymph nodes[23,24]. Preliminary findings in our laboratory suggest that lymphocytes may also migrate to the uterus in a hormone dependent fashion[19]. When pooled ^{51}Cr-tagged lymphocytes from the mesenteric lymph nodes, Peyer's patches, peripheral lymph nodes and para-aortic nodes were injected intravenously, an increase in radioactivity was observed in the uteri of estradiol-treated rats. Further work, however, is necessary to determine whether lymphocytes migrate to the uterus in the same selective way that they do in the mammary gland.

Estradiol also plays an important role in the movement of IgA into the uterine lumen. By analyzing the IgA in uteri and uterine fluid following estradiol treatment, we observed that the concentration of IgA in the uterine lumen was about 20x greater than that found in the uterus. This indicates that IgA moves against a concentration gradient and suggests that it may be transported into the uterine lumen. When these results are considered along with our immunofluorescent findings[20], it suggests that estradiol, by its action on epithelial cells in the uterus, may regulate IgA movement into the uterine lumen. In the absence of estradiol very little IgA was present in these cells. With hormone treatment, IgA accumulated within the epithelial cells at a time that coincided with the maximal build up of IgA in uterine secretions.

The data in table II showing that secretory component is present in the uterine lumen both during the estrous cycle and in response to estradiol treatment, suggests that secretory component might function as a transport protein to move polymeric IgA from the uterus into the lumen. The possibility that secretory component facilitates IgA transport by functioning as a receptor on epithelial cells receives support from several studies. Orlans et al.[10] and Socken et al.[9] reported that radiolabeled polymeric IgA binds to rat hepatocytes. Binding was inhibited, however, when either anti-secretory component or excess polymeric IgA was added. Fisher et al.[7] used the isolated perfused rat liver system to determine that radiolabeled polymeric IgA, but not monomeric IgA, binds to secretory component as it is transported into the bile space. In a more recent study, oligomeric, J-chain-containing immunoglobulins were observed to be transferred selectively from serum to colostrum[21]. The experiments reported here indicate that the presence of secretory component in uterine secretions is estradiol dependent and that its appearance coincides with the maximal accumulation of IgA in the uterine lumen. In other studies[20], we have found that IgA is associated with secretory component in the uterine lumen. These experiments as well as those cited earlier support the hypothesis that IgA transport into the lumen is regulated by the action of estradiol on uterine epithelial cells which contain secretory component.

The present studies indicate that estradiol regulates the movement of IgG in the uterus in a way that is distinctly different from IgA. This conclusion is based on two findings. First, immunofluorescent studies have failed to demonstrate either the presence of IgG-positive cells in the uterus or the accumulation of IgG in uterine epithelial cells following estradiol treatment; and second, that IgG does not accumulate in uterine secretions against a concentration gradient as does IgA. Studies are presently underway in our laboratory to establish the means whereby estradiol regulates the movement of IgG into the rat uterine lumen.

SUMMARY

The female genital tract is a part of the secretory immune system that functions to keep the body free from disease by working against bacterial invasion. In response to estradiol, the essential component in this system, IgA, accumulates in uterine secretions of ovariectomized rats. Evidence is presented

that estradiol has an effect on at least three parameters of the
uterine IgA response by increasing: 1) the amount of IgA and the
infiltration of IgA-positive lymphocytes into the uterine
endometrium and myometrium; 2) the movement of IgA from the
tissue into the uterine lumen, and 3) the amount of secretory
component present in the uteri of proestrus, and ovariectomized
rats treated with estradiol. These studies indicate that estradiol
plays an important role in regulating the uterine immune system.
Further, it suggests that estradiol may control lymphocyte
migration into the uterus as well as IgA transport into the
uterine lumen.

Acknowledgements. We are indebted to Dr. Herve Bazin of the
Universite Catholique De Louvain for his kind gift of IR22
immunocytoma material and to Dr. Brian Underdown of the University
of Toronto for his generous gift of antisera for rat secretory
component. This work was supported by Research Grant AI 13541
from the National Institutes of Health U.S.P.H.S.

REFERENCES

1. T.B. Tomasi, Jr., and J. Bienenstock, Secretory immunoglobulins,
      Adv. Immunol. 9:1 (1968).
2. M.E. Lamm, Cellular aspects of immunoglobulin A, Adv. Immunol.
      22:223 (1976).
3. R. Ganguly, and R.H. Waldman, Local immunity and local immune
      responses, Prog. Allergy 27:1 (1980).
4. T.S. Bistany, and T.B. Tomasi, Jr., Serum and secretory
      immunoglobulins of the rat, Immunochemistry 7:453 (1970).
5. D.J. Stechschulte, and K.F. Austen, Immunoglobulins of rat
      colostrum, J. Immunol. 104:1052 (1970).
6. R.S. Labib, and T.B. Tomasi, Jr., Secretory immunoglobulin A,
      in: "CRC Handbook Series in Clinical Laboratory Science,
      Section F: Immunology, vol· 1" (A. Baumgarten, and
      F.F. Richards) eds., CRC Press, West Palm Beach (1978).
7. M. Fisher, B. Nagy, H. Bazin, and B. Underdown, Biliary
      transport of IgA: role of secretory component, Proc. Natl.
      Acad. Sci. U.S.A. 76:2008 (1979).
8. S. Crago, R. Kulhevy, S. Prince, and J. Mestecky, Secretory
      component on epithelial cells is a surface receptor for
      polymeric immunoglobulins, J. Exp. Med. 147:1832 (1978).
9. D.J. Socken, K.N. Jeejeebhoy, H. Bazin, and B.J. Underdown,
      Identification of secretory component as an IgA receptor
      on rat hepatocytes, J. Exp. Med. 50:1538 (1979).
10. E. Orlans, J. Peppard, J.F. Fry, R.N. Hinton, and B.M. Mullock,
      Secretory component as the receptor for polymeric IgA on
      rat hepatocytes, J. Exp. Med. 150:1577 (1979).

11. R.H. Waldman, J.M. Cruz, and D.S. Rowe, Immunoglobulin levels
     and antibody to candida albicans in human cervicovaginal
     secretions, Clin. Exp. Immunol. 9:427 (1971).
12. C.R. Wira, and C.P. Sandoe, Sex hormone regulation of IgA and
     IgG in rat uterine secretions, Nature 268:534 (1977).
13. D.R. Tourville, S.S. Ogra, J. Lippes, and T.B. Tomasi, Jr.,
     The human female reproductive tract: immunohistological
     localization of λA, λG, λM, "secretory piece", and
     lactoferrin, Am. J. Obstet. Gynec. 108:1102 (1970).
14. R. Rebello, F.H.Y. Green, and H. Fox, A study of the secretory
     immune system of the female genital tract, Brit. J. Obstet.
     Gynec. 82:812 (1975).
15. R.H. Waldman, J.M. Cruz, and D.S. Rowe, Intravaginal
     immunization of humans with Candida albicans, J. Immunol.
     109:662 (1972).
16. E.J. Chipperfield, and B.A. Evans, The influence of local
     infection on immunoglobulin formation in the human
     endocervix, Clin. Exp. Immunol. 11:219 (1972).
17. C.R. Wira, and C.P. Sandoe, Hormonal regulation of immuno-
     globulins: influence of estradiol on immunoglobulins A and
     G in the rat uterus, Endocrinology 106:1020 (1980).
18. C.R. Wira, and C.P. Sandoe, Regulation by sex hormones of
     immunoglobulins in rat uterine and vaginal secretions, in:
     Secretory Immunity and Infection: "Proceedings of the
     International Symposium on the Secretory Immune System and
     Carrier Immunity." J.R. McGhee, J. Mestecky, and J.L. Babb,
     eds.) Plenum Press, N.Y. (1978).
19. C.R. Wira, E. Hyde, C.P. Sandoe, D. Sullivan, and S. Spencer,
     Cellular aspects of the rat uterine IgA response to
     estradiol and progesterone, J. Steroid Biochem. 12:451
     (1980).
20. C.R. Wira, D.A. Sullivan, and C.P. Sandoe, (unpublished
     observation).
21. J.F. Halsey, B.H. Johnson, and J.J. Cebra, Transport of
     immunoglobulins from serum into colostrum. J. Exp. Med.
     151:767 (1980).
22. M.E. Lamm, P. Weisz-Carrington, M.D. Roux, M. McWilliams and
     J.M. Phillips-Quagliata, Development of the IgA System in
     the Mammary gland, in: "Secretory Immunity and Infection:
     Proceedings of the International Symposium on the Secretory
     Immune System and Carrier Immunity." J.R. McGhee, J.
     Mestecky, and J.L. Babb, eds.) Plenum Press, N.Y. (1978).
23. M.E. Roux, M. McWilliams, J.M. Phillips-Quagliata, P. Weisz-
     Carrington and M.E. Lamm, Origin in IgA-secreting plasma
     cells in the mammary gland, J. Exp. Med. 146:1311 (1977).
24. P. Weisz-Carrington, M.E. Roux, M. McWilliams, J.M. Phillips-
     Quagliata and M.E. Lamm, Hormonal induction of the secretory
     immune system in the mammary gland, Proc. Nat. Acad. Sci.
     75:2928 (1978).

THE SEARCH FOR PROGESTERONE-DEPENDENT PROTEINS SECRETED BY HUMAN ENDOMETRIUM

David T. MacLaughlin, Paul E. Sylvan and George S. Richardson

Vincent Memorial and Mass. General Hospitals; Dept. Obstet. & Gynec., Harvard Medical School, Boston, MA

INTRODUCTION

It has been generally agreed that the mechanism of steroid hormone action in human endometrium is similar to the model developed from studies in a variety of experimental animals (1-6). Briefly outlined, the model has three main features: 1) steroids bind to hormone and tissue-specific intracellular receptors with high affinity resulting in an "activated" steroid-receptor complex; 2) this complex translocates to the nucleus and binds to specific "acceptor" and "effector" sites on the genome; 3) binding induces the synthesis of messenger ribonucleic acids that are processed, transported to the cytoplasm and translated into proteins that alter cell function. A complete definition of a steroid hormone receptor, therefore, should not only include data on binding kinetics for the receptor-steroid interaction but also a direct correlation with the control of some known biological activity in the target tissue.

The value of measuring specific gene products of steroid hormones in addition to the receptors themselves, particularly in the area of the clinical management of neoplasias, is best illustrated by the following observations. Human breast cancers that do not contain detectable levels of estradiol receptor do not respond to various endocrine manipulations. The presence of such receptors, on the other hand, is correlated with significant improvement with hormonal therapy in only 60% of the cases (7). Similarly, the presence of glucocorticoid receptors in cultured hepatocytes or lymphoma cells does not mean that they will respond to glucocorticoids. In some instances "defective receptors" do not translate to the nucleus; in others receptors are present and

113

translocation occurs but the response still fails (8,9). If
receptor measurements were the sole method of analysis in such
cases, the results would prove to be misleading. Whether such
peculiarities of sex steroid receptor dynamics exist in human
endometrial carcinoma remains to be seen.

Direct relationships between sex steroid receptors and the
control of specific cellular functions have been described for a
number of systems including the induced protein (IP) in rat uterus
(10), avidin (11), and ovalbumin (12) in chick oviduct, low density
lypoprotein of chicken liver (13), $\alpha 2$ μg globulin of rat liver (14),
and perhaps uteroglobin from the rabbit uterus (15) to name a few.
Although "receptors" for estradiol (16-26), progesterone (22,27-34)
and perhaps testosterone (35-37) have been described in normal and
abnormal human endometrium, few correlations between these
receptors and a known biologic activity have been reported. Among
the best characterized are the appearance of estradiol dehydrogenase
in response to progestins (38-40) and the control of receptor levels
by estrogens and progestins (41-43). More recently, Maslar and
Riddick (44) have presented evidence that immunoreactive prolactin
is synthesized and released by the human endometrium in response
to progesterone. Further evidence for prolactin secretion is
provided by the report of Golander et al (45) in which incubations
of decidua obtained at cesarean section produced prolactin-like
material.

The cellular functions that have been implicated as being
under estrogenic and/or progestational (and presumably receptor-
mediated) control in the human endometrium are manifested by
products that are of two kinds: intracellular and secretory. The
intracellular metabolic activities, in addition to those mentioned
above, include the control of certain enzymes of carbohydrate,
protein, steroid and prostaglandin synthesis and degradation (46-
57). These provide energy early in the endometrial cycle in the
form of adenosine triphosphate (ATP) and reduced enzyme cofactors
such as nicotinamide-adenosine diphosphate (NADPH), perhaps for
use later on in the synthesis of new macromolecules and the
metabolism of steroids.

Secretion of materials by the endometrial glands appears to
be largely under the control of progesterone. Histochemical
studies suggest that endometrial secretions contain glycogen, glycoproteins, nucleic acid, lipids, hydrolytic enzymes, and possibly
alkaline and acid phosphatases (46,49-51). In other studies it has
been reported that the secretory fluid consists mainly of serum
proteins (58-63). Still others have reported the presence of
proteins, in addition to those from blood, that appear to be
secretory phase-specific (61,62,64). Conflicting results have also
appeared concerning the identification of a uteroglobin-like (15)
protein in human uterine fluid (63,65,66).

   The question of which products can be termed "receptor-dependent" gene products in either the intracellular or secretory compartments of human endometrium is by no means clear. As part of our continuing studies into the mechanism of action of progesterone on human endometrium, we have recognized the need for identifying gene-products for this steroid, and have undertaken a detailed analysis of uterine-luminal fluid in search of such a protein. The results of our initial studies (67,68) are presented in this paper.

MATERIALS AND METHODS

   Collection of Uterine Luminal Fluid. Samples of human uterine luminal washings were obtained under sterile conditions by means of the Gravlee negative pressure technique (69) from young women under anesthesia mainly for the purpose of tubal ligation. The washings, obtained in 0.15 M glycine, were centrifuged at 4 C at 850 g for 30-60 minutes to remove cells and other particulate matter, desalted by dialysis against distilled water for 24-48 hours at 4 C or by Sephadex G-25 (1 x 50 cm) chromatography in distilled water, and concentrated by lyophilization. All preparations were stored at -20 to -80 C.

   Collection of Sera. Sera were prepared from blood collected from patients from whom uterine washings were obtained at the time of the procedure. A portion of each serum sample was frozen at -20 to -80 C and the remainder desalted in the same manner as the luminal wash samples.

   Histological Evaluation of Endometrium. Tissue specimens obtained immediately after the washes were performed were reviewed according to the scheme of Noyes et al (70) by our Pathology Department without prior knowledge of the experimental results.

   Protein Determinations. The protein content of desalted washes and sera was estimated using the sensitive and nondestructive optical technique of Waddell (71). Sephadex G-25 and G-200 (see below) eluates were monitored for protein by the Waddell technique also, and occasionally pooled, concentrated fractions were analyzed further by the method of Lowry et al (72). Bovine serum albumin (BSA) was used as the standard for both techniques.

   Polyacrylamide Gel Electrophoresis. Two types of electrophoretic runs were performed in this study. The first method employed was that of Davis (73) using 7.5% acrylamide gels in a Gilson disc gel electrophoresis apparatus. Minor alterations in the technique included the omission of the stacking gel. The gels were stained with Coomassie Brilliant Blue or Amido-Schwarts 10-B (Sigma) overnight prior to electrophoretic destaining.

In subsequent studies sodium dodecyl-sulfate (SDS) polyacryl-amide gel electrophoresis was carried out in 10% acrylamide essentially according to the method of Weber and Osborn (74). The samples were incubated at 37 C for 2 hours prior to the run. These gels were stained with either Coomassie Brilliant Blue or periodic acid-Schiff (PAS) reagent by the technique of Zacharius et al (75). In all cases the dye marker used was bromphenol blue and the length of the gels and the location of the dye band were measured before and after staining and destaining. The length of the runs, current applied and sample composition are listed in the legends to the figures.

Column Chromatography. Samples of uterine wash protein or serum in 0.5 ml of Tris-EDTA buffer (Tris-hydroxymethyl-amino-methane; EDTA-disodium (ethylene-dinitrilo-tetracetate); (10 mM, 1.5 mM, pH 8.0) were run over a Sephadex G-200 (superfine) column (1 x 25 cm) (Pharmacia) equilibrated with the appropriate buffer at 4 C. Fractions of 0.5 ml were collected using a Gilson micro-fractionator. The protein elution profile was monitored using the Waddell technique and the fractions were pooled by size, desalted, and concentrated by lyophilization.

Sucrose Gradient Centrifugation. Samples (200 μl) of uterine wash proteins or bovine serum albumin were layered onto linear sucrose gradients (5 ml, 5-15% w/v) and centrifuged for 18 hours, 4 C, 300,000 x g in a Beckman L3-50 ultracentrifuge equipped with a swinging bucket rotor. At the end of the run, fractions were collected dropwise from the bottom of the polyallomer tubes and analysed for protein using the Waddell technique.

RESULTS

Characterization of Uterine Luminal Washes. Each wash procedure was carried out using 10 ml of the glycine buffer. The average volume of the washes collected was 9.01 mls containing an average protein content of 7.29 mg (Table I). No significant difference was noted between the washes of proliferative and secretory endometria with respect to the volume or protein content.

TABLE I

VOLUME AND PROTEIN CONTENT OF UTERINE LUMINAL WASHES

	Volume (mls)*	Protein (mg)**
All samples	9.01 ± .91	7.29 ± .02
Proliferative samples	8.53 ± 1.57	7.71 ± 3.45
Secretory samples	9.39 ± 1.12	6.97 ± 3.20

*Volume in mls ± S.E.M.
**Protein by Waddell method ± S.E.M.

Polyacrylamide Gel Electrophoresis of Sera and Luminal Washes.
Analysis of either proliferative or secretory-phase luminal washes
by standard polyacrylamide gel electrophoresis revealed a protein
profile after staining that was indistinguishable from that seen
with serum (Figure 1). In some cases, fewer bands were seen in
the wash material than in serum, but the bands that were present
were also seen in serum samples. Because of the complexity of the
protein banding patterns and the possibility that proteins unique
to the luminal washes might be obscured by contaminating serum,
the washes and sera were fractionated by molecular size before
further analysis.

Column Chromatography. Representative elution profiles of
Sephadex G-200 column chromatography of proliferative and secretory
uterine washes and their corresponding sera are shown in Figure 2.
The Waddell protein peak, termed peak III, that eluted between 15
and 18 mls, was present only in the washes of secretory endometrium
(Figure 2B). No such peak was seen in the accompanying serum
profile from the same patient or in the uterine washings or serum
from a different patient in the proliferative phase (Figure 2A).
In all, 21 uterine washes (8 proliferative, 11 secretory, 2
inactive) and 9 sera (4 proliferative, 4 secretory, 1 inactive)
were examined in this manner. The results of these experiments
are summarized in Table II.

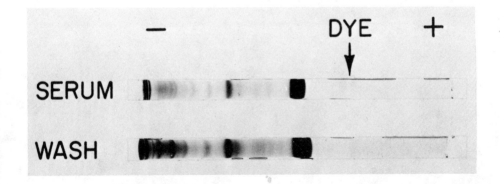

Figure 1. Polyacrylamide (7.5%) gel electrophoresis of dialyzed
and lyophilized serum (140 µg) and Gravlee wash (100 µg)
proteins. The electrophoresis run was for 60 min, 4 MA/
gel at room temperature followed by staining with Amido-
Schwartz 10-B. The dye marker was bromphenol blue.

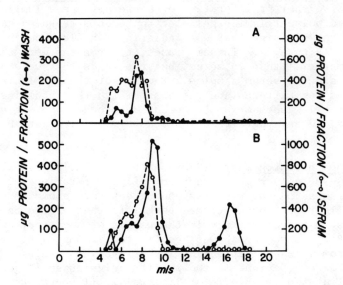

Figure 2.   A) Sephadex G-200 (superfine) 1 x 25 cm column chromatography of 1.0 mg of proliferative wash protein (•-•)
and serum (o--o) from the same patient, a composite
figure.   Elution buffer - Tris-EDTA, 0.5 ml fractions,
protein estimated by the Waddell technique (void volume
4 mls, retention volume ∼20 mls).
B) Column chromatography of 2.5 mg of secretory wash
protein (•-•) and serum (o--o) from the same patient.
A composite figure.   Conditions as above.

TABLE II

'PEAK III' IN WASHES AND SERA

	Sera		Washes	
	(-)	(+)	(-)	(+)
Proliferative	4	0	7	1[1]
Secretory	4	0	1	10[2]
Inactive	1	0	2	0
Total	9	0	10	11

[1]18% of recovered protein in 'Peak III'
[2]25-65% of recovered protein in 'Peak III'

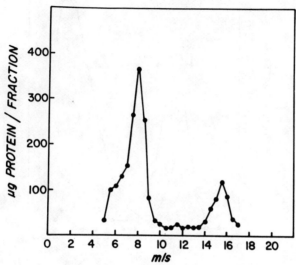

Figure 3. Sephadex G-200 column chromatography of an equal mixture
           of serum and wash protein (1 mg each) from the same
           patient. Column conditions as in Figure 2.

Serum contaminations did not affect the presence of peak III. When
equal quantities of protein from serum and uterine washings known
to contain peak III were mixed and chromatographed over a Sephadex
G-200 column, the peak appeared at the expected locations and in
the predicted amount (Figure 3).

   Sucrose Gradients. The apparent low molecular weight of the
peak III material was confirmed by ultracentrifugation on a 5-15%
(w/v) linear sucrose gradient (Figure 4). Dialyzed, lyophilized
and reconstituted peak III material remained near the top of the
gradient. Similar low molecular weight material was observed in
an unfractionated wash preparation known to contain peak III.
Note also that the higher molecular weight fraction from Sephadex
chromatography, peak II, (8-10 mls of elution) contained
essentially no peak III-like material.

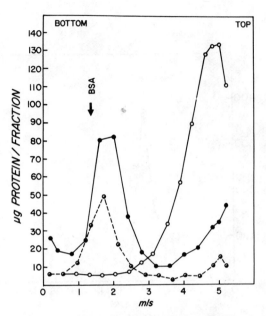

Figure 4.   Sucrose density gradient ultracentrifugation. Bovine
serum albumin, BSA (arrow), secretory Sephadex G-200
peak III (o-o), unfractionated secretory wash protein
(●--●), and secretory Sephadex G-200 peak II protein
(◐--◐).   Each sample 500 μg protein by Waddell.

Protein Measurement of Peak III Material. The Waddell measurements of protein in peak III were confirmed by Lowry protein
measurements of the same material. Estimates of peak III protein
obtained independently by these two techniques agreed extremely
well (r = .984, y = 1.3x - 22.33, p < 0.001). (Figure 5).

Polyacrylamide Gel Electrophoresis of Fractionated Wash
Proteins. Samples of secretory phase Sephadex G-200 peak I (6-
8 mls), II (8-10 mls) and III (15-18 mls) material were desalted
separately by dialysis or Sephadex G-25 column chromatography in
distilled water and concentrated by lyophilization. Figure 6 shows
a representative set of stained protein profiles for peak I, II

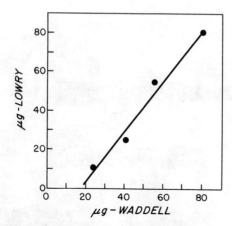

Figure 5.   Correlation between protein values for four preparations
            of Sephadex G-200 peak III material determined by the
            methods of Lowry et al (72) and Waddell (71).

and III material. As expected, peaks I and II show a considerable
overlap of similar proteins with peak I having more of the slower
moving components (Figures 6I and II). A portion of the peak III
material co-migrated with proteins seen in the peak I and II
fractions (Figure 6III, large arrow). Another faster moving but
more diffuse area of staining was occasionally seen but its
significance is as yet unclear (small arrow).

    Peak III material was also subjected to SDS polyacrylamide gel
electrophoresis and stained with Coomassie Blue or periodic-acid
Schiff (PAS) reagent. The protein staining of these gels revealed
one major and four minor bands in this system (Figure 7A). Only
the major band, however, was evident when the gels were stained
with PAS (Figure 7B). Based on comparisons with the relative
mobilities of the protein standards run on companion gels, the
apparent molecular weight of the major band was 69,000, while the
minor bands exhibited molecular weight values ranging from 88,000
to 17,500.

DISCUSSION

    It is clear from these initial studies (Figure 1) and from
the work of others (58-64) that the uterine luminal fluid

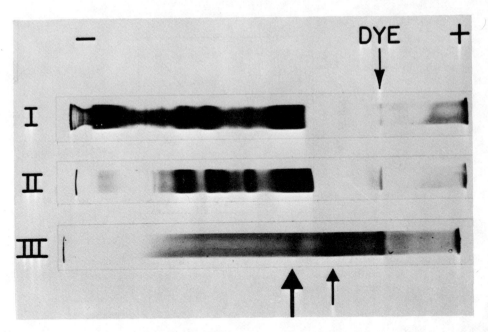

Figure 6.   Polyacrylamide (10%) gel electrophoresis of dialyzed and
            lyophilized Sephadex G-200 peak I (elution volume 4-6
            mls, 140 µg) I, Peak II (elution volume 7-10 mls, 100 µg)
            II, and peak III (elution volume 16-18 mls, 10 µg) III,
            of a secretory-phase uterine wash sample. The run was
            for 60 min, 4 MA/gel, at room temperature followed by
            staining with Coomassie Brilliant Blue. The dye marker
            was bromphenol blue.

collection from humans contains a considerable amount of serum
protein. It was also clear that electrophoretic analyses of whole
washes and sera were inadequate to identify wash-specific material.
Our objective, therefore, was to simplify the comparison between
washes and sera by fractionating the proteins contained in such
preparations according to their molecular size before further
analysis. The first step in the fractionation scheme was Sephadex
G-200 column chromatography. As can be seen in Figure 2, this
simple step reveals a "low molecular weight" fraction that appears
to be unique to secretory phase wash material. The apparent low
molecular weight of peak III material relative to the other
proteins in these preparations is confirmed by its location in
sucrose gradient ultracentrifugation (Figure 4). Standard polyacrylamide gel electrophoresis of peak III from secretory wash
preparations shows that it co-migrates with proteins seen in the
larger molecular weight fractions (G-200 peaks I and II) in this
system (Figure 6). This may explain why no "unique" luminal wash
proteins could be demonstrated when unfractionated material was

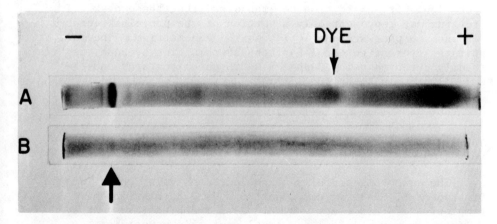

Figure 7. S D S polyacrylamide (10%) gel electrophoresis of 10 µg
of dialyzed and lyophilized peak III material from a
secretory-phase wash. The gels were stained with either
Coomassie Brilliant Blue, A, or PAS stain, B. The
arrow indicates the position of the major staining
component in each gel. The dye marker was bromphenol
blue. The run was for 1 hour, 20 MA/gel.

examined by disc electrophoresis. As can be seen from Figure 1,
many serum proteins also migrate in the area of peak III, but as
shown in Figure 3, serum proteins apparently do not interact with
peak III proteins. SDS disc gel electrophoresis, on the other hand,
shows that peak III contains a major and four minor bands of protein
(Figure 7A) exhibiting apparent molecular weights, with one
possible exception, that are discordant with what one would expect
based on the elution profile from Sephadex G-200 column chromatography. This paradox may be explained in part by the apparent
glycoprotein nature implied by the positive PAS staining of the
major band (Figure 7B). Abnormal electrophoretic behavior is
known to occur with glycoproteins in SDS gels. Conversely, the
proteins in the peak III fraction may be interacting with the
Sephadex beads during the column run, thereby retarding their
movement through the gel matrix. The reason for the lack of
agreement between the properties of peak III on Sephadex columns
and sucrose gradients and the SDS gel electrophoresis is currently
under investigation.

In conclusion, human uterine luminal fluid contains a group
of proteins not present in serum that are detectable chiefly in
the secretory phase of the menstrual cycle. It has not yet been
established that these "peak III" proteins are progesterone-
dependent, and this important point is currently under investigation. The indirect evidence, however, suggests that these
proteins may be progesterone-induced products of human endometrial

secretion. It should also be emphasized that these peak III
proteins may represent only a portion of the proteins secreted in
response to progesterone action on the endometrium. They are of
primary interest to our laboratory at this time because they are
readily detected using Sephadex G-200 chromatography and the
Waddell protein technique (71).

ACKNOWLEDGEMENTS

This work was supported by USPHS Grant CA 18678, American
Cancer Society (NY) Grant PDT-138, and the Vincent Fund.

The authors gratefully acknowledge the valuable assistance of
Dr. Robert E. Scully, Jean Stuart and Jane Anthony in the
completion of this study. We are also indebted to Ms. Nancy
Delaney for her skillful preparation of this manuscript.

REFERENCES

1. Baulieu, E.-E. Steroid receptors and hormone receptivity.
    New approaches in pharmacology and therapeutics. J. Amer.
    Med. Assoc. 234:404, 1975.

2. Baulieu, E.-E., Atger, M., Best-Belpomme, M., Corvoll, P.,
    Courvalin, J.-C., Mester, J., Milgrom, E., Robel, P.,
    Rochefort, H. and DeCatalogne, D. Steroid hormone receptors.
    Vitamins and Hormones 33:649, 1975.

3. Chan, L. and O'Malley, B.W. Mechanism of action of the sex
    steroid hormones (first of three parts). N.Eng. J. Med. 294:
    1322, 1976.

4. Chan, L. and O'Malley, B.W. Mechanism of action of the sex
    steroid hormones (second of three parts). N.Eng. J. Med.
    294:1372, 1976.

5. Chan, L. and O'Malley, B.W. Mechanism of action of the sex
    steroid hormones (third of three parts). N.Eng. J. Med.
    294:1430, 1976.

6. Clark, J.H., Hsueh, A.J.W. and Peck, E.J., Jr. Regulation of
    estrogen receptor replenishment by progesterone. Ann. NY
    Acad. Sci. 286:161, 1977.

7. McGuire, W.L., Carbone, P.P. and Vollmer, E.P. (eds.), In:
    Estrogen Receptors in Human Breast Cancer, Raven Press, New
    York, 1975.

8. Sibley, C.H. and Tomkins, G.M. Mechanism of steroid
    resistance. Cell 2:221, 1974.

9. Thompson, E.B. The cellular actions of glucocorticoids in
    relation to human neoplasms. In: Current Topics in
    Endocrinology 4:114, 1974.

10. Notides, A. and Gorski, J. Estrogen induced synthesis of a
    specific uterine protein. Proc. Natl. Acad. Sci. USA 56:
    230, 1966.

11. Korenman, S.G. and O'Malley, B.W. Progesterone action:
    regulation of avidin biosynthesis by hen oviduct in vivo and
    in vitro. Endocrinology 83:11, 1968.

12. Oka, T. and Schimke, R.T. Interaction of estrogen and
    progesterone in chick oviduct development. II. Effects of
    estrogen and progesterone on tubular gland cell function.
    J. Biol. Chem. 43:123, 1969.

13. Chan, L., Jackson, R.L. and O'Malley, B.W.   Synthesis of very
    low density lipoproteins in the cockerel: effects of
    estrogen.   J. Clin. Invest.   58:386, 1976.

14. Roy, A.K. and Neuhaus, O.W.   Proof of the hepatic synthesis
    of a sex dependent protein in the rat.   Biochem. Biophys.
    Acta   127:82, 1966.

15. Beier, H.M.   Uteroglobin - a hormone sensitive endometrial
    protein involved in blastocyst development.   Biochem.
    Biophys. Acta   160:289, 1968.

16. Tseng, L. and Gurpide, E.   Nuclear concentration of estradiol
    in superfused slices of human endometrium.   Am. J. Obs. Gynec.
    114:995, 1972.

17. Tseng, L., Stolee, A. and Gurpide, E.   Quantitative studies
    on the uptake and metabolism of estrogens and progesterone
    by human endometrium.   Endocrinology   90:390, 1972.

18. Crocker, S.G., Milton, P.J. and King, R.J.B.   Uptake of
    (6,7-^{3}H) oestradiol-17β by normal and abnormal human endo-
    metrium.   J. Endocrinol.   62:145, 1974.

19. Evans, L.H., Martin, J.D. and Hähnel, R.   Estrogen receptor
    concentration in normal and pathological human uterine
    tissues.   J. Clin. Endocrinol. Metab.   38:23, 1974.

20. Hähnel, R., Twaddle, E. and Bundle, L.   Influence of enzymes
    on the estrogen receptor of human uterus and breast carcinoma.
    Steroids   24:489, 1974.

21. Tseng, L. and Gurpide, E.   Nuclear concentration of estriol
    in superfused human endometrium: competition with estradiol.
    J. Ster. Biochem.   5:273, 1974.

22. Bayard, F., Damilano, S., Robel, P. and Baulieu, E.-E.
    Estradiol and progesterone receptors in human endometrium
    during the menstrual cycle.   C.R. Acad. Sci. D (Paris)   281:
    1341, 1975.

23. Hunter, R.E. and Jordan, V.C.   Detection of the 8S oestrogen-
    binding component in human endometrium during the menstrual
    cycle.   J. Endocrinol.   65:757, 1975.

24. Muechler, E.K., Flickinger, G.L., Mangan, C.E. and Mikhail,
    G.   Estradiol binding by human endometrial tissue.   Gynecol.
    Oncol.   3:244, 1975.

25. Puukka, M.J., Kontula, K.K., Kauppila, A.J.I., Janne, O.A. and Vihko, R.K. Estrogen receptor in human myoma tissue. Mol. Cell Endocrinol. 6:35, 1976.

26. Ratajczak, T. and Hähnel, R. Chromatographic and other properties of the estrogen receptor from human myometrium. J. Ster. Biochem. 7:185, 1976.

27. Wiest, W.G. and Rao, B.R. Progesterone binding proteins in rabbit uterus and human endometrium. In: Advances in the Biosciences, Vol. 7, Pergamon Press, Viehweg, 1971, p. 251.

28. Haukkamaa, M. and Luukkainen, T. The cytoplasmic progesterone receptor of human endometrium during the menstrual cycle. J. Ster. Biochem. 5:447, 1974.

29. Rao, B.R., Wiest, W.G. and Allen, W.M. Progesterone "receptor" in human endometrium. Endocrinology 95:1275, 1974.

30. Young, P.C.M. and Cleary, R.E. Characterization and properties of progesterone-binding components in human endometrium. J. Clin. Endocrinol. Metab. 39:425, 1974.

31. Pollow, K., Lübbert, H., Boquoi, E., Kreuzer, G. and Pollow, B. Characterization and comparison of receptors for 17β-estradiol and progesterone in human proliferative endometrium and endometrial carcinoma. Endocrinology 96:319, 1975.

32. Bayard, F., Damilano, S., Robel, P. and Baulieu, E.-E. Variations in the estradiol and progesterone receptor in human endometrium during the menstrual cycle. Ann. Endocrinol. (Paris) 37:93, 1976.

33. MacLaughlin, D.T. and Richardson, G.S. Progesterone binding by normal and abnormal human endometrium. J. Clin. Endocrinol. Metab. 52:667, 1976.

34. Pollow, K., Schmidt-Gollwitzer, M. and Nevinny-Stickel, J. Progesterone receptors in normal human endometrium and endometrial carcinoma. In: Progesterone Receptors in Normal and Neoplastic Tissues. (W.L. McGuire, J.P. Raynaud and E.-E. Baulieu, eds.), Raven Press, NY, 1977, p. 313-318 (p. 29).

35. Yudaev, N.A., Pokrovsky, B.V., Asribekova, M.K. and Maltzev, A.V. Characteristics of testosterone binding components of human uterus endometrium cytoplasm and their interaction with cytoplasm. Biochem. (Moscow) 40:1123, 1975.

36. Muechler, E.V. and Kohler, D.   Dihydrotestosterone binding
     by human endometrium. Gyn. Invest. 8:104, 1977, Abst. 162.

37. MacLaughlin, D.T. and Richardson, G.S.   Specificity of
     medroxyprogesterone acetate binding in human endometrium:
     Interaction with testosterone and progesterone binding sites.
     J. Ster. Biochem. 10:371, 1979.

38. Tseng, L. and Gurpide, E.   Estradiol and 20α-dihydropro-
     gesterone dehydrogenase activities in human endometrium during
     the menstrual cycle. Endocrinology 94:419, 1974.

39. Tseng, L. and Gurpide, E.   Induction of human endometrial
     estradiol dehydrogenase by progestins. Endocrinology 97:
     826, 1975.

40. Pollow, K., Lübbert, H., Boquoi, E., Kreutzer, G., Jeske, R.
     and Pollow, B.   Studies of 17β hydroxysteroid dehydrogenase
     in human endometrium and endometrial carcinoma. I. Sub-
     cellular distributions and variations of specific enzyme
     activity. Acta Endocrinologica 79:134, 1975.

41. Janne, O., Kontula, E., Luukkainen, T. and Vihko, R.
     Oestrogen-induced progesterone receptor in human uterus.
     J. Steroid Biochem. 6:501, 1975.

42. Tseng, L. and Gurpide, E.   Effects of progestins on estradiol
     receptor levels in human endometrium. J. Clin. Endocrinol.
     Metab. 41:402, 1975.

43. Janne, O., Kontula, K. and Vihko, R.   Progestin receptors in
     human tissues: Concentrations and binding kinetics. J.
     Steroid Biochem. 7:1061, 1976.

44. Maslar, I.A. and Riddick, D.H.   Prolactin production in human
     endometrium during the normal menstrual cycle. Am. J. Obs.
     Gynec. 135:751, 1979.

45. Golander, A., Jurley, T., Barrett, J. and Handwerger, S.
     Synthesis of prolactin by human decidua in vitro. J.
     Endocrinol. 82:263, 1979.

46. McKay, D.G., Hertig, A.T., Bardawil, W.A. and Velardo, J.T.
     Histochemical observations on the endometrium. I. Normal
     endometrium. Obstet. Gynecol. 8:22, 1956.

47. Pickles, V.R., Hall, W.J., Best, f.A. and Smith, G.   Prosta-
     glandins in endometrium and menstrual fluid from normal and
     dysmenorrheic subjects. J. Obstet. Gynec. Br. Commwlth.
     72:185, 1965.

48. Wilson, E.   Induction of malate dehydrogenase by oestradiol-
     17β in the human endometrium.   Nature   215:758, 1967.

49. Csermely, T., Demers, L.M. and Hughes, E.C.   Organ culture of
     human endometrium.   Effects of progesterone.   Obs. Gynec.
     34:252, 1969.

50. Hughes, E.C., Demers, L.M., Csermely, T. and Jones, D.B.
     Organ culture of human endometrium.   Effects of ovarian
     steroids.   Am. J. Obs. Gynec.   109:707, 1969.

51. Schmidt-Mattheisen, H.   Histochemistry of the effects of
     gestagens on the human endometrium.   In: International
     Encyclopedia of Pharmacology and Therapy, Secretion 48, Vol.
     1, Taush, M., Ed., Pergamon Press, Oxford, 1971, p. 457.

52. Tseng, L., Stolee, H. and Gurpide, E.   Ouantitative studies
     on the uptake and metabolism of estrogens and progesterone
     by human endometrium.   Endocrinology   90:390, 1972.

53. Spellman, C.M., Fottrell, P.F., Baynes, S., O'Dwyer, E.M.
     and Clinch, J.D.   A study of some enzymes and isoenzymes of
     carbohydrate metabolism in human endometrium during the
     menstrual cycle.   Clin. Chim. Acta   48:259, 1973.

54. Downie, J., Poyser, N.L. and Wunderlich, M.   Levels of
     prostaglandins in human endometrium during the menstrual
     cycle.   Journal of Physiology   236:465, 1974.

55. Shapiro, S.A. and Hagerman, D.D.   Protein and RNA synthesis
     in human proliferative endometrium in organ culture and the
     effect of progesterone.   J. Endocrinology   62:663, 1974.

56. Pollow, K., Lübbert, H., Boquoi, E. and Pollow, B.   Proges-
     terone metabolism in normal human endometrium during the
     menstrual cycle and in endometrial carcinoma.   J. Clin. Endo.
     Metab.   41:729, 1975.

57. Singh, E.J., Baccarini, I.M. and Suzpan, F.P.   Levels of
     prostaglandins F2α and E2 in human endometrium during the
     menstrual cycle.   Am. J. Obs. Gynec.   121:1003, 1975.

58. Bernstein, G.S., Aladjem, F. and Chen, S.   Proteins in human
     endometrial washings.   A preliminary report.   Fert. Ster.
     22:722, 1971.

59. Beier, H.N. and Hellwig-Beier, K.   Specific secretory protein
     of the female genital tract.   Acta Endocrinol. Suppl.   180:
     404, 1973.

60. Garcea, N., Caruso, A. and Compiani, A. Protein content of
     human uterine secretion. Acta Eur. Fertil. 4:11, 1973.

61. Wolf, D.P. and Mastroianni, L., Jr. Protein composition of
     human uterine fluid. Fert. Ster. 26:240, 1975.

62. Hirsch, P.J., Ferguson, I.L.C. and King, R.J.B. Protein
     composition of human endometrium and its secretion at
     different stages of the menstrual cycle. Ann. NY Acad. Sci.
     286:233, 1977.

63. Voss, H.J. and Beato, M. Human uterine fluid proteins: gel
     electrophoretic pattern and progesterone binding properties.
     Fert. Ster. 28:972, 1977.

64. Roberts, G.P., Parker, J.M. and Henderson, S.R. Proteins in
     human uterine fluid. J. Reprod. Fert. 48:153, 1976.

65. Shirai, E., Iizuka, R. and Notake, Y. Analysis of human
     uterine fluid protein. Fert. Ster. 23:522, 1972.

66. Daniel, J.C. A blastokinin-like component from the human
     uterus. Fert. Ster. 24:326, 1973.

67. Sylvan, P.E., MacLaughlin, D.T., Richardson, G.S., Scully,
     R.E. and Nikrui, N. A low molecular weight protein if human
     uterine luminal fluid in the luteal phase. A progesterone
     induced product? Abst. 557, 61st Annual Meeting of the
     Endocrine Society, 1979.

68. Sylvan, P.E., MacLaughlin, D.T., Richardson, G.S., Scully,
     R.E. and Nikrui, N. Human luminal fluid proteins associated
     with secretory phase endometrium: progesterone-induced
     products? Biol. Reprod., submitted.

69. Gravlee, L.E. Jet irrigation method for the diagnosis of
     endometrial carcinoma. Obstet. Gynecol. 34:168, 1969.

70. Noyes, A.T., Hertig, A.T. and Rock, J. Dating the
     endometrial biopsy. Fert. Ster. 1:3, 1950.

71. Waddell, W.J. A simple ultraviolet spectrophotometric method
     for the determination of protein. J. Lab. Clin. Med. 48:
     311, 1956.

72. Lowry, O.H., Rosebrough, N.J., Farr, A.L. and Randall, R.J.
     Protein measurement with Folin-phenol reagent. J. Biol.
     Chem. 193:265, 1951.

73. Davis, B.J. Disc electrophoresis. II. Method and appli-
     cation to human serum proteins. Ann. NY Acad. Sci. 121:
     404, 1964.

74. Weber, K. and Osborn, M. The reliability of molecular weight
     determination by dodecyl sulfate-polyacrylamide gel electro-
     phoresis. J. Biol. Chem. 244:4406, 1969.

75. Zacharius, R.M., Zell, T.E., Mornson, J.H. and Woodlock, J.L.
     Glycoprotein staining following electrophoresis on acrylamide
     gels. Anal. Biochem. 30:148, 1969.

ESTROGEN REGULATION OF GROWTH AND SPECIFIC PROTEIN SYNTHESIS IN HUMAN BREAST CANCER CELLS IN TISSUE CULTURE

Dean P. Edwards, David J. Adams and William L. McGuire

University of Texas Health Science Center
Department of Medicine
7703 Floyd Curl Drive
San Antonio, TX 78284

INTRODUCTION

Successful endocrine therapy in breast cancer has been theorized to be dependent upon retention by the tumor of at least part of the cell's differentiated endocrine functions (1). Estrogen receptors (ER) therefore have been measured extensively in breast tumor biopsies in numerous laboratories as a potential marker of a functional endocrine system. Accordingly, tumors containing ER are much more likely to respond to endocrine therapies than tumors without ER (2). ER alone however is not a totally reliable marker of tumor sensitivity to hormones since certain tumors containing ER do not respond to endocrine manipulations. This is not surprising however, considering that binding of the hormone to the estrogen receptor is only the first step in a complex biochemical pathway leading to the physiological effect of estrogens (3). Any number of points in the pathway may conceivably be missing or defective. For this reason, we hypothesized that an end product of estrogen stimulation would improve the reliability of ER as a marker of hormone-responsive tumor growth (4). Progesterone receptor (PgR) is a likely candidate since it has been shown to be regulated by estrogens in animal mammary tumor models (5, 6) and in human breast cancer cells in tissue culture (7). Simultaneous measurement of PgR and ER in fact does improve the reliability of ER measurement alone in predicting patient response to endocrine therapies (8).

There is some evidence however, that estrogen stimulation of PgR and tumor cell growth may involve separate pathways. For instance, PgR is regulated by estrogens in the hormone-independent MTW 9B transplantable mammary tumor (9), and we have also observed that growth of at least 2 DMBA rat mammary tumors was independent of estrogen, while PgR in these tumors remained under estrogen control (5). There is a clear

133

need, therefore, to identify additional end products of estrogen action in breast tumor cells which might serve as markers of the hormone-responsiveness of tumor growth. This article deals with our approach to identifying new protein markers of estrogen action and with the question of whether PgR regulation is dependent upon estrogen stimulated cell growth. As a model for study, we have utilized MCF-7 human breast cancer cells in tissue culture.

EFFECTS OF ESTROGEN AND ANTIESTROGEN ON GROWTH OF HUMAN BREAST CANCER CELLS IN LONG TERM TISSUE CULTURE.

The MCF-7 human breast cancer cell line is not dependent upon estrogens for growth or long term survival, yet these cells do contain a functional ER and are responsive to estrogens in that PgR is strictly regulated by estrogens (7). Though proliferation of MCF-7 cells is not reproducibly stimulated by addition of estradiol to the growth medium (10, 11), cell growth is paradoxically inhibited with antiestrogens such as tamoxifen and nafoxidine (10, 12). A typical growth curve, showing the

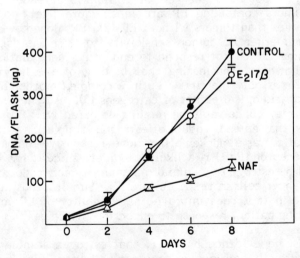

Figure 1. Effects of estradiol and nafoxidine on growth of MCF-7 cells: E_2 17β, estradiol (0.1 nM), Naf, nafoxidine (1.0 uM). Total DNA per flask was measured at the times indicated by the diphenylamine method of Burton (13). (reproduced from reference 10).

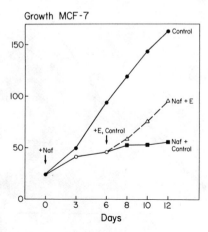

Figure 2. Antiestrogen effect on cell growth and reversal with estradiol: Naf, nafoxidine (1.0 uM). Nafoxidine inhibited cells were changed either to control medium or medium containing estradiol (10 nM).

effects of estradiol and nafoxidine on the growth rate is illustrated in Figure 1. MCF-7 cells are routinely grown in Eagle's minimum essential medium (MEM) supplemented with 5% calf serum stripped of endogenous steroids by treatment with dextran coated charcoal (7). There is concern that charcoal stripping leaves residual endogenous estrogens which may obscure the effects of added estrogens. It is not likely, however, that significant amounts of endogenous estrogens remain in the charcoal treated calf serum, because estradiol exchange assays have shown that estrogen receptor in MCF-7 cells grown in this medium are not occupied with hormone (14). It is nevertheless a possibility that other growth factors present in calf serum, which are not removed by the charcoal treatment may mask the stimulatory effect of estradiol on cell growth. To unequivocally establish the role of estrogens in MCF-7 cell growth, studies with a chemically defined medium for this cell line will be required.

One indication that the ER system in MCF-7 cells is involved in regulation of cell growth is that growth inhibition caused by antiestrogens can be rapidly reversed by subsequent incubation of the cells with estrogens (10, 12, 15). As shown in Figure 2, cell growth is nearly arrested by 6 days incubation with nafoxidine (1 uM). Inhibition is maintained even if nafoxidine is removed and replaced with control medium, but is rapidly reversed by subsequent incubation with estradiol (10 nM). Because antiestrogens such as tamoxifen and nafoxidine bind to MCF-7 cytosol ER and promote translocation to the nucleus (16), it seems likely that

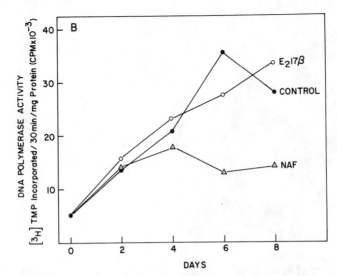

Figure 3. Effects of estradiol and nafoxidine on MCF-7 cytosol DNA polymerase activity: E$_2$ 17β, estradiol (0.1 nM), Naf, nafoxidine (1.0 uM). DNA polymerase activity was measured as the rate of incorporation of (^{3}H)-thymidine-5'-triphosphate (15 uM, with a specific activity of 1,900-2,000 cpm/pmole) into an acid insoluble product in the presence of 0.1 mM deoxyribonucleotide triphosphates (dATP, dCTP, dGTP), 5 mM MgCl$_2$, 2 mM ATP and calf thymus DNA as the template-primer. Enzyme activity is expressed as the cpm incorporated in 30 min at 30°C per mg of cytosol protein. (adapted from reference 10).

antiestrogen inhibition and subsequent reversal with estradiol are acting through the ER. One major interest in our laboratory has been the study of molecular mechanisms underlying estrogen-mediated breast tumor cell proliferation. Since estrogen-rescue from antiestrogen growth inhibition is the only condition under which estrogens are able to stimulate growth of MCF-7 cells, we have examined under these growth conditions, certain biochemical parameters including DNA polymerase activity, relative rates of protein synthesis and PgR content.

ESTROGEN AND ANTIESTROGEN MODULATION OF DNA POLYMERASE ACTIVITY

The majority of DNA polymerase activity in MCF-7 cells is contained in the cytosol fraction. This cytosol enzyme displays several properties characteristic of DNA polymerase α described in other tissues (10). Since DNA polymerase α has been correlated with the proliferative state in a number of other systems (17), we chose to measure only cytosol DNA

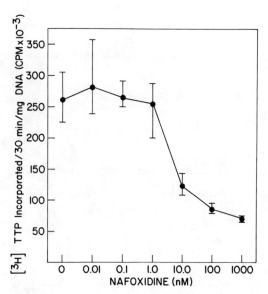

Figure 4. Dose effect of nafoxidine on cytosol DNA polymerase in MCF-7. (reproduced from reference 10).

polymerase activity in these studies. Incubation of cells with estradiol does not affect DNA polymerase activity relative to controls (Figure 3); repeated experiments failed to show a significant stimulation of DNA polymerase activity in response to any estradiol dose tested. Despite the failure to observe an estrogen response, nafoxidine growth inhibition is undoubtedly accompanied by a reduction in cytosol levels of DNA polymerase activity. Figure 4 shows the effect of increasing concentrations of nafoxidine on cytosol DNA polymerase activity. Decreases in enzyme activity in response to increasing doses of nafoxidine are paralleled by decreases in total DNA content per flask. Because enzyme activity is expressed in units per mg of DNA, the effect of nafoxidine is not a result of there being fewer cells, rather, nafoxidine has caused a reduction in enzyme activity per cell.

Antiestrogen suppression of cytosol DNA polymerase activity is reversed by estradiol in a dose dependent manner (Figure 5). Of the two antiestrogens tested, nafoxidine appears to be more effective than tamoxifen in suppressing cytosol DNA polymerase activity. Growth and enzyme inhibition caused by tamoxifen is gradually reversed by estradiol doses between 0.01 nM and 100 nM while slightly more estradiol was required to begin reversal in nafoxidine-inhibited cells. The difference in sensitivity of DNA polymerase to nafoxidine compared to tamoxifen is probably due to their differing affinities for the estrogen receptor (16). Reversal of antiestrogen inhibition of DNA polymerase activity by estradiol doses parallels stimulation of cell growth (DNA/flask).

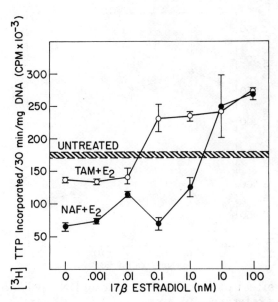

Figure 5. Estradiol stimulation of cytosol DNA polymerase activity in antiestrogen-suppressed cells. Cells were pretreated for 6 days with antiestrogen, 1.0 uM TAM (tamoxifen) or 1.0 uM Naf (nafoxidine) and then changed to medium containing estradiol for an additional 4 days. (reproduced from reference 10).

Stimulation of DNA polymerase activity in antiestrogen-suppressed cells is hormone specific. At higher doses, less biologically active estrogens such as estriol (1.0 uM), 17α-estradiol (1.0 uM), and estrone (0.1 uM), are as effective as 17β-estradiol (0.01 uM) in reversing nafoxidine suppression of cytosol DNA polymerase activity. Testosterone, progesterone, cortisol and insulin at 1.0 uM concentrations have no effect on DNA polymerase activity.

The rate of estradiol reversal of antiestrogen inhibition of DNA polymerase activity is shown in Figure 6. No significant increase in either growth or DNA polymerase activity was observed for the first 24 hr. A doubling in enzyme activity occurred by day 2 and a 4-fold maximal stimulation (over zero time) was observed after 4 days exposure to estradiol. This increase in enzyme activity was paralleled by increases in total DNA per flask. Enzyme activity in cells maintained on nafoxidine for the entire incubation period was unchanged. The time course, magnitude, dose dependency and hormone specificity of the estrogen response in these antiestrogen-inhibited MCF-7 cells is similar to estrogen-stimulated changes in cellular proliferation and DNA polymerase activity described in other estrogen target tissues (18-21).

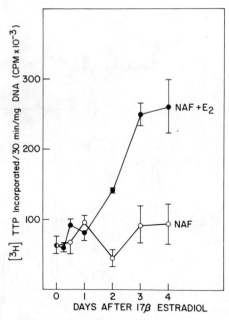

Figure 6. Time course of estrogen reversal of DNA polymerase inhibition by nafoxidine. MCF-7 cells pretreated for 6 days with nafoxidine were either changed to medium containing 10 nM estradiol (NAF +E$_2$) or continued on nafoxidine (NAF). (reproduced from ref 10) .

ESTROGEN REGULATION OF SPECIFIC PROTEIN SYNTHESIS

To determine whether estrogens might stimulate synthesis of a specific protein or proteins during the period of rescue from antiestrogen growth inhibition, we have analyzed the relative rates of synthesis of MCF-7 cell proteins by a double isotope method of labeling intracellular proteins (22). Estrogen-rescued cells were pulsed in vivo for 2 hr with (^{3}H)-leucine. Nafoxidine pretreated cells, switched to control medium and grown for the same length of time as an estrogen served as treatment controls and were also pulsed for 2 hr with (^{3}H)-leucine. Nafoxidine-pretreated cells used as the reference were pulsed with (^{14}C)-leucine. Equal numbers of cells from the reference group and treatment groups were mixed, homogenized and centrifuged at 105,000 xg. Aliquots of the supernatant were then submitted to SDS-polyacrylamide gel electrophoresis. Figure 7 shows a profile of the ^{3}H and ^{14}C counts in each gel slice of proteins analyzed after 4 days incubation of nafoxidine-inhibited cells with estradiol (10 nM). A pronounced increase in the ^{3}H/^{14}C ratio over baseline was detected at a molecular weight of about 24,000. A distinct but smaller increase was detected at a molecular weight of about 36,000. Data from several independent experiments gave a mean value of 24,183 (range, 23,202-26,467) and 35,510 (range, 34,455-37,638) molecular weights, respectively, for these ratio peaks. No substantial or consistent

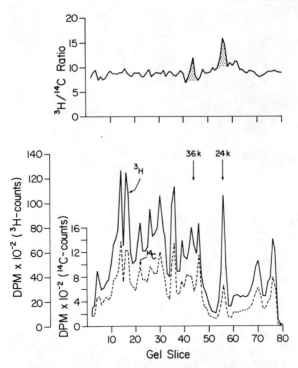

Figure 7. SDS-electrophoresis in 10% polyacrylamide of proteins syn-thesized by nafoxidine-treated cells and cells rescued from nafoxidine inhibition by estradiol. Nafoxidine-pretreated cells served as controls and were labeled for 2 hr with (^{14}C)-leucine (2.5 u Ci/ml of medium at a specific activity of >300 mCi/mmol), while 4 day estrogen-rescued cells were labeled for 2 hr with (^{3}H)-leucine (10 uCi/ml of medium at a specific activity of >110 Ci/mmol). Equal numbers of control and estrogen-rescued cells were mixed together and homogenized, then cytosols were prepared and run on SDS-gels. The arrows indicate the positions and molecular weight estimates of the prominent ^{3}H/^{14}C ratio peaks relative to the Rf of protein standards. The upper panel shows the ^{3}H/^{14}C ratio in each gel slice. The lower panel shows the total dpm in each gel slice in both ^{3}H and ^{14}C channels. (reproduced from reference 22).

increase over the basal ratio was observed in the rest of the gel. Control experiments have shown that ratio peaks are not detectable when relative rates of protein synthesis are compared between nafoxidine-inhibited cells labeled with (^{3}H) or (^{14}C)-leucine (Figure 8, middle panel) or when compared between nafoxidine-inhibited cells and nafoxidine-blocked cells changed to control medium (Figure 8, lower panel). The 4 day estrogen-rescued group of cells from the same cell plating was included for comparison (Figure 8, upper panel).

One important concern in these experiments is that we have analyzed the relative rates of synthesis of proteins between two populations of cells which are harvested at very different stages of cell growth.   Anti-estrogen-pretreated cells have been blocked at mid growth and remain low density cultures as opposed to estrogen-rescued cells which by day 4 of treatment have at least doubled their number and reached confluence. We thought it essential, therefore, to compare the relative rates of synthesis of proteins in untreated cells at various stages of cell growth with that in nafoxidine-blocked cells.   Nafoxidine-inhibited cells at mid growth were

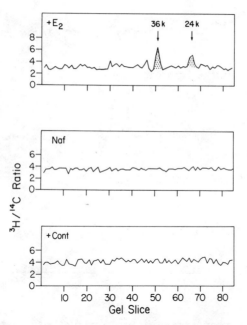

Figure 8. SDS-gel electrophoresis of double labeled MCF-7 cytosol proteins. Upper panel: The experimental protocol was the same as described in Figure 7.   This is an identical but independent experiment.   Middle panel:Cytosol proteins from two groups of nafoxidine-treated cells were labeled with (^{3}H) or (^{14}C)-leucine, mixed and run on the same gel.Lower panel: Nafoxidine-pretreated cells were either continued for an additional 4 days on nafoxidine and labeled with (^{14}C)-leucine or changed to control medium for 4 days and then labeled with (^{3}H)-leucine. (reproduced from reference 22).

labeled with (^{14}C)-leucine and mixed either with (^{3}H)-leucine labeled proteins from untreated cells or with (^{3}H)-leucine labeled proteins from untreated cells which had grown past confluence. Aliquots of the mixed proteins were then submitted to SDS-polyacrylamide gel electrophoresis. No ^{3}H/^{14}C ratio peaks were detected when comparing protein synthesis rates between nafoxidine-inhibited cells with untreated cells from low density cultures (Figure 9, upper panel). Three very distinct ratio peaks, however, were detected when proteins from nafoxidine-blocked cells were

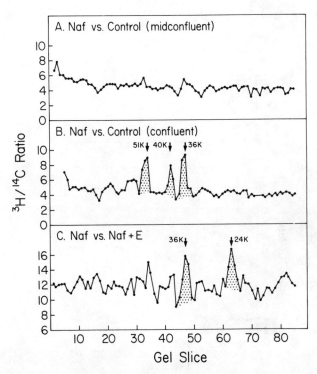

Figure 9. Comparison of rates of protein synthesis between untreated MCF-7 cells at different stages of growth. MCF-7 cells pretreated with nafoxidine for 6 days served as reference cells and were labeled for 2 hr with (^{14}C)-leucine. Untreated cells at the same cell density as nafoxidine inhibited cells (low cell density) and untreated post-confluent cells served as the treatment groups and were labeled for 2 hr with (^{3}H)-leucine. Equal aliquots of cytosol proteins from treatment and reference groups were mixed and electrophoresed on SDS-polyacrylamide gels. For comparison, cells labeled for 2 hr with (^{3}H)-leucine after 4 day rescue by estradiol from nafoxidine inhibition were also included. (Naf vs. Naf +E).

mixed and co-electrophoresed with proteins from post-confluent untreated cells (Figure 9, middle panel). One of these peaks has a molecular weight of 36,000. For comparison, nafoxidine-inhibited cells and estrogen-rescued cells from the same cell plating as the above were also analyzed (Figure 9, lower panel). This experiment indicates that there are indeed quantitative differences in the rates of synthesis of certain proteins between untreated cells in the two stages of growth. In particular, the ratio peak at 36,000 molecular weight obtained after 4 days of estrogen-rescue can be produced independent of estrogen stimulation. Small differences in protein synthesis rates between cells in the two stages of growth may also account for the

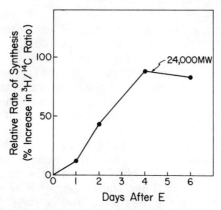

Figure 10. Time course of estrogen-stimulated synthesis of the 24,000 molecular weight protein. The protocol for this experiment is the same as described in Figure 7, with the exception of the time of estradiol treatment. Relative rates of protein synthesis were determined as the percent increase in the $^3H/^{14}C$ ratio in SDS-gels over baseline at the 24,000 molecular weight band.

fluctuations in the $H/^{14}C$ baseline often observed on SDS-gels of proteins analyzed after 4 days of estrogen rescue as shown in Figure 9 (lower panel). We find, therefore, that an increased rate of synthesis of the specific 24,000 molecular weight protein is not simply a reflection of increased growth rate or the stage of cell growth. Increased synthesis occurs only during estrogen rescue of antiestrogen growth inhibition, suggesting that this protein is regulated specifically by estrogens.

Under conditions of rescue from nafoxidine growth inhibition, estrogen affects protein synthesis in two stages. The baseline $^3H/^{14}C$ ratio increases by as much as 2-4 fold by 24 hr treatment with estradiol, which we interpret as an early increase in general protein synthesis. This occurs prior to stimulation of cell division. By the 4th day of estrogen treatment, this general stimulation has decayed as evidenced by the baseline $^3H/^{14}C$ ratio returning to values observed prior to incubation with estradiol. At this time, however, the relative rate of synthesis of the 24,000 molecular weight protein remains elevated. Figure 10 shows the time course of this stimulation. The magnitude of stimulation was estimated by measuring the percent increase in the $^3H/^{14}C$ ratio in the protein band at 24,000 molecular weight over the baseline value. Baseline was determined as the cumulative average of $^3H/^{14}C$ in each gel slice. The relative rate of synthesis is changed very little after 1 day of estrogen treatment, but gradually increases between day 1 and day 6. The maximal percent increase in the $^3H/^{14}C$ ratio above baseline is reached by day 4 and is about 90% in this experiment.

We have examined the hormone specificity and dose response of the selective stimulation of the 24,000 molecular weight protein. Only estrogenic steroids were able to stimulate the relative rate of synthesis of this protein, whereas progesterone (1.0 uM), cortisol (1.0 uM) and DHT (1.0 and 0.10 uM) did not. No induced ratio peak was detected below 1.0 nM estradiol. Likewise, reversal of antiestrogen growth inhibition requires concentrations of estradiol of 1.0 nM or greater. At 1.0 nM estradiol, the degree of stimulation of the 24,000 molecular weight protein is about 50% that obtained at 10 nM. Concentrations above 10 nM give about the same degree of stimulation. To test the generality of the anti-estrogen-pretreatment, cells were inhibited with the antiestrogens tam-oxifen (1.0 uM) or CI-628 (1.0 uM) and then changed to medium containing estradiol (10 nM) and grown for an additional 4 days. In both cases, estrogen promoted reversal of growth inhibition and gave selective stim-ulation in the rate of synthesis of a 24,000 molecular weight protein.

We have estimated the magnitude of specific protein stimulation by monitoring changes in the rates of uptake of radiolabeled leucine. This method, however, only gives a minimum estimate because extraneous proteins may contribute to the total counts contained in each protein band in the gel. Coomassie-stained SDS-gels of cytosol proteins show a prominent band at the Rf for 24,000 molecular weight proteins. We have determined by directly cutting out and counting this band that it contains the estrogen-induced ratio peak. The intensity of this stained band and the relative number of counts incorporated into protein contained in this band (Figure 7) indicate that the 24,000 molecular weight protein may represent a significant amount (>1%) of the total intracellular protein.

We do not know the nature or identity of the 24,000 molecular weight protein. The molecular weight is different from that of the rat uterine induced protein (23) and the time course of induction is much slower (24). The milk protein casein (25) has a molecular weight of about 24,000, however synthesis of casein by MCF-7 cells has not been demonstrated.

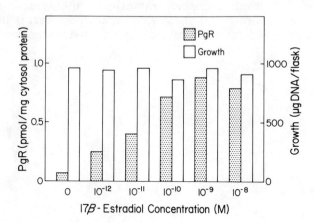

Figure 11. Growth and stimulation of PgR in cells treated with estradiol. PgR was measured by incubating cytosol from each treatment group for 4 hr at 4° C with 20 nM (^{3}H)-R5020 alone or with a 100 fold excess of unlabeled R5020. Free ligand was separated with dextran coated charcoal.

Westley and Rochefort (26), recently demonstrated that estrogens induce MCF-7 cell secretory proteins, the principal one being a 46,000 molecular weight band on SDS-polyacrylamide gels. Estradiol has also been shown to induce the production of plasminogen activator by MCF-7 cells (27). Induced plasminogen activator is released almost entirely into the culture medium (virtually no enzyme activity is detected intracellularly) and stimulated production occurs under conditions where growth of the cells is not stimulated by estradiol. It is unlikely, therefore, that either of these estrogen-induced MCF-7 cell proteins are the same protein detected in our studies. Plasminogen activator and the 46,000 molecular weight protein described by Westley and Rochefort (27) may in fact be the same protein since both are released into the culture medium and the time course of their inductions is similar.

ESTROGEN REGULATION OF PgR: LACK OF DEPENDENCE ON
GROWTH STIMULATION.

PgR in MCF-7 cells is strictly regulated by estradiol (7). However,
the question arises as to whether PgR as an end product of estrogen action
is necessarily linked to estrogen-stimulated tumor cell growth. As shown
in Figure 11, PgR levels increase dramatically in response to increasing
doses of estradiol. Growth of these same cells, however, is not influenced
by estradiol. PgR induction therefore has occured under conditions where

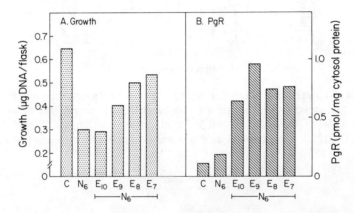

Figure 12. Estrogen stimulation of growth and PgR in nafoxidine-pretreated cells. Cells were pretreated with 1.0 uM nafoxidine
(N_6) and then changed to medium containing estradiol (E_{10}, 0.1 nM, E_9, 1.0
nM, E_8, 10 nM, E_7, 100 nM).

cell growth is not stimulated by estradiol. This does not constitute proof
but suggests that estrogen stimulation of PgR and of cell growth may
involve independent mechanisms. Because cell division of antiestrogen-inhibited cells can be stimulated with estradiol, we have compared the PgR response to estradiol in nafoxidine-pretreated cells with
that in untreated cells. As shown in Figure 12, estradiol is as effective in
stimulating PgR in nafoxidine-pretreated cells as it is in untreated cells.
Under these conditions however, cell growth is stimulated by estradiol.

Estradiol at 0.1 nM, however, has stimulated PgR in nafoxidine-pretreated cells but at this dose is unable to promote growth stimulation. The dissociation of estrogen effects at this concentration provides further evidence that estrogen regulation of PgR and tumor cell growth may involve separate mechanisms.

SUMMARY

Taking advantage of the fact that estrogens can stimulate proliferation of antiestrogen-inhibited MCF-7 cells has enabled us to study molecular events involved in steroid-mediated growth of tumor cells, using a breast cancer cell line which otherwise is affected very little in its growth by estrogens. Under these growth conditions, estradiol stimulates DNA polymerase activity in a manner analogous with reported estrogen effects on enzyme activity in normal target tissues. We also observed dissociation of estrogen effects on cell growth and PgR stimulation, indicating that PgR induction and estrogen-mediated cell division may involve separate control mechanisms. The relative rate of synthesis of a specific 24,000 molecular weight protein is also increased under these conditions of estrogen-stimulated cell growth. Since increased synthesis of the 24,000 molecular weight protein was determined not to be a reflection of different stages of cell growth, we suggest that this protein is regulated specifically by estrogens and that it may be a marker of estrogen stimulated growth of human breast tumor cells.

ACKNOWLEDGMENTS

1.   NIH Grant, CA 11378
2.   NIH Contract, CB 23862
3.   ACS, BC 23
4.   NIH Training Grant, CA 09042
5.   NIH Training Grant HD 07139

REFERENCES

1.   E. V. Jensen, G. E. Block, S. Smith, K. Kyser, and E. R. DeSombre, Estrogen receptors and breast cancer response to adrenalectomy, Natl. Cancer Inst. Monographs 34:55 (1971).
2.   W. L. McGuire, P. P. Carbone, M. E. Sears, and G. C. Escher, Estrogen receptors in human breast cancer: An overview, in: "Estrogen receptors in human breast cancer," W. L. McGuire, P. P. Carbone, and E. P. Vollmer, eds., p.1., Raven Press, New York (1975).
3.   B. S. Katzenellenbogen and J. Gorski, Estrogen action on syntheses of macromolecules in target cells, in: "Biochemical Actions of Hormones," G. Litwack, ed., p. 187, Academic Press, New York (1975).

4. W. L. McGuire and K. B. Horwitz, Progesterone receptors in breast cancer, in: "Hormones, Receptors and Breast Cancer," W. L. McGuire, ed., p. 31, Raven Press, New York (1978).

5. K. B. Horwitz and W. L. McGuire, Progesterone and progesterone receptors in experimental breast cancer, Cancer Res. 37:1733 (1977).

6. A. J. M. Koenders, A. Geurts-Moespot, S. J. Zolinger, and T. J. Benraad, Progesterone and estradiol receptors in DMBA-induced mammary tumors before and after ovariectomy and after subsequent estradiol administration, in: "Progesterone Receptors in Normal and Neoplastic Tissues," W. L. McGuire, J. P. Raynaud, and E. E. Baulier, eds. p. 71, Raven Press, New York (1977).

7. K. B. Horwitz and W. L. McGuire, Estrogen control of progesterone receptor in human breast cancer, J. Biol. Chem. 253:2223 (1978).

8. D. P. Edwards, G. C. Chamness, and W. L. McGuire, Estrogen and progesterone receptor proteins in breast cancer, Biochemica et Biophysica Acta 560:457 (1979).

9. I. Margot, R. J. Milholland, and F. Rosen, Mammary cancer: Selective action of the estrogen receptor complex, Science 203:361 (1979).

10. D. P. Edwards, S. R. Murthy, and W. L. McGuire, Estrogen and antiestrogen effects on DNA polymerase in human breast cancer, Cancer Res., in press (1980).

11. S. Jozan, C. Moure, M. Gillois, and F. Bayard, Effects of estrone on cell proliferation of a human breast cancer (MCF-7) in long term tissue culture, J. Steroid Biochem. 10:341 (1979).

12. M. Lippman, G. Bolan, and K. Huff, The effects of estrogens and antiestrogens on hormone-responsive human breast cancer in long term tissue culture, Cancer Res. 38:4595 (1976).

13. K. Burton, A study of conditions and mechanisms of the diphenylamine reaction for the colorimetric estimation of DNA. Biochem. J. 62:315 (1956).

14. D. T. Zava and W. L. McGuire, Estrogen receptor: Unoccupied sites in nuclei of a human breast cancer cell line, J. Biol. Chem. 252:3703 (1977).

15. D. T. Zava and W. L. McGuire, Androgen action through estrogen receptor in a human breast cancer cell line, Endocrinology 103:624 (1978).

16. K. B. Horwitz and W. L. McGuire, Nuclear mechanisms of estrogen action: Effects of estradiol and antiestrogen on cytoplasmic and nuclear estrogen receptors and nuclear receptor processing, J. Biol. Chem. 253:8185 (1978).

17. A. Weissbach, Eukaryotic DNA polymerases, Ann. Rev. Biochem. 46:25 (1977).

18. J. N. Harris and J. Gorski, Estrogen stimulation of DNA-dependent DNA polymerase activity in immature rat uterus, Mol. Cell. Endocrinol. 10:293 (1978).

19. H. J. Rohde, W. E. G. Muller, and R. K. Zahn, Alterations of DNA-dependent DNA polymerase activities in the immature quail oviduct in response to estrogen stimulation, Nuclei Acid Res. 2:2101 (1975).

20. R. L. Sutherland, M.-C. Legeau, P. H. Schmelck, and E. E. Baulieu, Synergistic and antagonistic effects of progesterone and estrogen on estrogen receptor concentration and DNA polymerase activity in chick oviduct, FEBS Letters 79:253 (1977).

21. M. D. Walker, A. M. Kaye, and B. R. Fridlender, Age-dependent stimulation by estradiol-17β of DNA polymerase α in immature rat uterus, FEBS Letters 92:25 (1978).

22. D. P. Edwards, D. J. Adams, N. Savage, and W. L. McGuire, Estrogen induced synthesis of specific proteins in human breast cancer cells, Biochem. Biophys. Res. Comm., in press (1980).

23. M. D. Walker, I. Gozes, A. M. Kaye, N. Reiss, and U. Z. Littauer, The estrogen-induced protein: Quantitation by autoradiography of poly-acrylamide gels, J. Steroid Biochem. 7:1083 (1976).

24. B. S. Katzenellenbogen and J. Gorski, Estrogen action in vitro: Induction of the synthesis of a specific uterine protein, J. Biol. Chem. 247:1299 (1972).

25. M. L. Groves and W. G. Gordon, The major component of human casein: A protein phosphorylated at different levels, Arch. Biochem. Biophys. 140:47 (1970).

26. B. Westley and H. Rochefort, Estradiol induced proteins in the MCF-7 human breast cancer cell line, Biochem. Biophys. Res. Comm. 90:410 (1979).

27. W. B. Butler, W. L. Kirkland, and T. L. Jorgensen, Induction of plasminogen activator by estrogen in a human breast cancer cell line (MCF-7), Biochem. Biophys. Res. Comm. 90:1328 (1979).

REGULATION OF PITUITARY GROWTH AND PROLACTIN GENE EXPRESSION BY ESTROGEN

Mara E. Lieberman[1], Richard A. Maurer[2], Philippa Claude[3],
Julie Wiklund[1], Nancy Wertz[1], and Jack Gorski[1]

Departments of Biochemistry and Animal Science[1] and Regional Primate Research Center[3], University of Wisconsin Madison, WI 53706 and Department of Physiology and Biophysics[2], University of Iowa, Iowa City, IA 52242

INTRODUCTION

Prolactin is synthesized and secreted by a morphologically and functionally distinct group of cells in the pituitary gland. The relative abundance and secretory activity of the mammotrophic cells is highly influenced by the prevailing endocrine milieu. Various lines of evidence indicate that estrogen is a major regulator of prolactin synthesis and secretion. In female rats, the sharp rise in serum prolactin levels at puberty and the cyclic release of prolactin is associated with the preovulatory surge of estradiol (1, 2). Administration of estrogen to prepubertal rats leads to increased serum levels of prolactin (3,4). Treatment of rats with estrogens was shown to result in increased pituitary DNA synthesis (5-8), hyperplasia and hypertrophy of mammotrophs (9), increased incorporation of radiolabeled precursors into prolactin (7, 10, 11), and increased cellular content of prolactin messenger RNA (12, 13).

Studies attempting to identify the site of action suggest that estrogen acts directly on the pituitary gland as well as indirectly through the hypothalamus by influencing the production of stimulatory and inhibitory factors which modulate prolactin release (14-16). In support of a direct action, it was reported that pituitary fragments incubated with 2 μM estradiol produced increased amounts of prolactin (17). A direct effect was also reported in a clonal strain of pituitary tumor cells with physiological concentrations of estradiol (18, 19). However, the stimulatory effect of estrogen on prolactin synthesis could no longer

be elicited in later generations of the same cell line (20). The
high dose of estrogen required to obtain a response coupled with
the difficulties inherent in the maintenance of organ cultures,
and the apparent change with time in the functional characteristics
of pituitary tumor cells limit the desirability of these systems
as models to study regulation of prolactin synthesis by estrogens.

In recent years, primary cultures of pituitary cells which
retain responsiveness to physiological concentrations of estradiol
have been developed (21,22). Using monolayer cultures of dispersed rat pituitary cells as the experimental model, we carried
out studies in an effort to clarify the site of estrogen action,
and to gain an understanding about some of the molecular events
involved in the regulation of prolactin synthesis.

Effects of estrogen on prolactin synthesis.

The pattern of proteins synthesized by pituitary cells cultured in steroid-free medium or in medium containing 10 nM estradiol was examined by the double label technique. Analysis of the
gel revealed that treatment of cells with estrogen for 5 days resulted in a highly increased ratio of radioactivity in the area of
the gel that corresponds to the migration of prolactin whereas
the ratio was relatively constant in other areas of the gel (Fig.
1). The results suggest that estradiol specifically stimulates
the incorporation of precursors into prolactin without appreci-
ably affecting the synthesis of other cellular proteins.

The rate of incorporation of the labeled precursor into prolactin was quantitated by immunoprecipitation of the cell extract
with an antiserum to prolactin. Analysis on gels of immunoprecipitates from cells pulse labeled for 1 h with (^{3}H)leucine showed
a single major ^{3}H-labeled peak that co-migrated with a (^{14}C)pro-
lactin standard (Fig. 2). It can be seen that estrogen caused a
marked increase in prolactin synthesis. We also established that
incorporation of the label into prolactin is linear for 4 h, and
that labeled prolactin is not detectable in the medium during the
1 h pulse (23). Thus, immunoprecipitation of the cell homogenates
provides a valid estimate of the total rate of prolactin synthesis.

The increase in prolactin synthesis was dose-dependent,
reaching an apparent maximum at a concentration of 10 nM estradiol (Fig. 3). Since the amount of steroid available to cells is
reduced in the growth medium that is supplemented with 17.5%
serum, the maximal effective dose in this system is probably
1-2 nM estradiol (cf. 24). The response was shown to be specific
for estrogenic hormones; at a concentration of 1 nM, estradiol,
diethylstilbestrol and estriol were stimulatory, whereas testosterone, 5α-dihydrotestosterone, progesterone and corticosterone

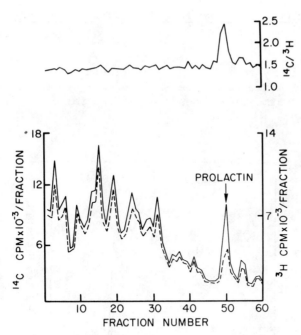

Fig. 1. Comparison between radiolabeled proteins from control
and estrogen-treated cells. Pituitary cells were cultured for 5
days in steroid-free (control) medium or in medium containing
10 nM estradiol. Cells were pulse labeled for 1 h with either
(^{3}H)leucine, 10 μCi/ml (control), or (^{14}C)leucine, 5 μCi/ml
(estrogen-treated). An aliquot of the cell extract from a control
and an estrogen-treated culture was combined and electrophoresed
on SDS-polyacrylamide gel. Dashed line, migration of radioactive
proteins from the control culture (^{3}H); solid line, radioactive
proteins from the estrogen-treated culture (^{14}C). Ratio of ^{14}C to
^{3}H is plotted at the top of the figure. The position of prolactin
was determined with authentic prolactin from the National Institute of Arthritis, Metabolism and Digestive Diseases. (Lieberman
et al., 1978[25]).

had no significant effect (25).

     The time course of induction of prolactin synthesis is shown
in Fig. 4. Exposure of cells to estradiol for 3 days resulted in
a highly increased rate of prolactin synthesis, reaching a 500%
increase over the control rate by day 7. Addition of estradiol on
day 3 rather than on day 1 resulted in a slight increase by day 4
and a highly increased rate of synthesis by day 7. Conversely,
cells exposed to estradiol for the initial 3 days continued to
synthesize increased amounts of prolactin, although at a somewhat
reduced rate (P <0.001).

Effects of estrogen on prolactin mRNA accumulation and mammotroph
cell proliferation.

The kinetics of the estrogen-induced response is consistent
with the possibility that increased prolactin synthesis is due to
proliferation of mammotrophs. Several investigators have reported
that estrogen treatment increased the incorporation of precursors

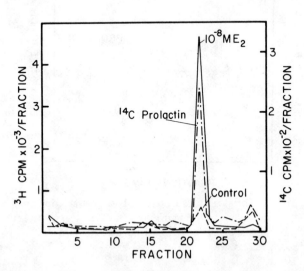

Fig. 2. Comparison between immunoprecipitable prolactin from control and estrogen-treated cells. Pituitary cells were cultured for
5 days in control medium or in medium containing 10 nM estradiol.
Cells were pulse labeled for 1 h with (^{3}H)leucine, 10 µCi/ml. Aliquots of the 10,000 x g supernatant of cell homogenates were immunoprecipitated with (^{14}C)prolactin carrier and antiserum to
prolactin and electrophoresed on SDS-polyacrylamide gels. (—)
Profile of ^{3}H-labeled immunoprecipitate from an estrogen-treated
culture. The peak of radioactivity coincides with the position of
(^{14}C)prolactin carrier (—·—). (---) Migration of ^{3}H-labeled immunoprecipitate from a control culture run in parallel (Lieberman
et al, 1978 [25]).

into pituitary DNA (5-8). In this system, we were unable to detect
estrogen-induced changes in DNA synthesis. When pituitary cells
were labeled with (^{3}H)thymidine, the radioactivity in cpm x 10^{-3}
of TCA precipitable material per µg DNA was 11±1.1 for controls
and 11.7±.9 for estrogen-treated cultures, while in replicate
cultures labeled with (^{3}H)leucine, prolactin synthesis was stimulated 3-fold. Autoradiographic studies revealed that the majority

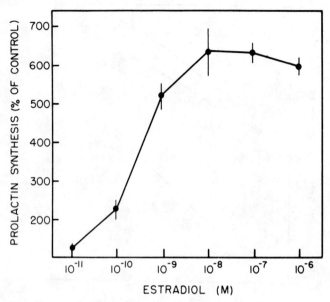

Fig. 3. Rate of prolactin synthesis as a function of estradiol
concentration. Pituitary cells were cultured for 5 days in control
medium or in medium containing estradiol at the concentrations indicated. Prolactin synthesis was quantitated by immunoprecipitation . Each point represents the mean ±SEM of four cultures (Lieberman et al., 1978 [25]).

of cells with labeled nuclei were fibroblasts (26). Since primary
cultures contain a mixed population of cells including rapidly
proliferating fibroblasts, a specific increase in a limited seg-
ment of secretory cells might not be detected by this method.

Another approach to address this question involved visual-
ization of mammotrophs by immunocytochemistry using the soluble
peroxidase-antiperoxidase method. We monitored prolactin synthesis and mammotroph cell population in control and estrogen-treated cultures that were exposed to specific inhibitors of DNA synthesis. The results of such an experiment are shown in Fig. 5.
Incorporation of (^{3}H)thymidine into DNA was not significantly different between control and estrogen-treated cultures within each
treatment group. In the absence of inhibitors, 3 days' treatment
with estradiol resulted in a 2.3-fold increase in prolactin synthesis and a 27% increase in the number of mammotrophs, compared
to controls. With .4 µM cytosine arabinoside, which inhibited DNA
synthesis by approximately 40% without affecting total protein
synthesis, prolactin production was stimulated 2-fold while the
number of mammotrophs increased by 11%, compared to controls.

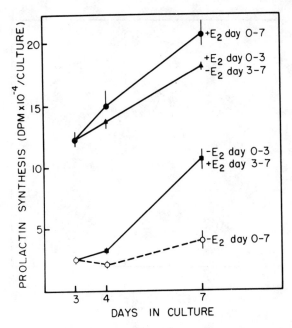

Fig. 4. Time course of induction of prolactin synthesis. Pituitary cells were cultured in control medium ($-E_2$), or in medium containing 10 nM estradiol ($+E_2$) for the periods indicated. Prolactin synthesis was quantitated by immunoprecipitation. Each point represents the mean ±SEM of four cultures (Lieberman et al., 1978[25]).

With 4 μM cytosine arabinoside or 1 and 10 mM hydroxyurea, which blocked DNA synthesis by 80 to 95% and also reduced the incorporation of (^{3}H)leucine into total protein by approximately 25%, prolactin synthesis was 145 to 160% of control values with little or no change in the number of mammotrophs. These results indicate that estrogen stimulates prolactin synthesis both by increasing the number of mammotrophs as well as their synthetic capacity.

We also examined the kinetics of estrogen-induced changes in prolactin synthesis, prolactin mRNA accumulation and mammotroph cell population (Fig. 6). Cultures treated with 10 nM estradiol for 1, 2 or 5 days contained 101, 113 and 132% of the number of mammotrophs present in control cultures. For the corresponding periods, prolactin synthesis was 94, 144 and 270% of controls and prolactin mRNA levels were 113, 160 and 327% of control values, respectively. Taken together, the data indicate that estradiol stimulates prolactin synthesis in cultured pituitary cells predominantly through an increase in prolactin mRNA per cell, and to a lesser extent, through increasing the number of prolactin

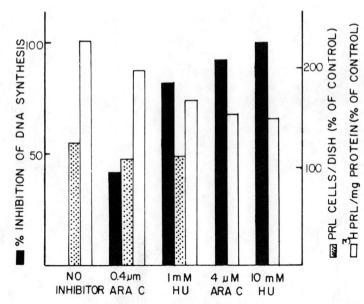

Fig. 5. Relationship between estrogen-induced prolactin synthesis
and mammotroph cell proliferation. Pituitary cells were cultured
for 3 days in control medium or in medium containing 10 nM estradiol with and without cytosine arabinoside (Ara C) or hydroxyurea
(HU) at the concentrations indicated (10 treatment groups). Incorporation of the labeled nucleotide into DNAase I sensitive TCA
precipitable material was determined after 16 h incubation with
(^{3}H)thymidine (5 μCi/ml). In replicate cultures prolactin synthesis was quantitated by immunoprecipitation. Mammotrophic cells
were identified by immunocytochemistry using anti-rat prolactin
(1:10,000 dilution) as the primary antibody (Lieberman et al.,
1980 [23]).

producing cells.

　　The time course and magnitude of the response observed in
cultured pituitary cells agree with in vivo data demonstrating
that treatment of rats with estradiol increased 3- to 5-fold the
incorporation of labeled precursors into prolactin and the accumulation of prolactin mRNA (12-14). A similar parallelism was
noted between in vivo and in vitro induction by estrogen of prolactin synthesis in sheep (27,28). Thus in the case of these two
species, a direct estrogen action on the pituitary may account
for all the increased capacity to synthesize prolactin.

Induction of pituitary tumors by diethylstilbestrol.

　　From the data presented, it is clear that one aspect of estrogen action on the pituitary involves prolactin cell replication.
Prolonged treatment with estrogens can lead to the development of
pituitary tumors in susceptible strains of rats and mice, which
secrete large amounts of prolactin (29, 30). In our hands, 8 weeks
of treatment with diethylstilbestrol resulted in a nearly 100%
incidence of pituitary tumors in the Fischer 344 strain of rats

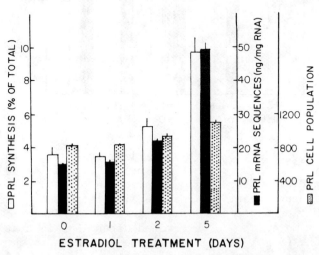

Fig. 6. Comparison of estrogen effects on prolactin synthesis,
prolactin mRNA accumulation and mammotroph cell population. Pituitary cells were cultured for 5 days in control medium or in medium
to which 10 nM estradiol was added for 1, 2 or 5 days. Prolactin
synthesis was quantitated by immunoprecipitation. Prolactin mRNA
content was assayed by hybridization of total cellular RNA to [3]H-
labeled prolactin cDNA. Mammotrophs were identified by immunocytochemistry. Each point represents the mean ± SEM of 3 cultures.
(Maurer and Lieberman, 1980 [33]).

while none of the Holtzman rats developed such tumors, although
the gain in uterine weight was similar in both strains (Fig. 7).
Shellabarger and coworkers also found strain differences in tumor
inducibility between ACI and Sprague-Dawley rats (31).

　　The effects of diethylstilbestrol implants on pituitary
weight, prolactin synthesis and DNA synthesis in Fischer 344 rats
is shown in Table I. When DES implants were present for 8 to 10

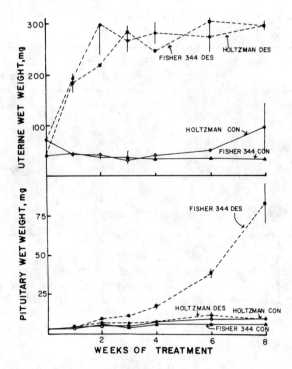

Fig. 7. Effect of DES on pituitary and uterine weights of Holtzman and Fischer 344 rats. Animals silastic tubing implants containing 5 mg DES or vehicle only. Mean ± SEM, four animals per point.

weeks, there was a dramatic increase in pituitary weight, prolactin and DNA synthesis. Cessation of treatment caused a sharp decline in pituitary weight and DNA synthesis, and a lesser decline in prolactin synthesis. We have shown that Holtzman rats are not totally unresponsive to the proliferative effects of estrogen (Figs. 5, 6 and cf. 7, 32). Wiklund et al. (32) showed that there was a 2-fold increase in DNA synthesis in pituitary nuclei of Holtzman rats after 2,3 or 4 daily injections of estradiol, but the rate of DNA synthesis declined after 7 days. By contrast, similar treatment of Fischer rats also increased DNA synthesis 2-fold, but this level was maintained even after 7 days. These results suggest that the Fischer 344 strain lacks the mechanism for shutting off estrogen-induced pituitary cell proliferation which is operative in the Holtzman strain. Current studies are aimed at characterizing the genetic factors involved in this phenomenon.

SUMMARY

We presented evidence that primary cultures of rat pituitary

Table I. Effects of DES on pituitary weight, prolactin synthesis
and DNA synthesis in Fischer 344 rats.

Treatment group	Pituitary weight (mg)	PRL synthesis (% of total)	DNA synthesis (cpm/µg DNA)
Sham implants (8-10 weeks)	8±.4	4±1	75±14
DES, 8 weeks	105±19	35±6	189±9
DES, 9 weeks	130±37	31±14	164±10
DES, 10 weeks	141±32	27±10	230±98
DES, 8 weeks withdrawn 1 week	72±14	24±5	101±12
Withdrawn 2 weeks	51±8	21±14	85±8

Fischer 344 male rats·received implants containing 5.0 mg diethylstilbestrol (DES) in silastic tubing or sham implants. Prolactin
synthesis was determined by SDS-polyacrylamide gel electrophoresis
of (^{3}H)leucine labeled pituitary tissue extracts. DNA synthesis
was estimated by incorporation of (^{3}H)dTTP into isolated pituitary
nuclei. Each value represents the mean ± SD of 2 to 4 pituitaries.

cells respond to estradiol by increased incorporation of precursors into prolactin. The response is specific for estrogenic
hormones and is maximal at physiological concentrations of estradiol. The time course and magnitude of the response in cultured
cells is in agreement with that observed under in vivo conditions,
suggesting that estrogen exerts its effect mainly through a direct
action on the pituitary gland. The data presented indicate that
estrogen stimulates prolactin synthesis predominantly through increased prolactin mRNA accumulation, and to a lesser extent,
through mammotroph cell proliferation. Chronic treatment with DES
caused sustained proliferation of pituitary cells leading to prolactin producing pituitary tumors in the Fischer 344 rat, but not
in the Holtzman rat. The genetic basis for these differences are
currently under investigation.

Acknowledgements

    We thank Bobbi Maurer and Mary Peretz for excellent technical
assistance. This work was supported in part by National Institutes
of Health Grant CA 18110, National Institutes of Health Training
Grant 5-T32-HDO 7007-03, Ford Foundation Grant 630-0505A, Iowa
State Cancer Registry, and American Cancer Society Grant NP-254.

REFERENCES

1. J. L. Voogt, C. L. Chen, and J. Meites, Serum and pituitary
    prolactin levels before, during, and after puberty in female
    rats, Am J Physiol 218:396 (1970).
2. J. D. Neill, M. E. Freeman, and S. A. Tillson, Control of the
    proestrous surge of prolactin and luteinizing hormone secretion
    by estrogens in the rat, Endocrinology 89:1448 (1971).
3. S. R. Ojeda and S. M. McCann, Development of dopaminergic and
    estrogenic control of prolactin release in the female rat,
    Endocrinology 95:1499 (1974).
4. W. W. Andrews and S. R. Ojeda, On the feedback actions of est-
    rogen on gonadotropin and prolactin release in infantile fe-
    male rats, Endocrinology 101:1517 (1977).
5. A. Mastro and W. C. Hymer, The effects of age and oestrone
    treatment on DNA polymerase activity in anterior pituitary
    glands of male rats, J Endocrinol 59:107 (1973).
6. C. Davies, J. Jacobi, H. M. Lloyd and J. D. Meares, DNA synthe-
    sis and the secretion of prolactin and growth hormone by the
    pituitary gland of the male rat: effects of diethylstilboestrol
    and 2-bromo-α-ergocryptine methanesulphonate, J Endocrinol
    61:411 (1974).
7. R. A. Maurer and J. Gorski, Effects of estradiol-17β and pimo-
    zide on prolactin synthesis in male and female rats,
    Endocrinology 101:76 (1977).
8. R. A. Maurer, Estrogen-induced prolactin and DNA synthesis in
    immature female rat pituitaries, Molec Cell Endocrinol 13:291
    (1979).
9. B. E. Gersten and B. L. Baker, Local action of intrahypophyseal
    implants of estrogen as revealed by staining with peroxidase-
    labeled antibody, Am J Anat 128:1 (1970).
10. K. Catt and B. Moffat, Isolation of internally labeled rat
    prolactin by preparative disc electrophoresis, Endocrinology
    80:324 (1967).
11. R. M. MacLeod, A. Abad, and L. L. Eidson, In vivo effect of
    sex hormones on the in vitro synthesis of prolactin and growth
    hormone in normal and pituitary tumor-bearing rats,
    Endocrinology 84:1475 (1969).
12. R. T. Stone, R. A. Maurer, and J. Gorski, Effect of estradiol-
    17β on preprolactin messenger ribonucleic acid activity in the
    rat pituitary gland, Biochemistry 16;4915 (1977).
13. R. Ryan, M. A. Shupnik, and J. Gorski, Effect of estrogen on
    preprolactin mRNA sequences, Biochemistry 18:2044 (1979).
14. S. Kanematsu and C. H. Sawyer, Effects of intrahypothalamic
    and intrahypophyseal estrogen implants on pituitary prolactin
    and lactation in the rabbit, Endocrinology 72:243 (1963).
15. V. D. Ramirez and S. M. McCann, Induction of prolactin secre-
    tion by implants of estrogen into the hypothalamo-hypophysial
    region of female rats, Endocrinology   75:206 (1964).

16. A. Ratner and J. Meites, Depletion of prolactin-inhibiting activity of the rat hypothalamus by estradiol or suckling stimulus, Endocrinology 75:377 (1964).

17. C. S. Nicoll and J. Meites, Estrogen stimulation of prolactin production by rat adenohypophisis in vitro, Endocrinology 70:272 (1962).

18. A. H. Tashjian, Jr., and R. F. Hoyt, Jr., Transient controls of organ specific functions in pituitary cells in culture, in: Molecular Genetics and Developmental Biology, M. Sussman, ed., Prentice Hall, Englewood Cliffs, New Jersey (1972).

19. E. Haug and K. M. Gautvik, Effects of sex steroids on prolactin secreting rat pituitary cells in culture, Endocrinology 99:1482 (1976).

20. P. S. Dannies, P. M. Yen, and A. H. Tashjian, Jr., Antiestrogenic compounds increase prolactin and growth hormone synthesis in clonal strains of rat pituitary cells, Endocrinology 101:1151 (1977).

21. W. L. Miller, M. M. Knight, H. J. Grimek, and J. Gorski, Estrogen regulation of follicle stimulating hormone in cell cultures of sheep pituitaries, Endocrinology 100:1306 (1977).

22. W. L. Miller, M. M. Knight and J. Gorski, Estrogen action in vitro: regulation of thyroid stimulating and other pituitary hormones in cell cultures, Endocrinology 101:1455 (1977).

23. M. E. Lieberman, P. Claude, R. A. Maurer, and J. Gorski, Relationship between estrogen-induced prolactin synthesis and mammotroph proliferation in cultured pituitary cells , Manuscript in preparation.

24. E. J. Pavlik and B. S. Katzenellenbogen, Human endometrial cells in primary tissue culture: estrogen interactions and modulation of cell proliferation, J Clin Endocrinol Metab 47:333 (1978).

25. M. E. Lieberman, R. A. Maurer, and J. Gorski, Estrogen control of prolactin synthesis in vitro, Proc Natl Acad Sci USA 75:5946 (1978).

26. P. Claude, M. E. Lieberman, R. A. Maurer, and J. Gorski, Morphological changes in estrogen-stimulated rat pituitary cells in culture, J Cell Biol 79:206A (1978) (Abstract HM 1260).

27. L. Vician, M. A. Shupnik, and J. Gorski, Effects of estrogen on primary ovine pituitary cell cultures: stimulation of prolactin secretion, synthesis and preprolactin messenger ribonucleic acid activity, Endocrinology 104:736 (1979).

28. M. A. Shupnik, L. A. Baxter, L. R. French, and J. Gorski, In vivo effects of estrogen on ovine pituitaries: prolactin and growth hormone biosynthesis and messenger ribonucleic acid translation, Endocrinology 104:729 (1979).

29. K. H. Clifton and R. K. Meyer, Mechanism of anterior pituitary tumor induction by estrogen, Anat Rec 125:65 (1956).

30. W. V. Gardner, Studies on ovarian and pituitary tumorigenesis, J Natl Cancer Inst 15:693 (1954).

31. S. Holtzman, J. P. Stone, and C. J. Shellabarger, Influence of diethylstilbestrol on prolactin cells of female ACI and Sprague-Dawley rats, Cancer Res 39:779 (1979).

32. J. Wiklund, N. Wertz, and J. Gorski, Diethylstilbestrol-induced pituitary growth and DNA synthesis: strain differences in response to chronic treatment, 62nd Annual Meeting of the Endocrine Society, Washington, D. C. (1980) (Abstract, in press).

33. R. A. Maurer and M. E. Lieberman, Comparison of estrogen effects on prolactin synthesis, prolactin mRNA accumulation and mammotroph cell population in cultured rat pituitary cells, 62nd Annual Meeting of the Endocrine Society, Washington, D.C. (1980) (Abstract, in press).

COMPARATIVE ANTIOESTROGEN ACTION

IN EXPERIMENTAL BREAST CANCER

V. Craig Jordan

Departments of Human Oncology & Pharmacology
Wisconsin Clinical Cancer Center
University of Wisconsin
600 Highland Avenue
Madison, WI 53792

INTRODUCTION

Tamoxifen (_trans_ 1-(4-β dimethylaminoethoxyphenyl)1,2
diphenylbut-1-ene) is a non-steroidal antioestrogen currently used
for the treatment of advanced breast cancer (1,2). Although
tamoxifen produces a variety of endocrine effects in pre- and
post-menopausal patients (Fig. 1) it is believed that its antitumour
effects are caused by blocking the oestrogen receptors found in
some breast tumours (3). Tamoxifen antagonises the direct effects
of oestrogen in tumour cells, however, it has been suggested that
tamoxifen can cause antitumour effects itself, through an oestrogen
receptor mediated mechanism (4).

Even though tamoxifen is an extremely effective anticancer
agent with low toxicity, it is important to explore the possibility
that related structures may be more effective or have properties
that may suggest special clinical applications. Unfortunately,
there is no single ideal laboratory model that can be utilized in
a screening and development program. The use of oestrogen receptor
binding assays and human breast cancer cell lines does not provide
any information on pharmacokinetic and metabolic factors;
transplantable spontaneously arising rat mammary tumours are often
not hormone dependent (5) and models using the mouse (nude-mice
with transplanted human tumours and spontaneously arising or
transplantable mouse mammary tumours) all suffer from the unusual
pharmacology of antioestrogens in this species (6).

The dimethylbenzanthracene (DMBA)-induced rat mammary carcin-

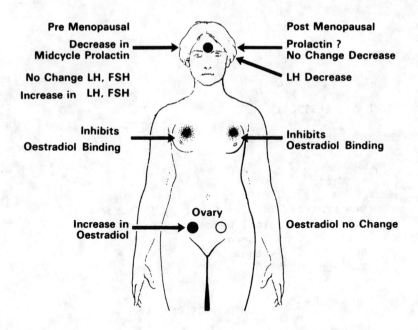

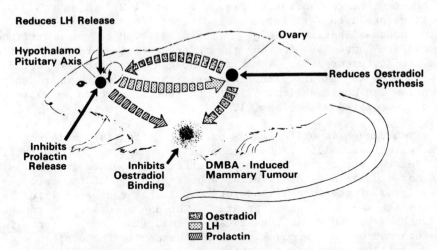

Fig. 1.   Comparative endocrine effects of tamoxifen in the pre-
          and post-menopausal woman with breast cancer and the
          mature rat with DMBA-induced mammary cancer.

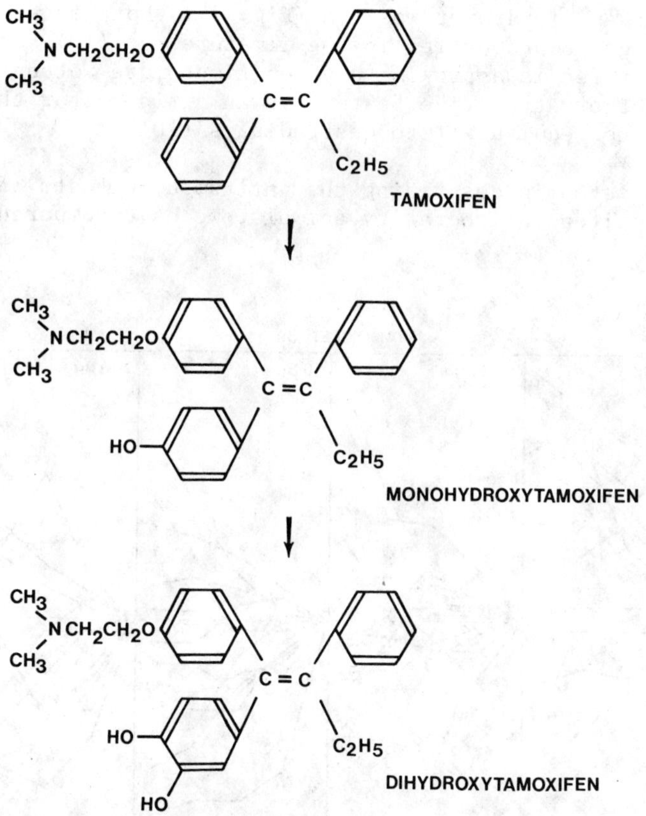

Fig. 2.   The oxidative metabolism of tamoxifen in the rat.

oma model has been studied extensively as a screen for potential
agents useful in the treatment of breast cancer (7,8). Antioestrogens are effective in controlling tumour growth (9). It is
now clear though, that unlike human breast cancer which is predominantly dependent upon the direct effects of oestrogen,
DMBA-induced mammary tumours are predominantly dependent upon
prolactin. It is, therefore, the ability of antioestrogens, like
tamoxifen, to modulate prolactin secretion by direct and indirect
mechanisms, that ultimately controls tumour homeostasis (Fig. 1).

    In our search for more potent antioestrogens with potential
antitumour properties we have focused our attention on monohydroxytamoxifen (10,11) as a basic structure that may be developed for
future clinical use (Fig. 2).

In the rat tamoxifen is metabolised (12) to monohydroxytamoxifen and then dihydroxytamoxifen (Fig. 2). Both metabolites
have antioestrogenic properties in the immature rat (10) but
monohydroxytamoxifen is approximately ten times more potent than
tamoxifen. Another attractive feature is an affinity for the
oestrogen receptor equivalent to oestradiol's (10).

As a first step in describing the antitumour effects of
monohydroxytamoxifen in laboratory animals, we have compared the

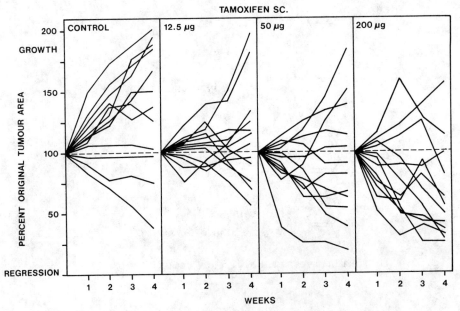

Fig. 3.   Effect of different daily doses of tamoxifen (sc in
          0.1 ml peanut oil) on the percentage growth or regression
          of DMBA-induced mammary tumours (100-150 days after
          DMBA). Controls were injected with vehicle alone.

dose-response effects with those of tamoxifen in the DMBA-induced
rat mammary carcinoma model. Unfortunately the use of animals
with established palpable tumours as an assay system is complicated by the heterogeneous response to antioestrogens (13-15). A
representative dose response experiment for tamoxifen is shown in
Fig. 3 to illustrate the problems involved.

We have devised a comparative assay system based upon the
treatment of animals with early microfoci of carcinogen trans-

formed breast cells by a one month course of antioestrogen therapy. The end point for the assay is the effectiveness of therapy in controlling the future development of tumours.

MATERIALS AND METHODS

Tamoxifen and monohydroxytamoxifen were gifts from ICI Ltd. (Pharmaceuticals Division) Macclesfield, UK. Each week fresh ethanolic solutions of tamoxifen and monohydroxytamoxifen were prepared. To prepare injection solutions the required volumes of antioestrogen solution were added to peanut oil and the ethanol evaporated under N_2 on a warm (60°) water bath. All s.c. injections were made in 0.1 ml peanut oil.

7,12 Dimethylbenz(a)anthracene (DMBA) was obtained from Sigma Chemicals. DMBA was dissolved in peanut oil by stirring for 16 hr at room temperature to yield a final concentration of 10 mg DMBA/ml.

Antitumour Activity

At 50 days of age, female Sprague Dawley rats were each given 20 mg DMBA by gavage. Three experiments were undertaken:

1) Four weeks after DMBA, animals were randomized into nine groups each of 15 rats. Treatments were instituted 30 days after DMBA for four weekly cycles (5 days per week). Four groups were injected sc with tamoxifen (0.2, 3, 50 or 800 µg daily) and four groups with monohydroxytamoxifen (0.012, 0.2, 3 or 50 µg daily). Controls received injections of peanut oil.

2) Four weeks after DMBA, animals were randomized into three groups each of twenty. Treatments were started 30 days after DMBA 5 days per week. One group was injected with tamoxifen (50 µg daily) for 30 days and another for 170 days.

3) Four weeks after DMBA, animals were randomized into 3 groups each of 20 rats. Treatments were started 30 days after DMBA, 5 days per week until 200 days after DMBA. Two groups were injected s.c. with monohydroxytamoxifen (3 or 50 µg daily) and controls were injected with peanut oil.

In all experiments animals were palpated weekly for tumours up to 200 days after DMBA. Where necessary animals with large and ulcerated tumours were killed prior to the end of experiments. In all cases, a sample of tumour tissue was taken for routine pathological identification.

In experiment 3, tumour areas (measured with calipers and calculated using the formula π x (length/2) x (width/2)) were determined every 2 weeks for 6 weeks starting 156 days after DMBA.

Effects of antioestrogens in ovariectomized rats

Female Sprague Dawley rats (100 days old) were ovariectomized under ether anesthesia and 14 days later were randomized into 25 groups each of five rats. Four major treatment groups each containing five of the groups of rats were selected for treatment with 4 cycles (5 days per week) of either tamoxifen (0.2 or 800 µg daily) or monohydroxytamoxifen (0.012 or 50 µg daily). Controls (5 groups) were injected with peanut oil. One of each of the groups was killed after 1 week of treatment, on the last day of treatment and 1, 3 and 5 weeks after the last day of treatment. Uteri were dissected out cleaned of adhering tissue and used for the determination of [^{3}H]oestradiol and [^{3}H]R5020 binding.

Determination of [^{3}H]oestradiol and [^{3}H]R5020 binding.

Each uterus was homogenized, with ice/water cooling, in 2 ml TED buffer (Tris 0.01 mole/l; EDTA 0.0015 mole/l and dithiothreitol 0.0005 mole/l, pH 7.4) using 2 x 10 sec bursts of an Ultraturrax tissue homogeniser. Homogenates were centrifuged (4°) at 2000 xg for 30 min. Supernatants were used to determine the binding of [6,7 ^{3}H]oestradiol-17β (42 Ci/mmole, Amersham) and [^{3}H]R5020 (dimethyl-19-norpregna-4,9 diene-3,20 dione-17α [17α methyl ^{3}H] (87 Ci/mmole, New England Nuclear). For [^{3}H]-oestradiol binding, uterine supernatants (150 µl) were added to 50 µl TED buffer or 50 µl TED buffer containing 5 x 10^{-6} mole/l diethylstilboestrol. Fifty microliters TED buffer containing 2.5 x 10^{-8} mole [^{3}H]oestradiol/l was added to each tube and the mixtures incubated at 0-4°C for 18 hrs. All samples were assayed in duplicate. Four hundred µl of a dextran coated charcoal suspension (1%) in TED was added to each tube and allowed to stand, with occasional shaking for 20 min at 0-4°C. Tubes were centrifuged at 2000 x g (4°C) for 10 min and 400 µl samples of the supernatants were used to determine the level of radioactivity.

To determine the binding of [^{3}H]R5020, 100 µl supernatant was added to either 100 µl TED containing 30% glycerol or 100 µl TED with 30% glycerol containing 3 x 10^{-6} mole norethindrone (Sigma Chemicals)/l. One hundred µl TED containing 3 x 10^{-8} [^{3}H]R5020/l was added to each tube and incubated at 0°C for 1 hr. Four hundred µl of a 0.25% dextran coated charcoal suspensions in TED buffer was

added to each tube at 0°C for 5 mins. Tubes were centrifuged at
2000 x g (4°C) for 3 min and 400 µl of supernatants were taken to
determine the level of radioactivity.

RESULTS AND DISCUSSION

The primary aim of the present study was to establish a
suitable assay system to evaluate the antitumour potential of the
potent antioestrogen monohydroxytamoxifen.

Carcinogenesis in breast tissue with DMBA is dependent on the
age of the animals (16) and the correct hormonal environment (17).
At the subcellular level prolactin-stimulated thymidine incorporation has been correlated with DMBA-induced carcinogenesis (18).
Although it is known (15) that the simultaneous administration of
tamoxifen and DMBA results in a reduction in tumour numbers, this
is a potentially poor assay for evaluating antitumour activity.
Tamoxifen inhibits oestrogen-stimulated rises in circulating
prolactin levels (19) and it is possible that breast tissue DNA
synthesis may be inhibited since antioestrogens have been found to

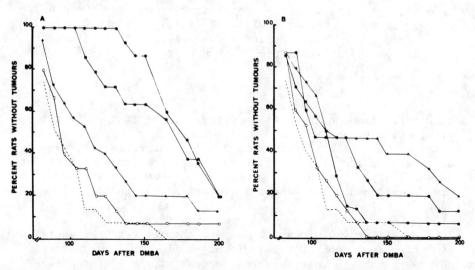

Fig. 4.   Effect of the administration of (A) tamoxifen (800 µg ● ;
           50 µg ■ ; 3 µg ▲ ; 0.2 µg O; daily) or (B) monohydroxy-
           tamoxifen (50 µg ● ; 3 µg ■ ; 0.2 µg ▲ ; 0.012 µg O;
           daily) between 30 and 60 days (5 times per week) after
           DMBA on the percentage of rats in groups without mammary
           tumours. Controls (----) were injected with peanut oil.
           Fifteen rats per group.

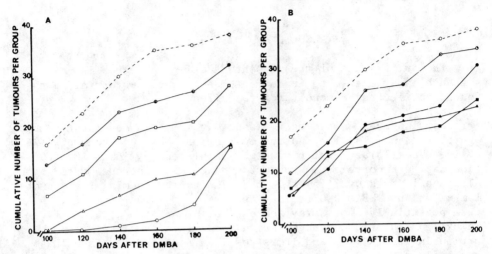

Fig. 5.   Cumulative number of mammary tumours after the adminis-
          tration of (A) tamoxifen (800 µg 0; 50 µg Δ ; 3 µg □ ;
          0.2 µg ⊘ daily) or (B) monohydroxytamoxifen (50 µg ▲ ;
          3 µg ●; 0.2 µg ■ ; 0.012 µg ⊘ daily) between 30 and 60
          days after DMBA.   Controls (0---0) received injections
          of peanut oil.   Fifteen rats per group.

inhibit cell division in other oestrogen target tissues of the rat
(11).   Therefore, under these conditions the process of carcinogenesis may be inhibited rather than malignant cells destroyed.
After consideration of these factors, all therapies were instituted
at least 28 days after DMBA administration when it was assumed that
carcinogenesis had occurred and microfoci of malignant cells were
present.

     In the first experiment to compare the antitumour properties
of tamoxifen and monohydroxytamoxifen, smaller daily doses of
monohydroxytamoxifen were selected because of its higher antioestrogen potency (10).   The administration of tamoxifen (0.2,
3, 50 or 800 µg daily) for four weekly cycles resulted in a
dose-related delay in the percentage of rats in groups without
tumours (Fig. 4a).   By contrast, treatment with monohydroxytamoxifen
(0.012, 0.2, 3 or 50 µg daily) did not produce a clear dose-related
inhibition of tumour appearance.   Although the various therapies
delayed the initial appearance of tumours, the majority of animals
had at least one palpable mammary tumour at 200 days after DMBA.

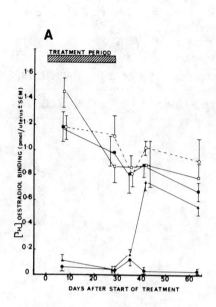

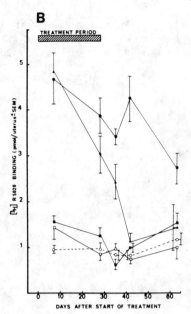

Fig. 6.   Effect of tamoxifen (800 µg ●; 0.2 µg ■ daily) or
monohydroxytamoxifen (50 µg ▲ ; 0.012 µg □ daily)
administered for 4 cycles of therapy 5 times per week on
ovariectomized rat (A) uterine [³H]oestradiol binding
(B) uterine [³H]R5020 binding. Controls (0---0) received
injections of peanut oil. Five rats in each group.

Similarly, the effect of tamoxifen on the total numbers of tumours
in treatment groups was dose related. Although monohydroxytamoxifen
was able to inhibit the appearance of mammary tumours, this effect
did not appear to be dose-related (Fig. 5).

   A comparison of the uterine effects of tamoxifen (800 µg or
0.2 µg daily) and monohydroxytamoxifen (50 or 0.012 µg daily) in
the ovariectomized rat showed that only the higher dose of each
compound was biologically active and the effects of tamoxifen
were more long-term than the effects of monohydroxytamoxifen.
During therapy tamoxifen (800 µg) and monohydroxytamoxifen (50 µg)
both increased the uterine binding of [³H]R5020 and completely
reduced the uterine binding of [³H]oestradiol (Fig. 6). However,
[³H]R5020 binding rapidly decreased during the 2 weeks after the
last injection of monohydroxytamoxifen and the binding of
[³H]oestradiol in the uterine cytosols increased. In contrast,
the uterine effects of tamoxifen (800 µg) were maintained until
the end of the experiment i.e., 5 weeks after the cessation of
therapy. From these data it seems that the antitumour effects

Table 1. Appearance and incidence of mammary tumours in groups
of rats treated with tamoxifen (50 μg daily) 30-60 days (Short
Course) or 30-200 days (Continuous Course) after DMBA.

Days after DMBA	CONTROL		SHORT COURSE		CONTINUOUS COURSE	
	% rats[1]	tumours[2]	% rats	tumours	% rats	tumours
100	65	26	40	12	10	3
120	65	26	40	12	10	3
140	85	29	50	14	10	3
160	100	43	65	18	10	2
180	100	44	75	28	10	2
200	100	44	75	28	10	2

1. % rats in groups with tumours. Twenty rats per group.
2. Cumulative total of tumours per group.

of either tamoxifen or monohydroxytamoxifen are related to their
relative biological half lives rather than their antioestrogenic
potency. It therefore seemed likely that the continued presence
of an antioestrogen might suppress tumour formation. This
suggestion was found to be valid when a short course of tamoxifen
therapy was compared with continuous therapy (Table 1). Although
a short course of therapy reduced tumour numbers, continuous
therapy allowed the majority of rats (90%) to remain tumour free.

It was also important to determine whether monohydroxytamoxifen could exert a sustained antitumour action after its
disappointing performance in the short course assay. Continuous
cycles of treatment with 3 μg monohydroxytamoxifen daily starting
30 days after DMBA resulted in a decrease in the cumulative number
of tumours (Fig. 7) and the individual tumour sizes measured at
163, 178, and 192 days after DMBA (Fig. 8). Fifty μg monohydroxytamoxifen daily was more effective in each of the recorded
parameters, however, a single tumour (F1 L2) in this group
continued to grow rapidly during therapy. Ovariectomy of the host
resulted in a progressive tumour reduction. Therefore, it appears
that the maintenance of high blood levels of a short acting
antioestrogen can effectively inhibit hormone dependent growth.
Clearly the prolonged biological activity of a compound like

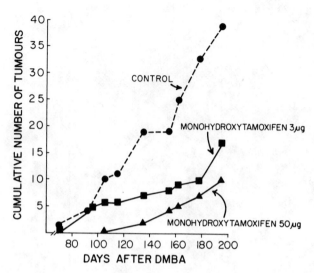

Fig. 7. Effect of continuous (5 times per week starting 30 days
         after DMBA) treatment with monohydroxytamoxifen (3 µg   ;
         50 µg   daily) on the cumulative number of DMBA-induced
         mammary tumours. Therapy was started 30 days after DMBA.
         Controls (0) were injected with peanut oil. Twenty rats
         per group.

tamoxifen appears to be very important as a criterion for
antitumour activity in this model.

SUMMARY AND CONCLUSIONS

     Although monohydroxytamoxifen is a more potent antioestrogen
than tamoxifen, tamoxifen appears to be a more potent antitumour
agent in the DMBA-induced rat mammary carcinoma model. Antitumour
effects in this model, or in fact the ability of an antioestrogen
to suppress the appearance of tumours, seem to be related to the
biological half life of the drug, such that tumour development is
best inhibited in the constant presence of the drug. Overall, it
seems clear that short course of antioestrogens do not destroy all

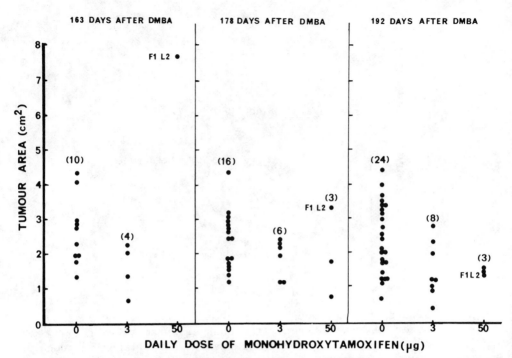

Fig. 8.   Areas of mammary tumours measured in controls or in groups
          treated continuously with either 3 μg or 50 μg monohydroxy-
          tamoxifen daily (5 times per week). The animal with
          tumour F1L2 was ovariectomized 163 days after DMBA. The
          numbers of tumours measured are shown in parentheses.
          Twenty rats per group.

the foci of hormone dependent DMBA induced tumour cells.

     These data are in marked contrast to the effects of anti-
oestrogens on human breast cancer cells maintained in long term
tissue culture (4).   This may be because it is generally believed
that human tumours are directly dependent upon oestrogen whereas
the rat tumour model is primarily dependent upon prolactin (Fig. 1).
Whether human breast cancer cells are protected from antioestrogen
action in vivo like rat tumour cells must await the completion of
clinical trials with tamoxifen as an adjuvant therapy following
mastectomy.

     The primary aim of the study was to evaluate the antitumour
actions of monohydroxytamoxifen.   The compound is active in the

DMBA-induced mammary tumour system but, in contrast to tamoxifen, it is short acting.

The question arises as to whether hydroxylated antioestrogens might have clinical applications. Monohydroxytamoxifen has been found to be ten times more potent than tamoxifen in experiments with the MCF7 human breast cancer cell line in vitro (Dr. H. Rochefort, Antioestrogen Workshop, Sydney, Australia 4-6th Feb. 1980). In its present form though, monohydroxytamoxifen does not appear to offer any therapeutic advantages over tamoxifen for long term treatment. In fact, it may be less effective since tolerance may develop sooner (cf. Fig. 7 & Table 1).

One area of potential application would be to use hydroxylated antioestrogens as cell cycle regulators for subsequent chemotherapy (Dr. C.B. Lazier, Antioestrogen Workshop, Sydney, Australia 4-6th Feb 1980). Tamoxifen would probably be less efficient in this regimen since several weeks are necessary to establish high blood levels. More important though, tamoxifen's long biological half-life might create problems of when to sequence the chemotherapy for individual patients.

In summary, the antioestrogen monohydroxytamoxifen is much more short acting than the parent compound tamoxifen and as such may have special applications in the clinic. Only careful pharmacokinetic studies in man will confirm the laboratory findings.

ACKNOWLEDGEMENTS

These studies could not have been undertaken at the Department of Pharmacology, University of Leeds, UK without the skilled help of Karen E. Allen and generous grants from ICI Ltd. (Pharmaceuticals Division) and the Yorkshire Cancer Research Campaign.

REFERENCES

1. Heel, R.C., Brogden, R.N., Speight, T.M. and Avery, G.S., Drugs 16: 1 (1978).
2. Mouridson, H.T., Palshoff, T., Patterson, J. and Battersby, L., Cancer Treat. Rev. 5: 131 (1978).
3. Jordan, V.C. and Koerner, S., Eur. J. Cancer 11: 205 (1975).
4. Lippman, M. and Bolan, G., Nature 256: 592 (1975).
5. Jordan, V.C., Dixon, B., Prestwich, G. and Furr, B.J.A., Eur. J. Cancer 15: 755 (1979).
6. Harper, M.J.K. and Walpole, A.L., J. Reprod. Fertil. 13: 101 (1967).

7. Griswold, D.P., Skipper, H.E., Laster, W.R., Wilcox, W.S. and
      Schabel, F.M., Cancer Res. 26: 2169 (1966).
8. Teller, M.N., Stock, C.C., Stohr, G., Merker, P.C., Kaufman,
      R.J., Escher, G.C. and Bowie, M., Cancer Res. 26: 245
      (1966).
9. Terenius, L., Eur. J. Cancer 7: 57 (1971).
10. Jordan, V.C., Collins, M.M., Rowsbey, L. and Prestwich, G.,
      J. Endocr. 75: 305 (1977).
11. Jordan, V.C. and Dix, C.J., J. Steroid Biochem. 11: 285
      (1979).
12. Fromson, J.M., Pearson, S. and Bramah, S., Xenobiotica 3:
      693 (1973).
13. DeSombre, E.R. and Arbogast, L.Y., Cancer Res. 34: 1971
      (1974).
14. Nicholson, R.I. and Golder, M.P., Eur. J. Cancer 11: 571
      (1975).
15. Jordan, V.C., Eur. J. Cancer 12: 419 (1976).
16. Huggins, C., Grand, L.C. and Brillantes, P., Nature 189: 204
      (1961).
17. Dao, T.L., Cancer Res. 22: 973 (1962).
18. Nagasawa, H., Yanai, R. and Taniguchi, H., Cancer Res. 36:
      2223 (1976).
19. Jordan, V.C. and Koerner, S., J. Endocr. 68: 305 (1976).

INHIBITION OF ESTROGEN BIOSYNTHESIS AND REGRESSION OF MAMMARY
TUMORS BY AROMATASE INHIBITORS

A.M.H. Brodie, H.J. Brodie, L. Romanoff, J.G. Williams,
K.I.H. Williams and J.T. Wu

Worcester Foundation for Experimental Biology, Shrewsbury, MA. 01545 & Dept. of Pharmacology, University of
Maryland Medical School, Baltimore, MD. 21201

INTRODUCTION

Aromatase inhibitors are potentially useful therapeutic
agents for patients with estrogen-dependent cancer. The rationale
for this approach is that compounds interacting with aromatizing
enzyme in all estrogen producing tissues could provide both
selective and effective inhibition. The conversion of androgens
to estrogens is a unique reaction in the biosynthesis of steroids
since it involves aromatization of the A ring of the steroid
molecule. This is the last series of steps in the biosynthetic
progression from cholesterol to the estrogens. Therefore,
compounds inhibiting the enzyme system mediating aromatization
would be expected to be more specific inhibitors of estrogen
biosynthesis than those influencing steps earlier in
steroidogenesis (Lipton and Santen, 1974; Levin et al., 1976). In
women, estrogens are produced primarily by the ovaries but
extragonadal tissues (Longcope et al., 1978; Hemsell et al., 1974)
such as fat, muscle and certain breast tumors (Miller et al., 1974;
de Thibault et al., 1974; Valera and Dao, 1978) also synthesize
estrogens which contribute to tumor growth. Thus, aromatase
inhibitors acting in all tissue sites may be more effective as well
as more specific than present methods for reducing estrogen
production.

STUDIES OF AROMATASE INHIBITORS IN VITRO

Utilizing the human placental and PMSG-primed, rat ovarian
microsomal system, we have previously evaluated steroid
derivatives for their ability to inhibit aromatization (Schwarzel

et al., 1973). The most promising were 17 keto-steroids, and while
substitution at Carbons 18 and 19 did not improve inhibitory
properties, substitution at carbon 4 and conjugation at carbons 1
and 6 were favorable modifications. The most active aromatase
inhibitors to date, all of which exhibit kinetics of competitive
inhibition of the enzyme (Schwarzel et al., 1973; Brodie et al.,
1977)   are   4-hydroxyandrostene—3,17dione   (4-OHA),   4-
acetoxyandrostene-3,17-dione   (4-acetoxyA)   and   1,4,6-
androstratriene-3,17-dione (ATD) (Table 1, Brodie, 1980).

To determine whether the compounds are specific to
aromatization we have studied their effects on other enzyme
systems in vitro. Incubation of ovarian microsomes with ^{3}H-
progesterone in the presence of 4-OHA had no effect on the
metabolic pathway between progesterone and androstenedione. The
metabolism of dehydroepiandrosterone to androstenedione was also
not affected by 4-OHA. We have recently studied the effect of 4-
OHA on 17β-hydroxy steroid dehydrogenase in ovarian microsomes and
find no inhibition by 4-OHA at 7μM, a concentration 10-fold higher
than that required to cause 80% inhibition of aromatase. However,
at 70μM concentration of 4-OHA, conversion of androstenedione to
testosterone was inhibited 78%. The conversion of androstenedione
to dihydrotestosterone (DHT) in human parenchymal tissue was
reported by Perel et al. (1979) to be inhibited also at a very high
concentration of 4-OHA (90 μM). It seems unlikely that the
inhibitor would be in such high concentrations in vivo that these
enzyme systems would be affected. Studies in rhesus monkeys
(Brodie et al., 1980) described below, support this view since the
interconversion of androstenedione to testosterone, of estrone to
estradiol or the conversion of androstenedione to DHT were not
modified by 4-OHA or 4-acetoxyA.

STUDIES OF ACTION OF AROMATASE INHIBITORS IN VIVO

4-OHA, 4-acetoxyA and ATD had no estrogenic or progestational
activities nor antihormonal activity compared to estrogen,
progesterone or testosterone as determined by bioassays. 4-OHA
and 4-acetoxyA had 1% the androgenic activity of testosterone,
while the activity of ATD was below detectable levels (Brodie et
al., 1977; Brodie et al., 1979a; Brodie et al., 1979b).

In studies to investigate whether the above compounds are
effective in vivo, female rats (225-250 g) were primed with 100 IU
pregnant mares' serum gonadotropin (PMSG) on alternate days for a
12-day period. On day 12, animals were injected SC with either a
single dose of 4-OHA (50 mg/kg bw) or vehicle only. Two rats from
each group were killed at 4, 12, 24, 48 and 72 hours after 4-OHA or
vehicle injection. Microsomes were prepared from the ovaries and
incubated with 1,2^{3}H-androstenedione. The conversion to ^{3}H-
estrogen was determined from tritiated water (Sitteri and

TABLE 1

COMPOUNDS EVALUATED FOR INHIBITION OF AROMATASE IN VITRO

COMPOUND[a]	CONCENTRATION (µM)	% Inhibition of Aromatization	
		HUMAN PLACENTA[b]	RAT OVARY[c]
Control		0	0
4-OHA	0.7	82	71
	2.1	91	88
	4.2	94	94
4-acetoxyA	0.7	81	39
	2.1	90	68
	4.2	–	78
ATD	0.7	69	75
	2.1	83	87
	4.2	93	93
A-trione	2.1	78	33
Teslac	4.2	2	22
Aminoglute- thimide	2.1	–	67
	4.2	–	80

[a]

4-OHA	4-hydroxyandrostene-3,17-dione
4-acetoxyA	4-acetoxyandrostene-3,17-dione
ATD	1,4,6-androstatriene-3,17-dione
A-trione	4-androstene-3,6,17-trione
Teslac	17α-oxo-D-homo-1,4-androstadiene-3,17-dione
Aminoglutethimide	3-(p-aminophenyl)-3-ethyl-2,6-piperidinedione

[b] Microsomes from 1g wet weight of human placental tissue incubated with test compound, $4^{14}C$-testosterone, 0.7µM androstenedione, and an NADPH generating system in 2.5 ml phosphate buffer (pH 7.4) for 30 mins. at 37°C under 95% O_2/5% Co_2. All are mean values.

[c] Microsomes equivalent to 50 mg rat ovarian tissue were incubated with test compound, $1,2^3H$-androstenedione, 0.7µM androstenedione and an NADPH generating system in 2.5 ml phosphate buffer (pH 7.4) for 30 mins. at 37°C under oxygen. All are mean value. (Reference Brodie, 1980)

Thompson, 1975) formed during aromatization (Brodie et al., 1969).
Inhibition of aromatization increased to 80% in about 12 hours and
then began to decline slowly from 90% inhibition 48 hours after
injection.   In similarly treated rats, peripheral blood samples
were collected at 18 hours after injection of 4-OHA and assayed for
steroid levels. The mean plasma estradiol was significantly lower
in 4-OHA-treated rats (161 $\pm$ 24 pg/ml) than in controls (316 $\pm$ 49
pg/ml). The percentage reduction was not as great as the reduction
in aromatization.   However, in rats treated with aromatase
inhibitors on proestrus there was a marked suppression (80-90%) of
ovarian estradiol secretion in samples collected 3 hours after
injection of inhibitor (Brodie et al., 1979b).   Our experiments
suggest that the reduction in plasma estrogen levels probably
resulted from aromatase inhibition rather than from a negative
feedback mechanism of aromatase inhibitor on LH and FSH since PMSG
injections would override potential changes in erdogenous
gonadotropins.

In the PMSG-primed rats, there was no significant difference
in peripheral plasma levels of progesterone, testosterone or
androstenedione in control and 4-OHA-treated rats (Brodie et al.,
1979a) confirming our in vitro results that enzymes involved in the
biosynthesis of these steroids are probably not inhibited by 4-
OHA.

Studies were undertaken in rhesus monkeys using the constant
infusion technique, to investigate the effect of 4-OHA and 4-
acetoxyA on peripheral aromatization (Brodie and Longcope, 1980).
Four male rhesus monkeys were injected with 4-OHA (50 mg/kg bw) at
1700 h on the day prior to and at 08:30 h on the day of a constant
infusion of 7-^{3}H-androstenedione (60 μCi) and 14-C-estrone (1.5
μCi).   Each monkey served as its own control (vehicle injected)
being infused one week before (2 animals) and one week after (2
animals) 4-OHA treatment.   Blood samples (5 ml) were withdrawn
during infusion from the brachial vein at 0,2.5,3 and 3.5 hours.
Following addition of recovery markers for androstenedione,
testosterone, dehydrotestosterone, estrone and estradiol, the
steroids were extracted and purified (Longcope et al., 1978). The
peripheral aromatization of androstenedione to estrone and
estradiol were inhibited in all 4 monkeys when treated with 4-OHA.
The percent conversion of androstenedione to estradiol was reduced
to an undetectable level in 3 out of 4 monkeys and inhibited by 77%
in the fourth.   In addition, in one of 2 monkeys treated with
silastic implants of 4-acetoxyA, peripheral aromatase   was
inhibited.   In the other animal in which there was no effect,
purulent fluid surrounded the   silastic implant and may have
retarded release of the inhibitor.

The interconversion of androstenedione to testosterone, of
estrone to estradiol and of androstenedione to dihydrotestosterone

were unaffected by 4-OHA treatment. These results substantiate our in vitro findings concerning the specificity of 4-OHA for aromatase. The enzymes involved in other steroid reactions do not appear to be inhibited in vivo by 4-OHA and 4-acetoxyA at the concentrations adequate for aromatase inhibition in vivo.

METABOLIC STUDIES WITH AROMATASE INHIBITORS

The metabolic clearance rates of both androstenedione and estrone in the above monkeys were not significantly affected by the inhibitor treatment, thus production and not clearance of estrogen is modified by 4-OHA or 4-acetoxyA.

In the same 4 monkeys injected with $6,7^3$H-4-OHA, pharmacokinetic studies indicate that the compound is cleared rapidly from the blood. 4-OHA· and a metabolite, 4-hydroxytestosterone, were isolated in small amounts (<2%) as both unconjugated and as glucuronide conjugates from monkey blood. No metabolism to testosterone was detected. In the rat the metabolic pattern was similar. Recently, 3-hydroxy-5-androstene-4,17-dione was identified as the major metabolite (20-50% of radioactivity) in rat blood. This compound was evaluated in vitro and was a poor inhibitor of aromatization (<10% of 4-OHA activity) (Brodie et al., 1980).

THE EFFECT OF AROMATASE INHIBITORS ON MAMMARY TUMORS

The effect of aromatase inhibitors upon mammary tumors was studied in rats, in which estrogen-dependent mammary tumors were induced with the carcinogen dimethylbenzanthracene (DMBA) (Huggins et al., 1961). Tumors developed in 6-8 weeks after the carcinogen was gavaged at 50-55 days of age and rats were selected for experiments when at least one tumor per rat was 2 cm in diameter. The tumors were measured in 2 dimensions with a caliper and the volume calculated ($4/3 \pi r_1^2$, r_2 where r_1 is the smaller radius (Desombre and Arbogast, 1974). Groups of rats were matched as closely as possible for number of animals, tumors and total volume of tumors. 4-OHA suspended in Klucil was administered twice daily SC. 4-acetoxyA and ATD were administered by silastic wafers placed subcutaneously and injections SC of 25 mg/kg/day. The total dose was similar to the injected dose of 4-OHA (50 mg/kg/day). This method was necessary for efficacy, possibly because of rapid clearance of the compounds from the blood as indicated by the monkey experiments with 4-OHA. All 3 compounds showed marked regression of mammary tumors in 4 weeks (Figs. 1 and 3). Over 90% of tumors regressed to less than half their original size (Brodie et al., 1977; Brodie et al., 1979a) with 4-acetoxyA, ATD (Fig. 1) and 4-OHA (Fig. 3). By contrast, 2 other aromatase inhibitors (Table 1) testololactone (teslac) (Sitteri and Thompson, 1975) and aminoglutethimide (Lipton and Santen, 1974) were much less effective. There was no significant tumor regression with testololactone (25 mg/kg/day) compared to controls. With aminoglutethimide injections (25 mg/kg/day), tumor growth was less than in controls but there was no decrease in the percentage change in mean tumor volume. However, both of these compounds are reported to have some clinical efficacy.

4-acetoxyA causes 65% of the tumors to regress completely. An additional number regressed to a very small size, no longer measureable but still palpable (Brodie et al., 1979b). In this experiment ovarian vein blood was collected at the end of 4 weeks of 4-acetoxyA treatment. Estrone and estradiol secretions were significantly reduced below basal levels for control animals

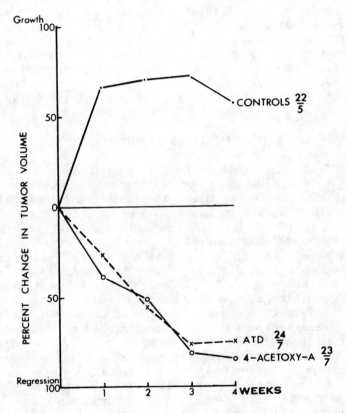

Fig. 1. Effect of aromatase inhibitors on DMBA-induced, rat mammary tumors. Rats (e.g., 7 with 24 tumors = 24/7) were implanted with silastic wafers with (or without, controls) 100 mg ATD or 4-acetoxyA and injected SC twice daily with 13 mg/kg bw (or vehicle, controls).

sampled on estrus or diestrus (Table 2). Gonadotropin levels in peripheral plasma were unaltered by 4-acetoxyA treatment. In view of the low estrogen secretion, increased gonadotropin as occurs after ovariectomy was anticipated. However, when ovariectomized rats were treated with 4-acetoxyA the expected elevation in LH or FSH was not observed, suggesting that the compound may directly affect gonadotropin release in addition to aromatase activity (Brodie, 1980b). Further studies of this effect on gonadotropins are in progress to determine to what extent this contributes to mammary tumor regression.

We have investigated the effect of combining 4-OHA treatment with other treatment modes on mammary tumor regression in the rat model. We envisaged that inhibition of estrogen production combined with inhibition of estrogen action might be more effective than either treatment alone. Anti-estrogen treatment has been shown to cause mammary tumor regression in DMBA-induced rat tumors (Jordan, 1976) and in women (Pearson et al., 1980). In our experiment, the combined treatment of 4-acetoxyA and the anti-estrogen, Tamoxifen (ICI 46,474) when given for 4 weeks was less effective than 4-OHA alone, but slightly greater than with Tamoxifen alone (Fig. 2, Brodie et al., 1979a). Mean ovarian secretion (347 ± 118 (SE) pg/10 min) was greater in tumor-bearing rats treated with Tamoxifen than the value for animals receiving the combined treatment (64 ± 27 (SE) pg/10 min). However, the difference was not significant in this experiment. Increased estradiol levels have also been shown in premenopausal women treated with Tamoxifen (Sherman et al., 1978). Although greater tumor regression may result from lower estrogen secretion in the combined treatment versus Tamoxifen alone, the anti-estrogen may have some "estrogenic" activity which might retard the full effect of the aromatase inhibitor (Fromson et al., 1973).

In another experiment, the effect of treatment with a cytotoxic agent following 4-OHA treatment was investigated. Since a cytotoxic agent kills growing cells exponentially by first order kinetics (DeVita, 1977), this type of agent may cause complete tumor regression when acting on tumors of a very small size. Thus, rats were first treated with 4-OHA injections to induce tumor regression (Fig. 3); within 4 weeks all except 2 tumors had decreased to less than 50% of their original size. Two other tumors that had ulcerated at the start of treatment healed completely. Adriamycin, a highly effective cytotoxic agent, was then administered biweekly SC for 4 weeks. Within 9 weeks, all of the 33 tumors except 1, had either regressed completely (36%) or could only be detected by palpation. The one remaining tumor of measurable dimensions had regressed 86%. This tumor and one other showed a variable pattern of response to 4-OHA and may have been hormone insensitive. Thus, although the cytotoxic agent caused

TABLE 2

THE EFFECT OF 4-acetoxyA ON PLASMA STEROID SECRETION AND GONADOTROPIN CONCENTRATIONS IN
RATS BEARING MAMMARY TUMORS INDUCED BY DMBA

†4-acetoxyA (mg/100g/day)	Estrone (pg/10 min)	Estradiol (pg/10 min)	Progesterone (ng/10 min)	LH (ng/ml)	FSH (ng/ml)	Prolactin (ng/ml)
0	159 $\pm$ 38	*167 $\pm$ 30	‡15.5 $\pm$ 5.5	37.6 $\pm$ 0.6	131 $\pm$ 0.7	83 $\pm$ 3.3
50	83 $\pm$ 18	*47 $\pm$ 17	5.5 $\pm$ 2.0	32.0 $\pm$ 6.0	120 $\pm$ 12	71 $\pm$ 17.1

* Significantly different (P < 0.05).

† Five rats in each group were injected sc twice daily for 4 weeks. Steroid hormones were measured in ovarian venous plasma collected 3 h after the last injection of 4-acetoxyA. Blood from control animals was collected on diestrus I. Gonadotropins were assayed in peripheral plasma taken immediately following the ovarian collection. Results reported as mean $\pm$ SE.

‡ Value from 4 rats.
(Reference Brodie et al, 1979b).

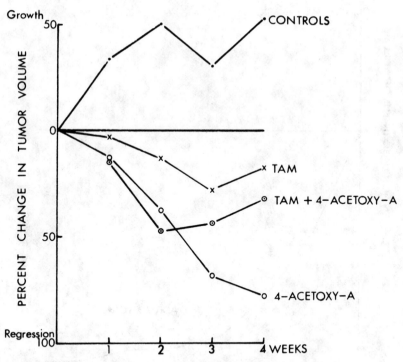

Fig. 2. Effect of 4-OHA SC injections (50 mg/kg/day) twice daily for 4 weeks followed by adriamycin i.p. injections (3 mg/kg bw) biweekly for 4 weeks (7 rats, 33 tumors).

some additional tumor regression, it did not produce complete regression in all tumors. Following cessation of treatment, several tumors grew back in a few weeks.

From studies of Osborne and McGuire (1979) and Pearson (1980) it now appears that patients with estrogen receptor positive tumors have a better prognosis than receptor negative patients and that ablative and additive hormone therapy produce remissions. Our studies show that aromatase inhibitors caused marked regression in mammary tumors in rats and that estrogen secretion was reduced. These findings together with our other evidence appear to be mediated, at least in part, by the inhibition of estrogen biosynthesis. In addition, we have demonstrated inhibition of ovarian and peripheral aromatization in vivo. Although the rat model with DMBA-induced tumors is limited in terms of its similarity to breast cancer, the marked regression of rat tumors with these aromatase inhibitors suggests that such compounds may have potential for breast cancer treatment.

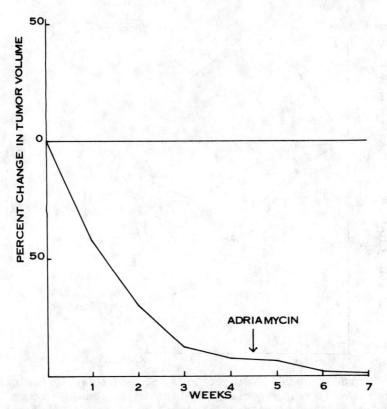

Fig. 3. Effect of combined anti-estrogen and aromatase inhibitor treatment on DMBA-induced, rat mammary tumors. Tamoxifen, ICI-46,474 (TAM): injections 200 g/rat/day. 4-AcetoxyA (4-acetoxy-4-androstene-3,17-dione): 100 mg wafers and injections 1.8 mg/rat/day (ref. Brodie et al., 1979a).

ACKNOWLEDGEMENTS. The assistance of Louise Hebert and Wesley Garrett were greatly appreciated. This work was supported by Contract NICHD 1-HD-0-2059 and grant CA-18595 from the National Institutes of Health.

REFERENCES

1.   Brodie, A. M. H., 1980, Recent advances in studies on estrogen biosynthesis -- a review article, J. Endocrinol. Invest., in press.
2.   Brodie, A. M. H., 1979, Inhibition of oestrogen biosynthesis; an approach to treatment of oestrogen-dependent cancer, in: "Proceedings of the First International Symposium on Hormones and Cancer," Rome, in press.

3. Brodie, A. M. H. and Longcope, C., 1980, Inhibition of peripheral aromatization by aromatase inhibitors, 4-hydroxy- and 4-acetoxy-androstenedione, Endocrinol., 106:19.

4. Brodie, H. J., Kripalani, K. J., and Possanza, G., 1969, Studies on the mechanism of estrogen biosynthesis VI. The stereochemistry of hydrogen elimination at C-2 during aromatization, J. Am. Chem. Soc., 91:1241.

5. Brodie, A. M. H., Marsh, D. A., Wu, J. T., and Brodie, H. J., 1979a, Aromatase inhibitors and their use in controlling estrogen-dependent processes, J. Steroid Biochem., 11:107.

6. Brodie, A. M. H., Marsh, D. A., and Brodie, H. J., 1979b, Aromatase inhibitors IV. Regression of hormone-dependent, mammary tumors in the rat with 4-acetoxy-4-androstene-3,17-dione, J. Steroid Biochem., 10:423.

7. Brodie, A. M. H., Schwarzel, W. C., Shaikh, A. A., and Brodie, H. J., 1977, The effect of an aromatase inhibitor, 4-hydroxy-4-androstene-3,17-dione, on estrogen-dependent processes in reproduction and breast cancer, Endocrinol., 100:1684.

8. Brodie, A. M. H., Wu, J. T., Marsh, D. A., and Brodie, H. J., 1979, Antifertility effects on an aromatase inhibitor, 1,4,6-androstatriene-3,17-dione, Endocrinol., 104:118.

9. Brodie, A. M. H., Wu, J. T., Romanoff, L., and Williams, K. I. H., 1980, Studies on the in vivo mechanism of action of 4-hydroxyandrostenedione, an aromatase inhibitor, The VI Internat. Congress Endocrinol., Melbourne, Abs. 530.

10. Desombre, E. R. and Arbogast, L. Y., 1974, Effect of the antiestrogen Cl628 in the growth of rat mammary tumors, Cancer Res., 34:1971.

11. De Thibault de Boesinghe, L., Lacroix, E., Eechante, W., and Leusen, I., 1974, Oestrogen synthesis by human breast carcinomas, Lancet, 2:1268.

12. DeVita, V. T., 1977, Surgery, radiotherapy and hormone therapy in early breast cancer, pp. 786-789, in: "Perspectives in the Treatment of Breast Cancer," Young, R. C., Moderator, Ann. Intern. Med., 86:784.

13. Fromson, J. M., Pearson, S., and Meek, S. B., 1973, Metabolism of Tamoxifen (ICI 46,474) 1. In laboratory animals, Xenobiotica, 3:693.

14. Hemsell, D. L., Grodin, M. M., Brenner, P. F., Sitteri, P. K., and McDonald, P. C., 1974, Plasma precursors of estrogen II. Correlation of the extent of conversion of plasma androstenedione to estrone with age, J. Clin. Endocrinol. Metab., 38:476.

15. Huggins, C., Grand, L. C., and Brillantes, F. P., 1961, Mammary cancer induced by a single feeding of polynuclear hydrocarbons and its extinction, Nature, 189:204.

16. Jordan, V. C., 1976, Antiestrogenic and anti-tumor properties
     of tamoxifen in laboratory animals, Cancer Treat. Rep.,
     60:1409.
17. Levin, J. M., Goldman, A. S., Rosato, F. E., and Rosato, E.
     E., 1976, Therapy of dimethylbenzanthracene-induced
     mammary carcinomas in the rat by selective inhibition of
     steroidogenesis, Cancer, 38:56.
18. Lipton, A. and Santen, R. J ., 1974, Medical adrenalectomy
     using aminoglutethimide and dexamethasone in advanced
     breast cancer, Cancer, 33:503.
19. Longcope, C., Pratt, J. H., Schneider, S. H., and Fineberg, S.
     E., 1978, Aromatization of androgens by muscle and
     adipose tissue in vivo, J. Clin. Endocrinol. Metab.,
     46:146.
20. Miller, W. R. and Forrest, A. P. M., 1974, Oestradiol
     synthesis by a human breast carcinoma, Lancet, 2:866.
21. Osborne, C. K. and McGuire, W. L., 1979, Therapy for cancer of
     the breast, current status on steroid hormone receptors,
     West. J. Med., 130:401.
22. Pearson, O. H., Manni, A.,Arafah, B., Marshall, J. S., and
     Hubay, C., 1980, Endocrine aspects of breast cancer, in:
     "The Proceedings of the Symposium on Hormones and
     Cancer, Worcester Foundation," in press.
23. Perel, E., Wilkins, D., and Killinger, D. W., 1979,
     Inhibition of androgen aromatization and interconversion
     by 4-hydroxy-androstenedione in breast tissue, 61st
     Endocrine Soc. Meeting, Abs. 303.
24. Schwarzel, W. C., Kruggel, W., and Brodie, H. J., 1973,
     Studies of the mechanism of estrogen synthesis VIII.
     The development of inhibitors of the enzyme system in
     human placenta, Endocrinol., 92:866.
25. Sherman, B. M., Chapler, F. K., Crickard, K., and Wycoff, D.,
     1978, Endocrine consequences of continuous antiestrogen
     therapy with Tamoxifen in premenopausal patients, J.
     Clin. Invest., 64:398.
26. Sitteri, P. K. and Thompson, E. A., 1975, Studies of human
     placental aromatase, J. Steroid Biochem., 61:317.
27. Valera, R. M. and Dao, T. L., 1978, Estrogen synthesis and
     estradiol binding by human mammary tumors, Cancer Res.,
     38:2429.

BIOLOGIC ACTIVITY OF THE IODOESTROGENS AND THEIR USE IN BREAST

CANCER

C. Longcope, T. Arunachalam, I. Rafkind, and E. Caspi

Worcester Foundation for Experimental Biology

Shrewsbury, Ma. 01545

SUMMARY

Several iodinated estrogens, 6-iodoestra-1,3,5(10),6-
tetraene-3,17β-diol (4), 16α-iodoestradiol (2) and 16β-iodo-
estradiol (3) were shown to displace ^{3}H-estradiol (1b) from the
uterine cytosol receptor by a competitive type of inhibition.
The three compounds translocated the cytosol receptor to the
nucleus in vitro and increased mouse uterine weight in vivo. In
all tests the relative activities were 16α-(2a) > 16β-(3a) > 6-
(4a). When the compounds were made with [^{125}I] the 16α-[^{125}I]-
iodoestradiol (2b) bound with high affinity, $K_d = 0.4 \times 10^{-10}$, to
the 8S cytosol receptor. No high affinity binding could be
demonstrated for the 6-[^{125}I]-iodoestratetraene (4b). In in vivo
experiments following the administration of 16α-[^{125}I]-iodoestra-
diol (2b) to rats, high levels of radioactivity were found in the
uterus, liver and thyroid but only in the liver and thyroid
following administration of 6-[^{125}I]-iodoestratetraene (4b).
After administration of (2b) to rats with DMBA-induced mammary
tumors, no tumor concentration of radioactivity could be detected
by imaging. When (4b) was administered similarly, radioactivity
could be detected in some of the tumors by imaging. The radioactivity was associated with non-specific 4S proteins.

INTRODUCTION

Studies on the dynamics of the interactions between estrogens
and their receptors have been carried out almost exclusively
using ^{3}H-estradiol as the probe (1,2,3,4). The use of this probe
has obviously been satisfactory and our current knowledge about
estrogen-receptor interactions has been gained from these studies.

However, ^{3}H is a weak β-emitting isotope which can be measured
only through scintillation counting and autoradiography, the
latter requiring long exposure periods.

Using ^{3}H-estradiol, Jensen showed that many breast cancers
contain a specific receptor for estradiol. He and others (5,6)
have shown a correlation between the presence of the estrogen
receptor in tumor cytosol and the subsequent response of the
patient to endocrine therapy. Currently, measurement of the
estrogen receptor is carried out in vitro, and it has not been
possible to do imaging or body scanning with ^{3}H-labeled estradiol
as the probe. Labeling estradiol with a strong gamma emitter
such as ^{131}I would permit imaging and other studies which are not
possible at the present time. For this and other reasons, we and
others (7,8,9,10,11) have tried for several years to develop γ-
ray emitting iodinated estrogenic analogs applicable to in vivo
studies.

2-Iodo, 4-iodo and 2,4-diiodo estradiol analogs were
prepared, but these compounds possessed minimal, if any, uterotropic activity (11). Katzenellenbogen has reported the labeling
of hexestrol and its analogs with ^{127}I and ^{131}I (8,12). The 3-
iodo-hexestrol (8) had a relative binding affinity 42% that of
estradiol for the estrogen receptor in rat uterine cytosol.
Although the [^{3}H]-3-iodohexestrol did bind to the 8S uterine
receptor, the majority of binding was to a 4S macromolecule and
this binding was abolished by iodo-hexestrol, but not estradiol.
While ^{3}H-iodo-hexestrol could be found in the nucleus after
incubation with rat uterus, most of the ^{3}H-iodo-hexestrol found
there appeared to be bound to a low affinity, high capacity
component. 3-Iodo-hexestrol possessed uterotropic activity when
injected into immature female mice. However, when [^{131}I]-3-iodo-
hexestrol was injected into ovariectomized rats, the liver was
noted to have as much radioactivity as the uterus and most of the
radioactivity was found in the small intestine and thyroid. This
compound was felt to be unsatisfactory for imaging or receptor
studies because of the large degree of non-specific binding (8).

Counsell et al. (9) have shown that 2-iodoestradiol has
little uterotropic activity and that [^{125}I]-16α-iodoestrone-3-
acetate undergoes considerable in vivo deiodination. Iodinated
clomiphene analogs were noted to undergo excessive deiodination
in vivo (9). In view of the reported presence of estradiol
receptors in the prostate (13) [^{125}I]-2-iodo and [^{125}I]-[2,4]-
diiodo estradiol have been tried as prostate-imaging agents (14).
These compounds were shown to undergo extensive deiodination and
non-specific binding despite initial claims to the contrary (15).

More recently, we (7) and Hochberg (10) have synthesized a
number of estradiol analogs labeled with ^{127}I and ^{125}I in rings A,

B and D. Certain of the compounds, particularly 16α-iodoestradiol
(2) and 6-iodoestra-1,3,5(10),6-tetraene-3,17β-diol (4), showed
interesting biological activities. The syntheses of the
iodinated estrogen analogs have been described previously (7,10),
and we now report on their biological activity.

METHODS

For the initial screening studies, we used [^{127}I]-labeled
analogs. The [^{127}I]-compounds were first tested for their
ability to displace ^{3}H-estradiol from uterine cytosol receptor
prepared from virgin adult female rabbits (7). To a series of
tubes were added incremental amounts of either nonradioactive
estradiol or nonradioactive iodinated steroid. Then 10,000 dpm of
2,4,6,7-^{3}H-estradiol (1b) (sp. act. 91.8 Ci/mmole) and cytosol
were added. Following a 16 h incubation at 4°C, the bound and
free steroids were separated with dextran-coated charcoal. The
tubes were then centrifuged and the ^{3}H-estradiol (1b) in the
supernatant was measured by liquid scintillation counting (7,16).
The relative binding affinities were calculated, using the
analysis of Rodbard (17).

For the investigation of the type of inhibition of binding,
the iodo-compounds with the strongest cross reactions (Fig. 1)
(2a), (3a) and (4a) were tested in standard inhibition assays.
To all but one of a series of tubes was added iodinated steroid
(2a), (3a) or (4a) at three concentrations, and to all the sets of
tubes were added uterine cytosol and incremental amounts of ^{3}H-
estradiol (1b). The tubes were incubated 16 h at 4°C. Subsequently, dextran-coated charcoal was added to all tubes, the
contents of which were mixed mechanically and allowed to incubate
for 20 min at 4°C. The tubes were then centrifuged, the supernatant removed and the radioactivity measured. The data were
analyzed for free and bound steroid and plotted using a double
reciprocal plot (18), from which the number of sites and the K_d
were calculated.

Subsequently, the compounds (2a), (3a) and (4a) were tested
using 10-30% sucrose gradients for their ability to displace the
8S bound ^{3}H-estradiol. Uterine cytosol was incubated for 15 min
with varying amounts (2a), (3a), (4a) or estradiol (1a). Then,
^{3}H-estradiol (1b) was added and the tubes incubated for 4 h at
4°C. The cytosol was removed and incubated for 20 min over a
charcoal pellet at 4°C, and the charcoal removed by centrifugation
at 3200 rpm. The supernatant was layered on sucrose gradients and
4-^{14}C-albumin in buffer added as an internal marker. The tubes
were centrifuged at 4°C at 297,000 xg for 16 1/3 h, and 0.1 ml
fractions were collected. The radioactivity in the fractions was
measured, and the counts per minute were plotted against tube
number. The 8S and 4S peaks were determined and the degree of

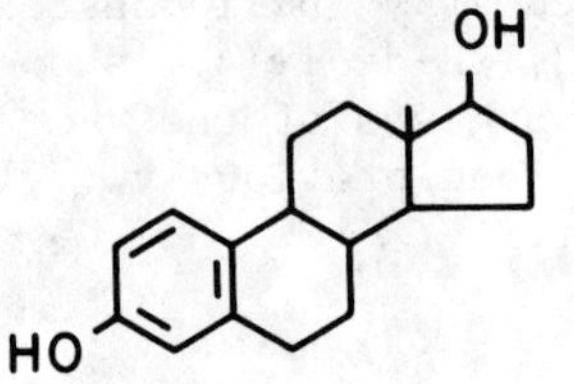

Fig. 1. Structures of estradiol-17β (1), 16α-iodoestradiol (2), 16β-iodoestradiol (3) and 6-iodo-estra-1,3,5 (10),6-tetraene-3,17β-diol (4).

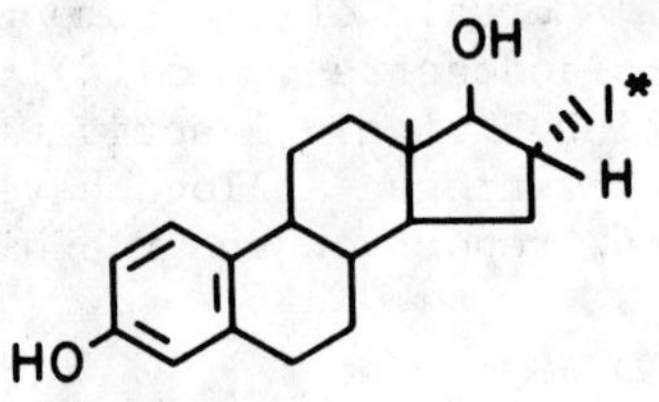

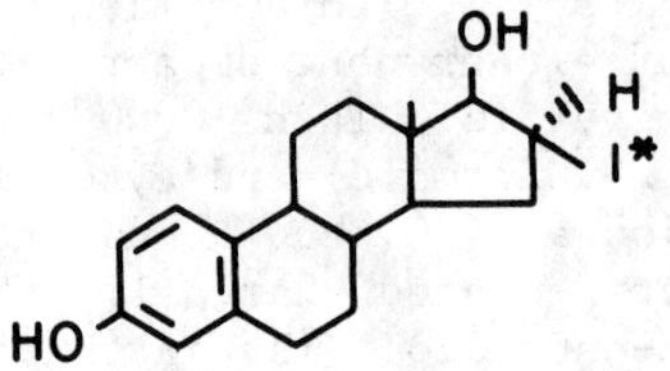

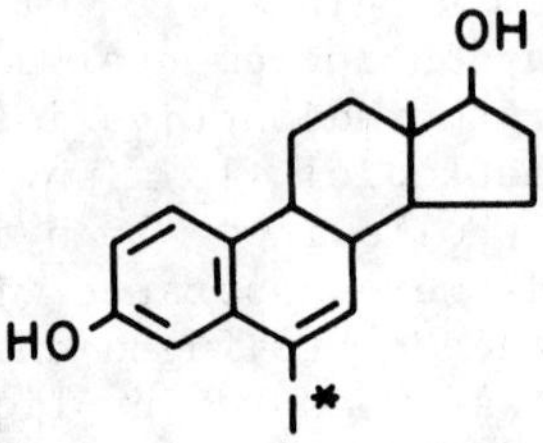

displacement by the iodinated estrogen calculated.

To determine whether compounds (2a), (3a) and (4a) could translocate cytosol receptor to the nucleus, the following series of experiments were carried out. Uteri from 21 day-old Sprague-Dawley rats were removed and placed in flasks; 3 uteri per flask. The flasks were incubated at 37°C for 1 h in the presence of estradiol, 10^{-10} - 10^{-7} M, or the iodinated estrogens (2a), (3a) or (4a), 10^{-9} - 10^{-7} M (19). At the termination of the experiment, the uteri were removed, homogenized and centrifuged. The resulting supernatants and nuclear pellets were separated and washed. The number of unfilled receptor sites in the cytosol and the filled and unfilled estrogen receptor sites in the nucleus were then measured (20).

We tested the biologic activity of the iodinated compounds (2a), (3a) and (4a) in vivo by determining their ability to increase the weight of the uterus of the immature mouse (21).

Solutions of the compounds (in 0.1 ml of ethanol) were injected into 20-21 day-old female mice daily for 3 days. On the 4th day, the mice were sacrificed, the uteri removed, cleaned and weighed.

To characterize better the interaction between the iodinated compounds and the uterine estrogen recentor, experiments were then carried out with [^{125}I]-substituted compounds. The [^{125}I]-16α-iodoestradiol (2b) and [^{125}I]-6-iodoestra-1,3,5(10),6-tetraene-3,17β-diol (4b) were incubated with rabbit uterine cytosol using the previously described dextran coated charcoal assay. The data for B/F and B were plotted using a Scatchard plot, and the K_d calculated.

To determine whether the [^{125}I]-iodo analogs were bound to the specific 8S receptor, [^{125}I]-16α-iodoestradiol (2b) and [^{125}I]-6-iodoestratetraene (4b) were incubated with rabbit uterine cytosol for 4 h at 4°C. Following treatment with dextran-coated charcoal, the cytosol was run on a sucrose gradient and centrifuged for 16 1/3 h at 297,000 xg and processed and analyzed as described above.

For in vivo distribution studies, Sprague-Dawley rats (200-250 g) were used. The rats were oophorectomized and, after two days, were injected with solutions of [^{125}I]-16α-iodoestradiol or [^{125}I]-6-iodo-estratetraene (0.5 μCi in 0.1 ml ethanol) with and without diethylstilbestrol (5 mg). The animals were sacrificed 6 h later, the tissues removed, weighed and the radioactivity determined in a gamma counter.

The [^{125}I]-6-iodoestratetraene (4b) and [^{125}I]-16α-iodo-estradiol (2b) were also tested as imaging agents. Fifty-two day old rats were administered DMBA, (25 mg in 2 ml peanut oil) and, over the course of the next 6-8 weeks, developed easily palpable mammary tumors. The tumorous rats were given [^{125}I]-6-iodo-estratetraene (4b) or [^{125}I]-16α-iodoestradiol (2b) (100 μCi) in ethanolic saline by subcutaneous injection. At varying times following the injection, the rats were scanned, using a gamma scanner.

RESULTS AND DISCUSSION

Although our overall purpose was to develop compounds which would be labeled with [^{125}I] or [^{131}I], we used [^{127}I]-substituted compounds for technical reasons for our initial experiments. A number of [^{127}I]-substituted compounds were synthesized and initially tested for their ability to cross-react with ^{3}H-estradiol (1b) for the uterine cytosol receptor. The results are shown in Tables 1, 2 and 3. All compounds containing iodine in the 2- or 17-position failed to cross-react with estradiol to any significant degree. Introduction of a 7α- or a 4-iodine atom gave compounds with weak cross-reacting abilities. The most active

Table 1. Relative Binding Affinity

Compound	Relative binding affinity[*]
Estra-1,3,5(10)-trien-3,17β-diol (1)	1.00
17α-Iodoestra-1,3,5(10)-triene-3-ol	0.01
17α-Iodoestra-1,3,5(10)-triene-3,16β-diol	0.01
17α-Iodoestra-1,3,5(10),6-tetraene-3-ol	< 0.001
17-Iodoestra-1,3,5(10),16-tetraene-3-ol	< 0.001
2-Iodoestra-1,3,5(10)-trien-3,17β-diol	< 0.001
2,6-Diiodoestra-1,3,5(10),6-tetraene-3,17β-diol	< 0.001
2,4,17-Triiodoestra-1,3,5(10),16-tetraene-3-ol	< 0.001
2,4,17α-Triiodoestra-1,3,5(10)-triene-3,16β-diol	< 0.001
4,17α-Diiodoestra-1,3,5(10)-triene-3,16β-diol	< 0.001

[*]calculated at $^B/Bo$ = 50% (17)

compounds were those with iodine in the 6- or the 16-position.
The 6-iodo-estratetraene (4a) cross-reacted $\sim$ 50%, and the 16β-
iodoestradiol (3a) $\sim$ 60% with estradiol for the uterine cytosol
receptor. The 16α-iodoestradiol cross-reacted 150-160% with ^{3}H-
estradiol, which is in accord with Hochberg's findings (10). It
is surprising that the large iodine atom in the 16α-position of
estradiol does not interfere, but enhances its ability to
cross-react with estradiol for the estrogen receptor. Both the
16α- (2a) and the 16β-iodo (3a) compounds cross-react with

Table 2. Relative Binding Affinity

Compound	Relative binding affinity[*]
Estradiol (1)	1.00
16α-Iodo-3-hydroxyestra-1,3,5(10)-trien-17-one	0.29
17α-Iodomethyl-estra-1,3,5(10)-trien-3,17β-diol	0.09
3-Acetoxy-16α-iodoestra-1,3,5(10)-trien-17-one	0.07
4-Iodo-3-hydroxy-estr-1,3,5(10),9(11)-tetraene-17-one	0.05
7α-Iodo-3,17α-diacetoxyestra-1,3,5(10)-triene-6-one	0.02
7α-Iodoestra-1,3,5(10)-triene-3,6β,17β-triol	0.02
7α-Iodo-3,6β,17β-trihydroxyestra-1,3,5(10)-triene-3,17-diacetate	0.01

[*]calculated at $^B/Bo$ = 50% (17)

Table 3. Relative Binding Affinity

Compound	Relative binding affinity*
Estradiol (1)	1.0
16α-Iodoestra-1,3,5(10)-triene-3,17β-diol (2)	1.60
16β-Iodoestra-1,3,5(10)-triene-3,17β-diol (3)	0.57
6-Iodoestra-1,3,5(10),6-tetraene-3,17β-diol (4)	0.49

*Calculated at $^B/Bo$ = 50% (17)

estradiol to a significantly greater degree than the respective 16-hydroxyestradiols, estriol (estra-1,3,5(10)-trien-3,16α,17β-triol), and epi-estriol (estra-1,3,5(10)-trien-3,16β,17β-triol) which cross-react only some 15-50% with estradiol (18) for the uterine cytosol receptor.

As shown in Fig. 2 and 3 when the type of inhibition exhibited by compounds (2a) and (4a) were examined the results were consistent with a competitive type inhibition of the binding of ^{3}H-estradiol (1b) with the uterine cytosol receptor. In each case the addition of increasing amounts of the iodinated compound resulted in a shift in the K_d for ^{3}H-estradiol (1b) binding to the cytosol receptor although the number of receptor sites remained unchanged.

In the presence of (2a), (3a) or (4a) the binding of ^{3}H-estradiol to the 8S cytosol receptor was inhibited almost completely (Fig. 4). This inhibition was brought about by concentrations of the iodinated estrogens (2a), (3a) or (4a) which were 5-10 times that of ^{3}H-estradiol.

One of the earliest steps in the transfer of estradiol from the circulating blood to the gene is the binding of estradiol to the cytosol receptor (2). Subsequently, the estrogen receptor complex is translocated to the nucleus (2). Having shown that (2a), (3a) and (4a) could displace ^{3}H-estradiol (1b) from the 8S cytosol receptor we were interested to see whether the iodinated compounds were capable of translocating the receptor to the nucleus. As shown in Table 4 the three iodinated compounds (2a), (3a) and (4a) were about equally active in this assay. It should appear that under these conditions, the 16α-iodoestradiol (2a) was no more active than the 6-iodo-estratetraene (4a) in translocating receptor. However, it is evident that estradiol is able to translocate receptors at lower concentrations than the iodinated estrogens.

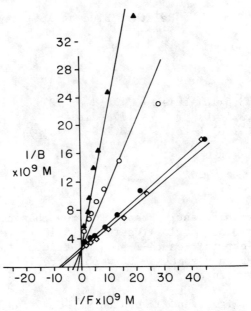

Fig. 2.   Double reciprocal plot (^{1}/B v ^{1}/F) for ^{3}H-estradiol
          binding to cytosol receptor in absence of ◇———◇ and
          presence of 16α–iodoestradiol (2a) 4 x 10^{-9} M ●———●,
          1.2 x 10^{-8} M o———o, and 2.0 x 10^{-8} M ▲———▲.

     The described in vitro experiments indicated possible
biologic activity for the compounds and, therefore, we undertook
to evaluate their activity in vivo to stimulate an increase in
uterine weight. The results of these tests indicated (Tables 5,
6) that the 16α (2a) is active in the amounts tested and does not
inhibit the activity of estradiol. The 6-iodo-estratetraene (4a),
although it increased uterine weight, is somewhat less active than
estradiol (1a) or 16α–iodoestradiol (2a). Since all compounds
were relatively equally active in most of the in vitro assays,
the difference noted in the in vivo assay may be due to faster
metabolism of the 6-iodotetraene or perhaps shorter residence
time in the nucleus (22). When the iodinated compounds (2a) or
(4a) were injected together with estradiol (1a) there was no
evidence for the iodinated compound inhibiting the activity of
estradiol.

     In summary, the above results indicate that [^{127}I]-iodo-
estrogens (2a), (3a) and (4a) are competitive inhibitors of the
binding of ^{3}H-estradiol (1b) to cytosol receptors; are capable of
translocating these receptors to the nucleus; and then residing
there long enough to stimulate uterine growth. These character-

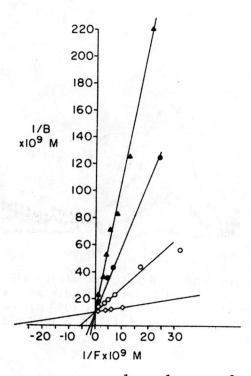

Fig. 3.   Double reciprocal plot (^{1}/B v ^{1}/F) for ^{3}H-estradiol
binding to cytosol receptor in absence of ◇————◇ and
presence of 6-iodo-estratetraene (4a) 4×10^{-9} M
●————●, 1.2×10^{-8} M o————o, and 2.0×10^{-8} M ▲————▲.

istics were also noted by Katzenellenbogen for the 3-iodo-
hexestrol (8), which was later shown to have extensive non-
specific binding.

In general, a compound to be useful as an imaging agent,
should show strong binding to the desired tissue(s) and much less
binding to surrounding tissues. We, therefore, tested the
utility of the idodestrogens (2b) and (4b) as imaging agents with
the use of [^{125}I]-labeled analogs. Our initial data suggested
compound (2b) would bind with somewhat higher affinity than
compound (4b) to the cytosol receptor.

When the data for ^{B}/F and B were examined, using a Scatchard
plot, the 16α-[^{125}I]-iodoestradiol (2b) (Fig. 5) bound with a K_d
of ∿ 0.4×10^{-10}, However, we were unable to demonstrate any
straight line relationship for ^{B}/F v B for the [^{125}I]-6-iodo-.
estratetraene (4b), suggesting that there was little high
affinity binding of that compound under the conditions of these
studies.

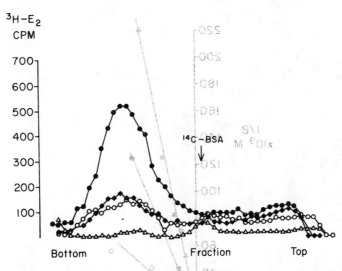

Fig. 4. Results of sucrose density gradients (10-30%) run in presence of ^{3}H-estradiol (1b) only ●——●, with added 6-iodo-estratetraene (4a) 4×10^{-8} M, ○——○, or with added 16α-iodoestradiol (2a) 6×10^{-8} M △——△, 2×10^{-8} M ◆——◆.

The results of the dextran coated charcoal assays were indicative of the results found using sucrose density gradients. The gradient with $[^{125}I]$-16α-iodoestradiol (2b) (Fig. 6) shows a peak of radioactivity in the 8S region which disappeared when DES, (400 nM) was present in the incubation. These results indicate binding of the $[^{125}I]$-16α-iodoestradiol (2b) to a high affinity, low capacity receptor. The gradient elution profile for the $[^{125}I]$-6-iodo-estratetraene (4b) (Fig. 7) reveals no 8S peak, but a large peak in the 4S region which is not displaceable by DES, indicating a high degree of non-specific binding. A similar elution profile was obtained in incubations with $[^{125}I]$-6-iodo-estratetraene (4b) in concentrations ranging from 0.2 to 20 nM. When carrier-free $[^{125}I_2]$ was incubated with rabbit uterine cytosol and run on sucrose gradients, no peak of activity could be found indicating that the radioactivity in the 4S peak was not due to molecular iodine. Incubation of $[^{125}I]$-6-iodo-estratetraene (4b) with rabbit uterine cytosol resulted in the chromatographic recovery of essentially all the radioactivity in the starting compound. The latter results show that no major metabolic transformation and/or deiodination of the 6-iodotetraene occurred

Table 4.   Translocation of Receptor, in vitro

		Cytosol fm/uterus*	Nuclear fm/uterus*
Control		601.0	132.5
Estradiol	10^{-9}M	173.5	488.6
	10^{-8}M	41.4	775.0
	10^{-7}M	69.7	832.4
16β–Iodoestradiol (1)	10^{-9}M	387.4	276.8
	10^{-7}M	126.0	772.4
	10^{-6}M	92.2	789.7
6–Iodoestra–1,3,5(10),6– tetraene–3,17β–diol (2a)	10^{-9}M	482.0	161.5
	10^{-8}M	156.4	666.6
	10^{-7}M	95.8	720.0
16α–Iodoestradiol (3a)	10^{-9}M	548.1	252.1
	10^{-7}M	83.3	629.4

during these experiments. It is probable that there is some specific 8S binding of (4b) and this binding would explain our cross-reaction and displacement data. However, the large amount of 4S binding interferes with our ability to demonstrate the small amount of specific 8S binding.

Previous studies with iodinated estrogens (8) had indicated that specific binding to target tissues was overshadowed by the large amount of non-specific binding to non-target tissues throughout the body.

However, as shown in Table 7, [^{125}I]-16α-iodoestradiol (2b) was bound in the uterus to a greater degree than in kidney or in fat. This binding, which was displaceable with the DES, demonstrates that there was specific binding in the uterus by (2b), although the degree of binding (0.02% of the dose per 100 mg of uterus) was rather low. It should be realized, however, that the amount of iodinated estrogen in the uterus is dependent not only on the number of its receptors but also its metabolism by extra-uterine tissues. As this latter metabolism increases the amount of iodinated estrogen available for uterine binding will be decreased. Extensive uptake by the liver was noted, indicating metabolism and perhaps some binding to the hepatic estrogen receptor (23). In contrast to Hochberg (10), we found appreciable deiodination of (2b) with considerable uptake of [125I] by the thyroid. For the tetraene (4b) no specific

Table 5. Effect of 6-Iodo-estratetraene on Uterus Weight of Immature Mice

Estradiol µg*	6-Iodo-estratetraene µg*	Uterus wt. mg	Uterus wt/body wt. mg/gm
–	–	9.27 ± 0.73	0.87 ± 0.08
0.02	–	15.34 ± 0.94	1.18 ± 0.04
0.04	–	28.59 ± 28.59	1.98 ± 0.15a
0.08	–	42.44 ± 3.28	2.84 ± 0.20a
–	1.0	18.90 ± 1.78	1.29 ± 0.08
–	3.0	14.93 ± 2.36	1.02 ± 0.14
–	6.0	16.80 ± 2.95	1.17 ± 0.16
–	9.0	19.64 ± 2.36	1.48 ± 0.24a
0.04	1.0	22.29 ± 1.04	1.58 ± 0.08a
0.04	3.0	32.34 ± 3.58	2.17 ± 0.22a
0.04	6.0	28.86 ± 1.35	2.05 ± 0.07a
0.04	9.0	34.42 ± 4.61	2.68 ± 0.34a

*Total dose given over 3 days. Administered daily in 0.2 ml subcutaneously.

a Groups so marked are significantly different (p < 0.05) from control.

Table 6. Effect of 16α-Iodoestradiol on Uterus Weight of Immature Mice

Estradiol μg*	16α-Iodoestradiol μg*	Uterus wt. mg	Uterus wt/body wt. mg/gm
-	-	12.00 ± 1.00	1.00 ± 0.08
0.02	-	23.83 ± 4.36	1.93 ± 0.26[a]
0.04	-	42.00 ± 3.08	3.14 ± 0.18[a]
0.08	-	53.50 ± 2.63	4.41 ± 0.06[a]
-	1.0	57.40 ± 3.65	4.73 ± 0.23[a]
-	3.0	67.16 ± 7.30	5.54 ± 0.36[a]
-	6.0	52.20 ± 5.90	4.60 ± 0.33[a]
-	9.0	61.00 ± 7.57	4.80 ± 0.40[a]
0.04	1.0	55.16 ± 9.58	4.83 ± 0.41[a]
0.04	3.0	48.60 ± 6.31	4.46 ± 0.29[a]
0.04	6.0	64.25 ± 3.52	5.07 ± 0.20[a]

*Total dose given over 3 days. Administered daily in 0.2 ml subcutaneously.

[a]Groups so marked are significantly different ($p < 0.05$) from control.

Table 7. Radioactivity in Tissues After Administration of 6-[125I]-Iodoestratetraene (4b) or 16α-[125I]-Iodoestradiol (2b) with and without Diethylstilbestrol (DES)

Tissue	6-[125I]-iodo-estratetraene (4b)		16α-[125I]-iodoestradiol (2b)	
	without DES	with DES	without DES	with DES
	cpm/100 mg tissue*		cpm/100 mg tissue*	
Uterus	38 ± 4	40 ± 3	403 ± 46	73 ± 2
Kidney	40 ± 2	49 ±	85 ± 8	71 ± 2
Liver	133 ± 13	162 ± 36	438 ± 17	418 ± 7
Fat	51 ± 12	36 ± 12	42 ± 12	53 ± 4
Thyroid	5565 ± 1427	5546 ± 348	4157 ± 1019	7424 ± 1081

*All results are given as the mean ± SE for each group, with 5 rats per group.

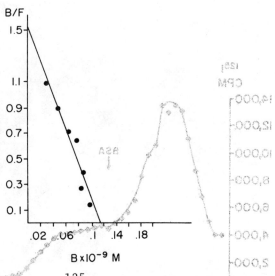

Fig. 5. The binding of 16α-[^{125}I]-iodoestriol (2b) to cytosol receptor as shown by Scatchard plot of $\overline{B}/F$ v B.

uptake into the uterus was observed, but radioactivity was present in the liver, as well as in the thyroid.

Although [^{125}I] is not a satisfactory agent for imaging purposes in the human, the sensitivity of present day equipment allowed us to evaluate the [^{125}I]-labeled compounds (2b) and (4b) as imaging agents in the rat.

Following their subcutaneous, intravenous or intraperitoneal injection into rats with DMBA-induced mammary tumors there was slow uptake of both compounds from the injection sites with most of the label appearing in the abdomen. The liver, G.I. tract, bladder, and probably the kidney (Fig. 8) are the organs containing the radioactivity. The uptake was considerable in these organs and persisted at least for 24 h. In several animals given [^{125}I]-6-iodo-estratetraene (4b), accumulation (uptake) of radioactivity in the tumor was noted. In Fig. 9 is shown the scan of two animals, one with no accumulation of radioactivity in the tumor and one with accumulation in a large tumor in the neck area. In one animal this radioactivity persisted in the tumor for up to 24 h. No [^{125}I]-radioactivity was detected in the thyroid by the scanner.

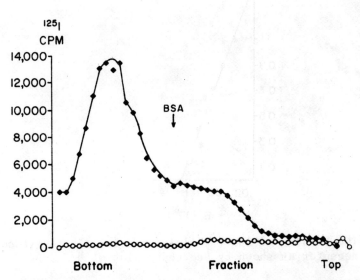

Fig. 6.   Result of sucrose density gradient following incubation
          of 16α-[125I]-iodoestradiol, 4 nM, alone, ◆——◆ , or
          with 400 nM diethylstilbestrol o——o with uterine
          cytosol. Cpm per fraction plotted against 0.1 ml
          fraction collected from gradient.

The localization of the [125I]-6-iodo-estratetraene (4b) in
several tumors may be due to high concentrations of non-specific
receptors in these particular tumors. In two tumors the number
of receptors was determined by conventional means after the
scanning was completed. Both tumors contained 8S receptors
although only one tumor had concentrated (4b) on the scan. The
[125I] peak was in the 4S region and could be demonstrated only
in the tumor which appeared to concentrate iodine.

Further studies on the possible usefulness of these compounds
as imaging agents are currently underway.

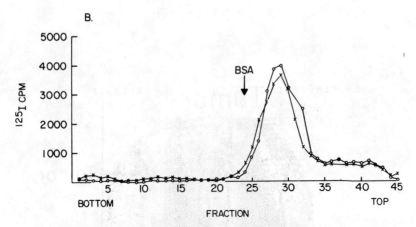

Fig. 7.   Result of sucrose density gradient following
          incubation of 6-[^{125}I]-iodo-estratetraene (4b), 4 nM,
          alone, o———o, or with 400 nM diethylstilbestrol
          x———x with uterine cytosol. Cpm per fraction
          plotted against 0.1 ml fraction collected from
          gradient.

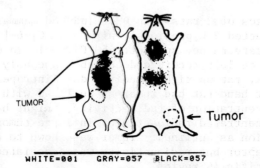

Fig. 8.   Images of two rats with DMBA induced mammary tumors
          injected with 100 µCi 16α-[^{125}I]-iodoestradiol, sp. act.
          250 Ci/mmol in 0.1 ml ethanol subcutaneously in posterior
          neck. Imaging was carried out 2 h after dose. Rat on
          left had two tumors and rat on right had one tumor as
          outlined. Neither tumor concentrated radioactivity.

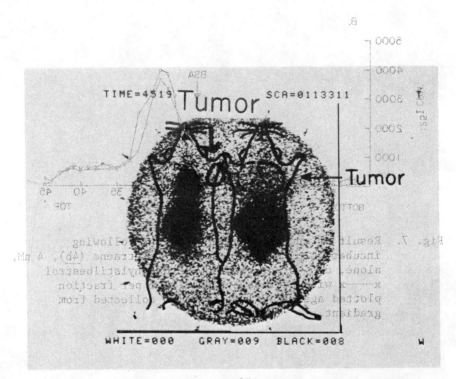

Fig. 9. Images of 2 rats with DMBA-induced mammary tumors
injected 2 h previously with 100 μCi 6-[^{125}I]-iodo-
estratetraene, sp. act. 250 Ci/mmole in 0.1 ml ethanol.
Rat on left received dose subcutaneously in posterior
neck, rat on right received dose intraperitoneally.
Left hand rat had tumor as outlined with no evidence of
concentration of radioactivity. Right hand rat
concentrated radioactivity in large tumor in neck
region as outlined. Tumor was shown to contain 8S
receptor but radioactivity was associated only with non-
specific 4S region.

ACKNOWLEDGMENTS

These studies were supported by Grant #CA-16464 from the National Cancer Institute and Grant #RD-16 from the American Cancer Society. The authors wish to thank Dr. Melvin Farmelant and the Nuclear Medicine Department of St. Vincent's Hospital, Worcester, Ma. for their assistance in the imaging experiments.

REFERENCES

1. E. V. Jensen and H. I. Jacobson, Basic guides to the mechanism of estrogen action, Recent Prog. Hormone Res. 18:387 (1962).

2. J. Gorski, D. Williams, G. Giannapoulos, and George Stancel, The continuing evolution of an estrogen-receptor model, Adv. Exp. Med. Biol. 36:1 (1973).

3. J. H. Clark and Ernest J. Peck, Jr., Steroid Hormone Action, Vol. 1, B. W. O'Malley and L. Birnbaumer, eds., Academic Press, New York (1977).

4. B. W. O'Malley, J. J. Tsai, and H. C. Towle, in: Receptors and Hormone Action, Vol. 1, B. W. O'Malley and L. Birnbaumer, eds., Academic Press, New York (1977).

5. E. V. Jensen, T. Z. Polley, S. Smith, G. E. Block, D. J. Ferguson, and E. R. DeSombre, in: Estrogen Receptors in Human Breast Cancer, W. L. McGuire, P. P. Carbone, and E. P. Vollmer, eds., Raven Press, New York (1975).

6. C. Kent Osborne and W. L. McGuire, The use of steroid hormone receptors in the treatment of human breast cancer: a review, Bull. Cancer (Paris) 66:203 (1979).

7. T. Arunachalam, C. Longcope, and E. Caspi, Iodoestrogens, syntheses, and interaction with uterine receptors, J. Biol. Chem. 254:5900 (1979).

8. J. A. Katzenellenbogen, H. M. Hsiung, K. E. Carlson, W. L. McGuire, R. J. Kraay, and B. S. Katzenellenbogen, Iodohexestrols. II. Characterization of the binding and estrogenic activity of iodinated hexestrol derivatives, in vitro and in vivo, Biochem. 14:1742 (1975).

9. R. E. Counsell, A. Buswink, N. Korn, M. Johnson, V. Ranade, and T. Yu, Radioiodinated estrogens and antiestrogens as potential imaging agents, in: Steroid Hormone Action and Cancer, K. M. J. Menon and J. R. Reel, eds., Plenum Press, New York (1976).

10. R. B. Hochberg, Iodine-121-labeled estradiol: a gamma-emitting analog of estradiol that binds to the estrogen receptor, Science 205:1138 (1979).

11. S. Albert, R. D. H. Heard, C. P. Leblond, and J. Saffran, Distribution and metabolism of iodo-α-estradiol labeled with radioactive iodine, J. Biol. Chem. 177:247 (1949).

12. J. A. Katzenellenbogen and H. M. Hsiung, Iodohexestrols. I.
    Synthesis and photoreactivity of iodinated hexestrol
    derivatives, Biochem. 14:1736 (1975).
13. R. J. B. King and W. I. P. Mainwaring, Steroid-Cell
    Interactions, University Park Press, Baltimore (1974).
14. K. Shida, J. Shimazaki, H. Kurihara, Y. Ito, H. Yamanaka,
    and N. Furuya, Uptake and scintiscanning of the prostate
    with ^{131}I-labeled estradiol phosphate, Int. J. Nucl. Med.
    Biol. 3: 86 (1976).
15. S. Ghanadian, S. L. Waters, M. L. Thakur, and G. D.
    Chisholm, Studies with radioactive iodine labelled
    oestrogens as prostate scanning agents, Int. J. Appl.
    Rad. Isotop. 26:343 (1975).
16. N. Nagai and C. Longcope, Estradiol-17β and estrone: Studies
    on their binding to rabbit uterine cytosol and their
    concentration in plasma, Steroids 17:631 (1971).
17. D. Rodbard, Mathematics of hormone-receptor interaction I.
    Basic principles, Adv. Exp. Med. Biol. 36: 289 (1973).
18. S. G. Korenman, Comparative binding affinity of estrogens and
    its relation to estrogenic potency, Steroids 13:163 (1969).
19. T. S. Ruh, and M. F. Ruh, The effect of antiestrogens on the
    nuclear binding of the estrogen receptor, Steroids 24:
    209 (1974).
20. J. Anderson, J. H. Clark, and E. J. Peck, Jr., Oestrogen and
    nuclear binding sites. Determination of specific sites by
    [^{3}H]oestradiol exchange, Biochem. J. 126:561 (1971).
21. B. L. Rubin, A. S. Dorman, L. Black, and R. I. Dorfman,
    Bioassay of estrogens using the mouse uterine response,
    Endocrinology 49:429 (1951).
22. J. H. Clark, E. J. Peck, Jr., J. W. Hardin and H. Eriksson,
    The biology and pharmacology of estrogen receptor binding:
    relationship to uterine growth, in: Receptors and Hormone
    Action, Vol. II, B. W. O'Malley and L. Birnbaumer, eds.,
    Academic Press, New York (1978).
23. A. J. Eisenfeld, R. F. Aten, G. K. Haselbacher, and K. Halpern,
    Specific macromolecular binding of estradiol in the
    mammalian liver supernatant, Biochem. Pharmacol. 26:919
    (1977).

PROLACTIN AND PROLACTIN RECEPTOR INTERACTIONS IN NORMAL AND NEOPLASTIC TISSUE

Paul A. Kelly, Jean Djiane and Lucile Turcot-Lemay

Department of Molecular Endocrinology,
Le Centre Hospitalier de l'Université Laval
Quebec G1V 4G2, Canada and
*Laboratoire de Physiologie de la Lactation
78350 Jouy-en-Josas, FRANCE

INTRODUCTION

The pituitary hormone, prolactin, has numerous reported actions, however, it is most commonly associated with its action in stimulating the development of the mammary gland and the ensuing lactation.

Prolactin initially binds to specific receptors on the plasma membrane of its target cell and elicits its action, by an as yet unknown mechanism (1, 2). Specific prolactin binding has been identified in crude membrane fractions of a number of tissues including mammary gland, mammary tumor, liver, kidney, adrenal, ovary, testis, prostate, seminal vesicle, uterus and choroid plexus of the brain (3-9).

In this chapter, we will describe the regulation of hormone receptors in a relatively new mammary tumor model system (nitroso-methylurea-induced mammary tumors) and describe the interaction of prolactin with its receptor and the down-regulation of prolactin receptors induced by prolactin in both in vivo and in vitro models.

PROLACTIN RECEPTORS IN MAMMARY GLANDS

The mammary gland is the primary target organ of prolactin. This tissue was in fact chosen for the development of a radioreceptor assay for lactogenic hormones (10). Prolactin receptors from the rabbit mammary gland were subsequently characterized (11),

211

solubilized and purified (12). One of the actions of prolactin in
the mammary gland is the production of milk proteins. In both rabbit (13) and rat (14) mammary gland, prolactin has been shown to
stimulate the production of casein messenger RNA. Antiserum prepared against purified prolactin receptors has been shown to inhibit
by more than 90% the binding of [^{125}I]prolactin to rabbit mammary tissue (15) as well as preventing the prolactin-induced synthesis of casein from rabbit mammary explants (16). These studies
demonstrate the functional importance of the binding of prolactin
to a specific receptor as the central event leading to hormone action.

Assay of Prolactin Receptors

For the quantification of receptor levels in a tissue, crude
plasma membrane fractions are prepared by differential centrifugation, and ovine prolactin is iodinated to a low specific activity
(40-80 µCi/µg). Prolactin binding is assayed by incubating receptors with labelled PRL in the absence or presence of excess unla-
belled PRL and is often reported as a percent of the total counts
added. In addition, saturation or displacement curves can be carried out on representative membrane preparations and the data transformed into Scatchard plots (17) which yield affinity constants and
binding capacities of the membranes.

In addition to the classical approach to measure prolactin receptors which involves differential centrifugation of a tissue homogenate and subsequent binding to the particulate membrane fraction, alternative approaches which utilize small biopsy determinations have emerged. Costlow et al. (18) reported prolactin binding
using 0.5 mm tissue slices of tumor tissue. Even smaller samples
can be utilized if frozen "microslices" are used (19). This involves cutting 20 µm slices of tumor on a cryostat and incubation of
approximately 8 slices (0.5 mm^2) with [^{125}I]-ovine prolactin
as described for membrane fractions (20). Ongoing studies in our
laboratory indicate that this technique is applicable to repeated
determinations in the same tumor (Turcot-Lemay and Kelly, unpublished observations) as well as for localization of receptors
using autoradiography (9).

Receptor Levels During Pregnancy and Lactation

The concept that hormone receptors are not static systems, but
change with the physiological state of the animal is important in
terms of the control of cellular activity. Recently, we measured
prolactin receptors in the mammary gland of rabbits which had been
pretreated for a 36-hour period with the dopamine agonist CB-154
(Sandoz, Basle, Switzerland) to lower circulating prolactin (21).
This technique was effective because the rabbit does not produce a
placental lactogen (22, 23). Measurement of receptor levels reveal-

ed a gradual increase in receptor concentration until day 22 followed by a decline until parturition, and a marked increase in early lactation (21). Prolactin binding to rat mammary gland decreased between day 30 to 100 of age in virgin glands. Binding was low during pregnancy and increased during early lactation and declined following removal of litters (24). It has been demonstrated, however, that by simply removing the ovaries and the uterus (including placentae) 24 hours prior to sacrifice, a marked increase in prolactin binding was observed, indicating that a large proportion of receptors are saturated by the high levels of circulating placental lactogen (25). PRL binding under these circumstances increases as pregnancy progresses and remains elevated during lactation. Other groups reported a peak of prolactin binding on day 2 of lactation after which receptor levels declined rapidly (26).

PROLACTIN RECEPTORS IN MAMMARY TUMORS

Binding sites for prolactin have been identified in the particulate membrane fraction of DMBA mammary tumors (7, 20). These binding sites are specific for prolactin or other lactogenic hormones and have an affinity similar to that of the mammary gland. We have previously reported that higher prolactin binding was observed

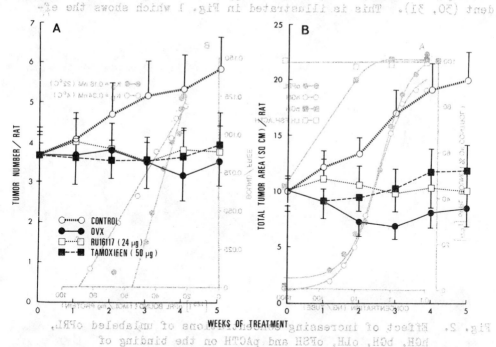

Fig. 1. Effect of daily 5-week treatment with RU16117 (24 μg) or tamoxifen (50 μg) or ovariectomy on (A) the number of NMU-induced mammary tumors per rat and (B) total tumor and (sq.cm) per animal (30).

in DMBA tumors which had shown the greater growth response to injected prolactin, indicating that the level of the receptor is important in determining the tissue response to prolactin (20).

In contrast to the importance of the pituitary to the maintaining of prolactin binding sites in rat liver (27, 28), there was only a slight reduction in prolactin receptors from tumors of hypophysectomized, DMBA-treated rats (18).

Holdaway and Friesen (19) reported that it was not possible to differentiate prolactin responsive from prolactin-independent tumors by prolactin receptor determination of biopsy samples, but that following either prolactin administration or prolactin suppression, prolactin responsive tumors had higher prolactin receptor levels. A combination of estradiol and prolactin receptor levels has also been reported to more accurately predict the responsiveness to endocrine ablation than either receptor levels alone (29).

In addition to DMBA-induced tumors, prolactin receptors as well as hormone receptors for estradiol and progesterone have been identified and characterized in nitrosomethylurea (NMU)-induced mammary tumors (30). These tumors appear to be hormonally dependent (30, 31). This is illustrated in Fig. 1 which shows the ef-

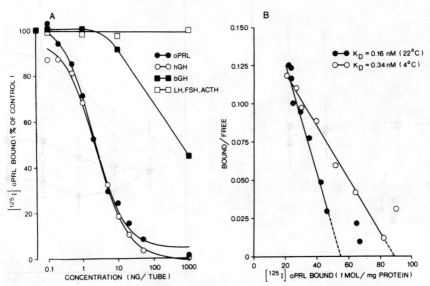

Fig. 2.   Effect of increasing concentrations of unlabeled oPRL,
          hGH, bGH, oLH, oFSH and pACTH on the binding of
          [^{125}I]oPRL to NMU-induced mammary tumor membranes. B.
          Scatchard analysis of PRL binding using increasing
          concentrations of unlabeled oPRL to displace the
          [^{125}I]oPRL from the receptors, at 4° and 22°C.

fect of ovariectomy or treatment with antiestrogens on growth of established tumors (118 days after NMU injection). Control rats show
a steady increase in the number of tumors per rat from 3.7 ± 0.7 to
5.8 ± 0.8 after 5 weeks (Fig. 1A). Ovariectomy and antiestrogen
(tamoxifen, RU16117) prevent further tumor growth, but fails to induce a regression of tumor growth as has been observed in DMBA-induced mammary tumors (32).

The specificity of $[^{125}I]$oPRL binding to a crude microsomal
fractions of NMU-induced mammary tumors is shown in Fig. 2A. Hormones with lactogenic activity such as oPRL and hGH are equipotent in
displacing the labeled hormone. Bovine GH causes a non-parallel
displacement of $[^{125}I]$oPRL which is evident only at higher concentrations. Other non-lactogenic hormones (LH, FSH, ACTH) do not
displace the labelled oPRL. Fig. 2B shows Scatchard analysis of PRL
binding which was carried out at 22°C for 18h and at 4°C for 48h,
using increasing concentrations of unlabeled oPRL to displace labeled oPRL from the receptor. Slightly different affinities are observed at the two temperatures (K_D = 0.16 at 22°C and K_D = 0.34 nM at
4°C).

Specific binding of $[^3H]$estradiol-17β, $[^3H]$R5020 and
$[^{125}I]$ovine PRL to NMU-induced tumors are shown in Table 1.
There is a significant decrease ($p < 0.01$) of $[^3H]$estradiol receptors in both the ovariectomized and tamoxifen treated groups however, the decrease observed in the RU16117-treated animals is not
statistically significant. Binding of $[^3H]$R5020 is significantly

Table 1. Effect of 5-week treatment with RU16117 or tamoxifen
on specific binding of $[^3H]$ E_2, $[^3H]$R5020 and
$[^{125}I]$oPRL to NMU-induced mammary tumors (30).

Group	Number of tumors	$[^3H]E_2$	Receptor levels $[^3H]$R5020	$[^{125}I]$oPRL
		pmol/g tissue		% specific binding
Control	49	1.2±0.2	5.1±1.0	6.4±0.5
OVX	32	0.6±0.1**	0.8±0.2*	4.3±1.5*
RU16117 (24 µg)	20	0.8±0.2	11.4±3.4**	5.0±0.8
Tamoxifen (50 µg)	33	0.2±0.03**	2.5±0.5	5.9±0.7

* $p < 0.05$ and **$p < 0.01$ compared to control group

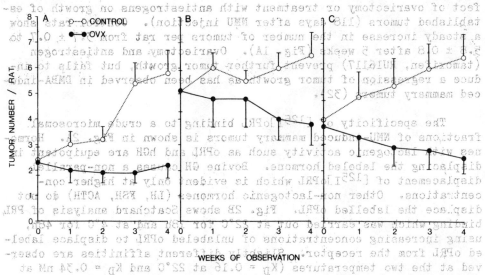

Fig. 3. Effect of ovariectomy on the number of NMU-induced mammary
tumors per rat in the first (A), second (B) and third (C),
4 week periods of observation (33).

reduced (p < 0.05) by ovariectomy and tamoxifen. RU16117 treatment
results in an increase in progesterone receptors. [125I]ovine
PRL receptors are not affected by the antiestrogen treatment, but
are significantly (p < 0.05) decreased by ovariectomy (30).

The effect of ovariectomy on tumor growth was examined in NMU-
treated rats, $2\frac{1}{2}$, $3\frac{1}{2}$ and $4\frac{1}{2}$ months after the first NMU injection.
Fig. 3 shows that ovariectomy performed at $2\frac{1}{2}$ months produced a
stabilization of tumor number (A), while at $3\frac{1}{2}$ (B) and $4\frac{1}{2}$ (C)
months, a slight regression of tumor number was apparent (33).

The effect of this treatment on hormone receptor levels in
these tumors is shown in Fig. 4. Estradiol receptors (Fig. 4A)
which range from 2.04 ± 0.18 to 2.24 ± 0.24 pmol/g tissue in control tumors during the first two treatment periods decline to 0.93
± 0.14 pmol/g tissue at the last time interval studied (p < 0.01).
Ovariectomy induces a significant (p < 0.01) 50% decline in E_2
receptors, regardless of the time at which OVX was performed. Fig.
4B illustrates the specific binding of [3H]R5020 during the three
periods of the study. The decrease of [3H]R5020 receptors in the
OVX groups is highly significant (p < 0.01) for the two first
groups of rats and slightly less (p < 0.05) for the third group.
Specific binding of [125I]ovine prolactin illustrated in Fig.
4C is also significantly reduced by OVX in the first (p < 0.05),
second and third (p < 0.01) periods of the experiment (33).

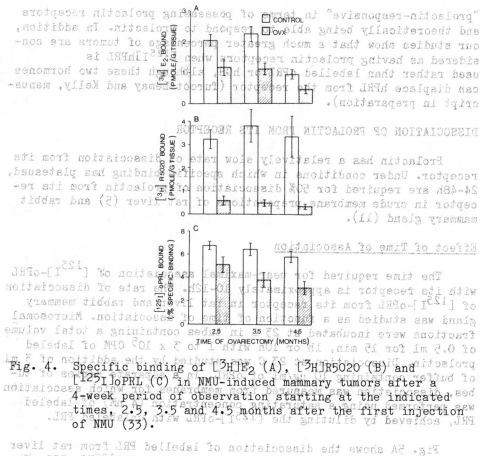

Fig. 4. Specific binding of [³H]E₂ (A), [³H]R5020 (B) and [¹²⁵I]oPRL (C) in NMU-induced mammary tumors after a 4-week period of observation starting at the indicated times, 2.5, 3.5 and 4.5 months after the first injection of NMU (33).

If prolactin does stimulate human mammary tumors, the tissue should contain prolactin receptors, as is the case for other prolactin responsive tissues as well as for experimental mammary tumors (3, 4, 6-8). Holdaway and Friesen (34) have reported specific binding of prolactin to human breast tumors. Specific binding of greater than 1% of the added radioactivity (which the authors considered significant) occurred in 8 of 41 tumors (19.5%). For one tumor, enough material was present to perform a Scatchard plot, and an affinity constant similar to that of other prolactin receptors was found (6, 20). More recently, another report appeared in which 27 of 83 tumors contained specific binding for prolactin of at least 1% (35).

In our laboratory, we have examined over 600 biopsies of human mammary carcinoma, both primary lesions and metastases (32). We feel the values above 0.5% reflect the presence of receptors. Our results indicate that slightly over 50% of the tumors are "prolactin-responsive" in terms of possessing prolactin receptors and theoretically being able to respond to prolactin. In addition, our studies show that a much greater percentage of tumors are considered as having prolactin receptors when [^{125}I]hPRL is used rather than labelled oPRL or hGH, although these two hormones can displace hPRL from the receptor (Turcot-Lemay and Kelly, manuscript in preparation).

DISSOCIATION OF PROLACTIN FROM ITS RECEPTOR

Prolactin has a relatively slow rate of dissociation from its receptor. Under conditions in which specific binding has plateaued, 24-48h are required for 50% dissociation of prolactin from its receptor in crude membrane preparations of rat liver (5) and rabbit mammary gland (11).

Effect of Time of Association

The time required for near-maximal association of [^{125}I]-oPRL with its receptor is approximately 10-12h. The rate of dissociation of [^{125}I]-oPRL from its receptor in rat liver and rabbit mammary gland was studied as a function of time of association. Microsomal fractions were incubated at 23 C in tubes containing a total volume of 0.5 ml for 15 min, 1h or 10h with 1 to 3 x 10^5 CPM of labeled prolactin. Dissociation at 23 C was studied by the addition of 3 ml of buffer containing 10 µg/ml of oPRL. In a separate series of tubes, dissociation was measured from membranes for which association was performed using a saturating concentration (4 nM) of labeled PRL, achieved by diluting the [^{125}I]-oPRL with unlabeled PRL.

Fig. 5A shows the dissociation of labelled PRL from rat liver microsomes using non-saturating concentrations of [^{125}I]-oPRL. The dissociation curves can be better fit in a computerized curve fitting model with two kinetic components, the faster component being 60 to 100 times more rapid than the slower component. For the shorter association times of 15 min and 1h, 50% dissociation is attained in the first hour, with maximal dissociation of 80-90% at 24-48h. For an association time of 10h, dissociation is slower due to a 5-fold reduction in the faster kinetic component, with maximal dissociation at 48h of only 53%. When association is performed in the presence of near-saturating concentrations of PRL (4 nM), a slightly larger percentage of the faster component is observed (Fig. 5B).

In contrast to rat liver, dissociation of [^{125}I]-oPRL from microsomal membrane fractions of rabbit mammary gland is less complete. The initial (first component) has a similar rate to that observed for rat liver, with however, the second component being irreversible. Maximal dissociation ranges between 25-40% (data not shown).

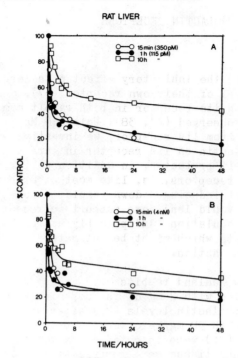

Fig. 5.   Dissociation of [^{125}I]oPRL from rat liver membranes.
Association was allowed to proceed for 15 min, 1h or 10h
in the presence of 1 to 3 x 10^5 CPM of labelled PRL.
Dissociation was initiated by the addition of 3 ml assay
buffer containing 10 µg/ml oPRL. Values are expressed as
a percentage of control (time 0) values.

In vitro desaturation using MgCl$_2$

Circulating levels of prolactin or placental lactogens are
often elevated, exceeding 1 µg/ml, therefore a certain fraction of
the prolactin receptors in target cells might be occupied by endogenous prolactin. Although the procedure of homogenization and
membrane fractionation offers the opportunity for prolactin to dissociate, a large portion of the prolactin remains bound to receptors due, in large part, to the low temperatures used and slow rate
of dissociation of prolactin from its receptor.

An in vitro desaturation technique to dissociate prolactin
from the receptor was developed (36). Magnesium chloride at a concentration of 3 to 5M is capable of removing 90-95% of the labelled
hormone from rabbit mammary gland or rat liver prolactin receptors.
When the receptors are re-exposed to fresh labelled prolactin,
they retain their ability to specifically bind the prolactin (36).

DOWN-REGULATION OF PROLACTIN RECEPTORS

<u>In Vivo</u>

     In contrast to the inhibitory effect of a large number of
hormones on the level of their own receptor (37), a stimulatory effect of prolactin on its receptor in both rabbit mammary gland and
rat liver has been observed (27, 38). Using 4M $MgCl_2$ to dissociate bound prolactin from its receptor, we investigated the short-
term action of prolactin on its receptor in target tissues with the
goal of evaluating if prolactin, in addition to its ability to up-
regulate prolactin receptors, is, like most other hormones, studied
thus far, capable of inducing a down-regulation of its own receptor. This in turn would lend some support to recent view (39) con-
tending that down-regulation (and possibly up regulation as well)
are ubiquitous events which might be intimately linked to the very
mechanism of hormone action.

     Lactating, New Zealand rabbits were injected every 12 hours
over a 36-hour period with 2 mg of the dopamine agonist, CB-154, to
lower circulating prolactin levels (21) after which the animals
were anesthesized with 50 mg/kg of sodium pentobarbital. Three mg
bovine prolactin (bPRL) were injected intravenously and 2 g biopsies of mammary gland tissue were removed at the indicated times
between 0 and 30 hours after prolactin injection.

     As illustrated in Fig. 6, injection of 3 mg of prolactin leads
to a maximal occupancy of free rabbit mammary gland prolactin receptors 15 min after the intravenous injection, corresponding to
periods just following maximal serum concentrations. The highest
serum levels are seen 1 min after injection with values rapidly de-
lining thereafter. Although saturating concentrations of circulating prolactin are present 15 min after injection, 20% of the prolactin receptors remain free to bind $[^{125}I]$oPRL. This could be
due to an inaccessibility of the receptors to the circulating prolactin or to some dissociation occuring while membranes were isolated from the tissues.

     Somewhat surprisingly, total prolactin receptor levels assayed
following <u>in vitro</u> desaturation with 4M $MgCl_2$ declined progressively up to 6 hours after the intravenous injection of prolactin and
returned to normal at 24 to 30 hours. The difference in total prolactin binding between time 0 and 6 hours was statistically significant (p < 0.01). A difference was observed between the pattern
of occupation (free receptors) and the down-regulation reflected by
total receptors. In addition, free receptors increased between 1
and 6 hours (40). A similar down-regulation of prolactin receptors
in rat liver was observed following injection of 1 mg oPRL into
ovariectomized, estrogen-treated rats (40).

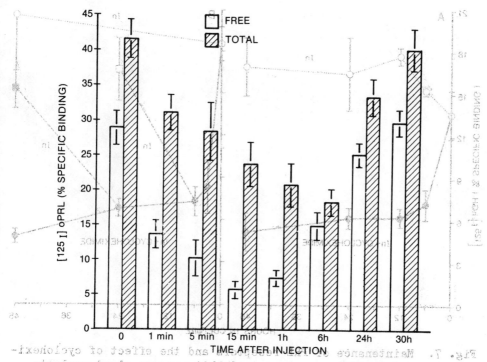

Fig. 6. Effect of an intravenous injection of 3 mg bovine PRL on PRL receptors in rabbit mammary glands. Biopsies (2 g) were removed at the indicated times after PRL injection from lactating rabbits. Free and total ($MgCl_2$-treated) PRL receptor levels were determined. Binding is expressed as a % of specific binding per 400 μg protein. Values are means ± SEM of 7 animals.

In Vitro

It has been well established that the mammary gland can be maintained in organ culture and responds well to hormones (41). In addition, mammary explants can be used as an experimental model to study the steps involved in the mechanisms of hormone action (13). The following studies were undertaken to verify the maintenance of PRL receptors in mammary glands in organ culture, to assess the apparent turnover of receptors and to describe the effect of large doses of prolactin on the levels of its own receptor.

Fig. 7A illustrates the maintenance of prolactin receptors in mammary gland explants cultured in the presence of insulin. Binding increases slightly up to 12h and remains constant up to 48h (42). Addition of cycloheximide (1 μg/ml) results in a rapid decline of binding during the first 6h which remains low until 48h.

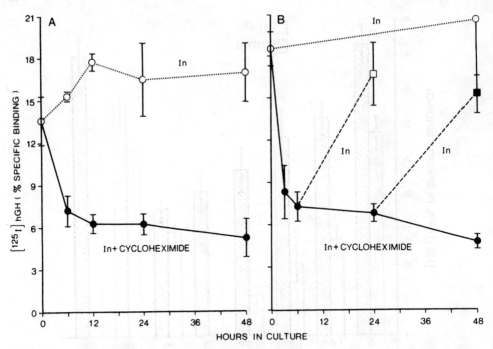

Fig. 7. Maintenance of PRL receptors and the effect of cycloheximide on PRL receptors in rabbit mammary gland explants.
A) Mammary explants were cultured for different times in
the presence of insulin (In) or In + cycloheximide. B)
Explants cultured in the presence of In + Cycloheximide
after which the media was changed at 6 or 24h and cycloheximide was removed. Values are means ± SEM of 3 cultures.
Prolactin binding was measured using [^{125}I]hGH which
binds to PRL receptors with an affinity equal to that of
PRL (42).

Fig. 7B shows another experiment and demonstrates the reversibility
of the effect of cycloheximide (1 µg/ml). In the presence of insulin only, the level of receptors is maintained up until 48h as
shown previously. The addition of cycloheximide results in a rapid
decrease of receptors which is almost maximal at 3h. Removal of cycloheximide from the culture medium at either 6h or 24h by replacement with a medium deficient in cycloheximide results in a return
of prolactin binding to near control levels 18-24 hours later (42).

A down-regulation of prolactin receptors in rabbit mammary
gland in organ culture has also been observed. Inclusion of PRL (5
µg/ml) in the incubation medium results in   80% saturation of free

receptors. The time-dependence of prolactin saturation and down-regulation of prolactin receptors in culture is shown in Fig. 8. Saturation is incomplete at 1h and is maximal at 24-48h. The pattern of the reduction of total prolactin receptors is different from that of free receptors with a maximal effect observed in explants cultured in the presence of prolactin for 48h (42).

For a number of polypeptide hormones, binding is followed by an internalization of the hormone-receptor complex (43, 44) after which the labelled ligands become associated with lysosomal components in the cells (44, 45). Lysosomotropic agents such as chloroquine, methylamine or ammonium chloride have been shown to reduce clustering for α_2-macroglobulin and epidermal growth factor (EGF) on cell surface of fibroblasts (46). [^{125}I]hCG has been internalized and is associated with lysosomes + rapidly degraded to monoiodotyrosine. This process of degradation could be inhibited by lysosomotropic agents (47).

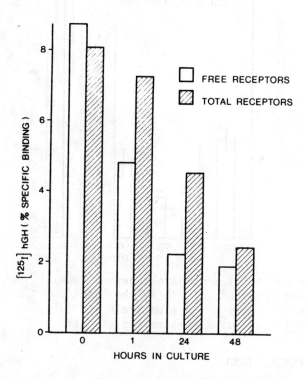

Fig. 8.   Time-course of the occupation of prolactin receptors and decline in total (MgCl$_2$-treated receptors in mammary explants cultured in the presence of In and PRL (5 μg/ml) for the indicated times. PRL binding was measured with [^{125}I]hGH (42).

In order to examine if the down-regulation of prolactin receptors in rabbit mammary gland involved a lysosomal-mediated step,
mammary explants were cultured in the presence of methylamine (20
mM). Fig. 9 shows PRL binding after 24 h in explant culture in the
presence of insulin. PRL induces a 53% down-regulation of total
PRL receptors. Methylamine alone markedly increases the basal level
of prolactin binding but almost completely reduces the ability of
prolactin to induce a down-regulation of its receptors. In addition to methylamine, chloraquine (100 µM) and ammonium chloride (10
mM) have similar effects in blocking prolactin-induced down-regulation of its receptor (48).

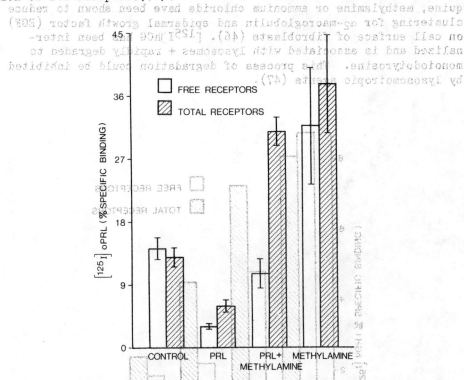

Fig. 9. Free and total prolactin receptor levels in mammary ex-
         plants cultured for 24h in the presence of insulin alone
         (control) or insulin plus prolactin (1 µg/ml) or methyla-
         mine (20 mM) or a combination of both.

SUMMARY AND CONCLUSIONS

In this chapter, we have attempted to describe prolactin receptor regulation and interactions. Prolactin receptors are abundant in normal mammary tissue as well as in a number of experimental mammary tumor models. An alternative to the DMBA-induced mammary tumor model is the NMU-induced mammary tumor. These tumors are

hormone-dependent to the extent that tumor growth is stopped by
ovariectomy or treatment with antiestrogens. Prolactin receptors
in NMU-induced tumors are reduced following ovariectomy of animals
with newly formed tumors (2½ months after NMU injection) or in
those animals with tumors present for longer periods.

In addition, have discussed the fate of prolactin and the prolactin receptor following hormone binding. The events involved in
the binding, internalization and cellular action of prolactin are
summarized in Fig. 10. Although the initial event of prolactin
action is the binding to receptors on the plasma membranes, data
are accumulating on the localization of prolactin and prolactin
receptors within the target cell (43, 49, 50). The fact that with
prolonged periods of incubation, microsomal membranes from rabbit
mammary gland and rat liver develop a slowly dissociable component,
implies that these membranes may retain at least some of the capacity of intact cells to internalize hormone and/or hormone receptor
complexes, which may represent an hetereogeneity or a compartmenta-
lization of prolactin receptors occuring subsequent to binding.

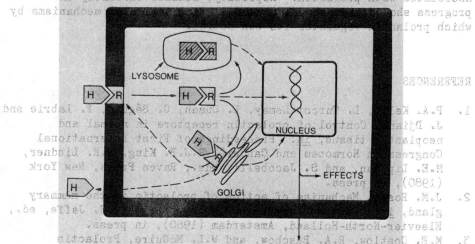

Fig. 10. Summary of possible mechanisms involved in the binding,
          internalization and cellular action of an hormone
                          (prolactin).

The regulation of prolactin receptor concentrations in various target tissues is complex. Prolactin has been clearly shown to have an up-regulatory or stimulatory activity on its own receptor level in both rabbit mammary gland and rat liver (28, 38). Following the development of a technique to remove endogenous prolactin from receptors without destroying receptors, we have been able to demonstrate a transient down-regulation of prolactin receptors both in vivo and in vitro. In addition, using mammary explants, we have shown that prolactin receptors appear to have a relatively rapid rate of turnover, based on the rate receptor replenishment following removal of cycloheximide.

Prolactin receptors have been localized within the purified Golgi fractions of rat liver. Following injection of [^{125}I] oPRL into female rats, radioactivity was localized in Golgi fractions (50). The radioactivity eluded from these fractions remained intact, as judged by its ability to bind fresh receptors. The involvement of lysosomes in hormone degradation, which has been clearly demonstrated for other peptide hormones is also suggested for prolactin therefore, one can postulate that following binding, prolactin is internalized after which some of the radioactivity is associated with Golgi elements and some with lysosomes. It is possible that the internalized prolactin receptor complex could act directly at the nuclear level to induce its action. Alternatively, a breakdown product from lysosomal degradation, or some altered form of prolactin or the prolactin receptor following association with the Golgi may interact with the nucleus to induce the actions associated with prolactin. Hopefully, studies currently in progress should shed some light on the intracellular mechanisms by which prolactin regulates its own action.

REFERENCES

1. P.A. Kelly, L. Turcot-Lemay, L. Cusan, C. Séguin, F. Labrie and J. Djiane, Control of prolactin receptors in normal and neoplastic tissue, in: "Proceedings of First International Congress on Hormones and Cancer", R.J.B. King, H.R. Lindner, M.E. Lippman, and S. Jacobelli, eds., Raven Press, New York (1980), in press.
2. J.M. Rosen, Mechanism of action of prolactin in the mammary gland, in: "Contemporary Endocrinology Series", R. Jaffe, ed., Elsevier-North-Holland, Amsterdam (1980), in press.
3. M.E. Costlow, R.A. Buschow, and W.L. McGuire, Prolactin receptors in an estrogen receptor-deficient mammary carcinoma, Science 184:85 (1974).
4. W.L. Frantz, J.H. MacIndoe, and R.W. Turkington, Prolactin receptors: characteristics of the particulate fraction binding activity. J. Endocrinol. 60:485 (1974).

5. P.A. Kelly, B.I. Posner, T. Tsushima, R.P.C. Shiu and H.G. Friesen, Tissue distribution and ontogeny of growth hormone and prolactin receptors. in: "Advances in Human Growth Hormone Research", S. Raiti, ed., General Printing Office, Washington, D.C., 567-584 (1974).

6. B.I. Posner, P.A. Kelly, R.P.C. Shiu and H.G. Friesen, Studies of insulin, growth hormone and prolactin binding: tissue distribution, species variation and characterization. Endocrinology 96:521 (1974).

7. R.W. Turkington, Prolactin receptors in mammary carcinoma cells. Cancer Res. 34:758 (1974).

8. R.J. Walsh, B.I. Posner, B.M. Kopriwa and J.R. Brawer, Prolactin binding sites in rat brain. Science 201:1041 (1978).

9. D. Dubé, P.A. Kelly and G. Pelletier, Comparative localization of prolactin binding sites in different rat tissues by immunohistochemistry, radioautography and radioreceptor assay, Mol. Cell. Endocrinol. In press.

10. R.P.C. Shiu, P.A. Kelly and H.G. Friesen, Radioreceptor assay for prolactin and other lactogenic hormones. Science 180: 968 (1973).

11. R.P.C. Shiu and H.G. Friesen, Properties of a prolactin receptor from the rabbit mammary gland. Biochem. J. 140:301 (1974).

12. R.P.C. Shiu and H.G. Friesen, Solubilization and purification of a prolactin receptor from the rabbit mammary gland. J. Biol. Chem. 249:7902 (1974).

13. E. Devinoy, L.M. Houdebine, and C. Delouis, Role of prolactin and glucocorticoids in the expression of casein genes in rabbit mammary gland organ culture. Quantification of casein mRNA. Biochim. Biophys. Acta 517:360 (1978).

14. R.J. Matusik, and J.M. Rosen, Prolactin induction of casein mRNA in organ culture: a model system for studying peptide hormone regulation of gene expression. J. Biol. Chem. 253:2343 (1978).

15. R.P.C. Shiu and H.G. Friesen, Interaction of cell-membrane prolactin receptor with its antibody. Biochem. J. 157:619.

16. R.P.C. Shiu and H.G. Friesen, Blockage of prolactin action by an antiserum to its receptors. Science 192:259 (1976).

17. G. Scatchard, The attraction of protein from small molecules and ions. Ann. N.Y. Acad. Sci. 51:660 (1949).

18. M.E. Costlow, R.A. Buschow, and W.L. McGuire, Prolactin receptors in 7,12-dimethylbenz(a)anthracene-induced mammary tumors following endocrine ablation. Cancer Res. 36:3941 (1976).

19. I.M. Holdaway and H.G. Friesen, Correlation between hormone binding and growth response of rat mammary tumor. Cancer Res. 36:1562 (1976).

20. P.A. Kelly, C. Bradley, R.P.C. Shiu, J. Meites and H.G. Friesen, Prolactin binding to rat mammary tumor tissue. Proc. Soc. Exp. Biol. Med. 146:816 (1974).

21. J. Djiane, P. Durand and P.A. Kelly, Evolution of prolactin receptors in rabbit mammary gland during pregnancy and lactation. Endocrinology 100:1348 (1977).

22. F. Talamantes, A comparative study on the occurrence of placental prolactin from different mammalian species. Gen. Comp. Endocrinol. 27:115 (1975).

23. P.A. Kelly, T. Tsushima, R.P.C. Shiu and H.G. Friesen, Lactogenic and growth hormone-like activities in pregnancy determined by radioreceptor assays. Endocrinology 99:765 (1976).

24. T.J. Hayden, R.C. Bonney and I.A. Forsyth, Ontogeny and control of prolactin receptors in the mammary gland and liver of virgin, pregnant and lactating rats. J. Endocrinol. 80:259 (1979).

25. H.H. Holcomb, M.E. Costlow, R.A. Buschow and W.L. McGuire, Prolactin binding in rat mammary gland during pregnancy and lactation. Biochim. Biophys. Acta 428: 104-112.

26. H.G. Bohnet, F. Gomez, and H.G. Friesen, Prolactin and estrogen binding sites in the mammary gland of the lactating and non-lactating rat, Endocrinology 101:1111 (1977).

27. P.A. Kelly, B.I. Posner, and H.G. Friesen, Effects of hypophysectomy, ovariectomy and cycloheximide on specific binding sites for lactogenic hormones in rat liver, Endocrinology 97:1408 (1975).

28. B.I. Posner, P.A. Kelly and H.G. Friesen, Prolactin receptors in rat liver: possible induction by prolactin, Science 187:57 (1975).

29. E.R. DeSombre, G.S. Kledzik, S. Marshall and J. Meites, Estrogen and prolactin receptor concentrations in rat mammary tumors and response to endocrine ablation. Cancer Res. 36:354 (1976).

30. L. Turcot-Lemay and P.A. Kelly, Characterization of estradiol, progesterone and prolactin receptors in nitrosomethylurea-induced mammary tumors and effect of antiestrogen treatment on the development and growth of these tumors. Cancer Res. In press.

31. P.M. Gullino, H.N. Pettigrew and F.H. Frantham, N-nitrosomethyl urea as mammary gland carcinogen in rats, J Natl Cancer Inst. 54:401 (1975).

32. P.A. Kelly, F. Labrie and J. Asselin, The role of prolactin in tumor development. in: Influences of Hormones in Tumor Development, J.A. Kellen and R. Hilf, eds., CRC Press, Boca Raton, Florida, (1979) pp. 157-194.

33. L. Turcot-Lemay and P.A. Kelly, The response to ovariectomy of N-nitrosomethylurea-induced mammary tumors in the rat. Submitted.

34. I.M. Holdaway and H.G. Friesen, Hormone binding by human mammary carcinoma. Cancer Res. 37: 1946 (1977).

35. R. Di Carlo and G. Muccioli, Prolactin receptor in human mammary carcinoma, Tumori. In Press. (1980).

36. P.A. Kelly, G. Leblanc, and J. Djiane, Estimation of total pro-

lactin binding sites after in vitro desaturation. Endocrinology 104:1631 (1979).

37. M.A. Lesniak, and J. Roth, Regulation of receptor concentration by homologous hormone: effect of human growth hormone on its receptor in IM-9 lymphocytes. J. Biol. Chem. 251:3720 (1976).

38. J. Djiane and P. Durand, Prolactin-progesterone antagonism in self-regulation of prolactin receptors in the mammary gland. Nature 266:641 (1977).

39. B.I. Posner, D. Raquidan, A. Josefsberg and J.M. Bergeron, Different regulation of insulin receptors in intracellular (Golgi) and plasma membranes from livers of obese and lean mice. Proc. Natl Acad. Sci. (USA) 75: 3302-3306.

40. J. Djiane, H. Clauser and P.A. Kelly, Rapid down-regulation of prolactin receptors in mammary gland and liver. Biochem. Biophys. Res. Commun. 90:1371-1378.

41. E.B. Barnawell, A comparative study of the response of mammary tissue from several mammalian species to hormones in vitro. J. Exp. Zool. 160:189 (1965).

42. J. Djiane, C. Delouis, and P.A. Kelly, Prolactin receptors in organ culture of rabbit mammary gland: effect of cycloheximide and prolactin. Proc. Soc. Exp. Biol. Med. 162:342 (1979).

43. J.J.M. Bergeron, B.I. Posner, Z. Josefsberg and R. Sikstrom, Intracellular polypeptide hormone receptors: the demonstration of specific binding sites for insulin and human growth hormone in Golgi fractions isolated from the liver of female rats. J. Biol. Chem. 253:4058 (1978).

44. P.M. Conn, M. Conti, J.P. Harwood, M.L. Dufau and K.J. Catt, Internalization of gonadotropin-receptor complex in ovarian luteal cells, Nature 274:598 (1978).

45. P. Gordon, J.L. Carpentier, S. Cohen, and L. Orci, Epidermal growth factor: morphological demonstration of binding, internalization and lysosomal association in human fibroblasts. Proc. Natl. Acad. Sci. USA 75:5025 (1978).

46. F.R. Maxfield, M.C. Willingham, P.J.A. Davies, and I. Pastan, Amines inhibit the dustering of α_2-macroglobulin and EGF on the fibroblast cell surface. Nature 277: 661 (1979).

47. M. Ascoli and D. Puett, Degradation of receptor-bound human chorio-gonadotropin by murine Leydig tumor cells. J. Biol. Chem. 253: 4892-4899.

48. J. Djiane, P.A. Kelly, and L.M. Houdebine, Effects of lysosomotropic agents, cytochalasin B and colchicine on the down-regulation of prolactin receptors in mammary gland explants. Mol. Cell. Endocrinol. (In press).

49. J.M. Nolin and R.J. Witorsch, Detection of endogenous immunoreactive prolactin in rat mammary epithelial cells during lactation. Endocrinology 99: 949 (1976).

50. Z. Josefsberg, B.I. Posner, B. Patel, and J.J.M. Bergeron, The uptake of prolactin into female rat liver: concentration of intact hormone in golgi apparatus. J. Biol. Chem. 254:209 (1979).

RETINOID BINDING IN NORMAL AND NEOPLASTIC MAMMARY TISSUE

Richard C. Moon and Rajendra G. Mehta

Life Sciences Division, IIT Research Institute
10 West 35th Street
Chicago, IL 60616

ABSTRACT

The inhibitory effect of dietary supplementation of certain retinoids on mammary carcinogenesis in the rat has been reported from our laboratory. Specific cytosolic retinoic acid binding proteins (cRABP) as well as retinol binding proteins sedimenting as 2S components have been detected in the mammary tissue during normal and neoplastic differentiation. Relatively higher levels of cRABP were observed in the mammary glands from pregnant animals as well as in ovarian hormone independent tumors; whereas in glands obtained from lactating rats and in hormone dependent tumors, lower levels of cRABP were evident. Exogenous treatment of such animals with estradiol-17β enhanced the levels of cRABP. The results indicate a possible correlation between endocrine and retinoid function in both normal and neoplastic differentiation of mammary tissue. [3H]retinoic acid-RABP complex, under appropriate conditions, translocates into the nucleus. Unbound [3H]retinoic acid, however, failed to associate with the nuclear sites. Additional studies indicate a possible selective inhibition of ovarian hormone independent tumors by the retinoids.

INTRODUCTION

Within recent years, several studies have shown that retinoids (vitamin A and its synthetic analogs) are effective inhibitors of chemically-induced carcinogenesis. Retinoids can prevent or reverse altered differentiation induced by vitamin A deficiency or treatment with chemical carcinogens in mouse prostate (1,2), hamster trachea (3,4), or mouse mammary gland (5) in organ culture. Earlier reports

from our laboratory have demonstrated that the incorporation of
various retinoids into the diet can inhibit *in vivo* carcinogenesis
of the urinary bladder and mammary gland (6-9). Moreover, the
retinoids are apparently organospecific; retinyl methyl ether,
retinyl acetate and 4-hydroxyphenyl retinamide effectively inhibit
mammary carcinogenesis while 13-*cis*-retinoic acid, ethyl retinamide
and 2-hydroxyethyl retinamide are effective chemopreventive agents
for the urinary bladder. Similarly, the naturally occurring
retinoids display a certain degree of specificity. Retinol functions
in vision, growth, reproduction and maintenance of differentiated.
epithelia whereas retinoic acid supports normal maintenance and
differentiation of epithelial tissues but can neither replace
retinol as a precursor of visual pigment (10) nor support reproduction.

The mechanism by which retinoids inhibit carcinogenesis is
poorly understood. However, several hypotheses have been suggested,
including stimulation of the host immune system (11), alterations
in synthesis of certain membrane glycoproteins (12,13), alterations
in RNA synthesis patterns (14,15), and suppression of DNA synthesis
(16-18).

The mediation of retinoid action by specific intracellular
retinoid binding proteins in a manner similar to that of steroid
hormones has been proposed (19,20). Two retinoid binding proteins
have been isolated, one binding specifically to retinol and the
other to retinoic acid. Cytosolic retinol binding protein (cRBP)
and cytosolic retinoic acid binding protein (cRABP) have been purified to homogeneity from rat liver (21) and testis (22), respectively.
Both proteins sediment in the 2S region on sucrose density gradients and have molecular weights of 14,600 daltons. However, the
tissue distribution and ligand specificities of these components are
quite different. Both binding proteins can migrate into the nucleus,
as has been shown for cRBP in rat liver (23) and cRABP in chick
embryonic skin (24).

Recently, we reported the presence of cRABP in both human breast
cancers and carcinogen-induced rat mammary tumors (25,26). In this
report we present the characterization of cytosolic retinoid binding
protein(s) and nuclear translocation of cRABP in mammary tissue
during normal and neoplastic differentiation.

MATERIALS AND METHODS

Treatment of Animals

Female Sprague-Dawley rats were obtained from ARS/Sprague-
Dawley, Madison, WI at 42 days of age and were housed 3 per cage
in a room maintained at 22 $\pm$ 1°C with 12 hr dark and light cycles.

At 50 days of age, rats were injected intravenously with a single dose of 5 mg N-methyl-N-nitrosourea (MNU) (Ash Stevens, Detroit, MI) dissolved in 0.9% saline (pH 5.0). One week after the carcinogen treatment rats were placed either on placebo diet or on diet supplemented with a retinoid. Animals were palpated for the presence of tumors twice weekly. At necropsy, all tumors were excised, a small piece was fixed in 10% buffered formalin for histopathological evaluation, and the remaining tumor tissue was frozen in liquid nitrogen and stored at -80°C in an ultrafreezer for retinoid binding protein analyses.

Ovarian hormone dependence of the tumors was determined by surgical ablation of the ovaries. When tumors reached a diameter of 2 cm the host rat was ovariectomized; tumors which decreased in size were designated as ovarian hormone dependent tumors. Some animals with regressing tumors were given 5 µg estradiol and 5 mg progesterone daily. Tumors which responded to this treatment and regrew to the original size were designated ovarian hormone responsive tumors. Tumors that did not regress upon ovariectomy were considered to be ovarian hormone independent.

Measurement of Retinoid Binding Proteins

Mammary tissues were minced and homogenized in 10 mM Tris buffer (pH 7.0) containing 1 mM dithiothreitol using a power driven Polytron homogenizer (Brinkman Instruments, Westbury, MA). Cytosol was prepared by centrifuging the homogenate at 105,000 x g for 30 min at 0°C, and retaining the supernatant. The protein concentration was measured by the procedure of Waddell (27). Aliquots of cytosol were reacted with 1×10^{-6} M [^{3}H]retinoic acid (S.A. 1.14 Ci/mmol). All other radioactive retinoids utilized in this study were used at 1 µM concentration. All reactions were accompanied by a parallel reaction containing both labeled retinoid and a 25-fold excess of unlabeled retinoid. Following the incubation, reactions were terminated by a brief treatment with dextran-coated charcoal solution to remove unbound retinoid. An aliquot of 0.2 ml was layered on a preformed 5-20% w/v sucrose gradient in Tris buffer and centrifuged at 65,000 rpm for 2 hr in a vertical tube rotor (DuPont Instruments Inc., Newtown, CT). Gradients were fractionated by puncturing the bottom of the tube and collecting 10 drop fractions. Radioactivity in each fraction was determined by scintillation counting. Myoglobin and hemoglobin were used as 2S and 4S markers, respectively.

Purification of Nuclei

Nuclei from the mammary tumors were purified according to the procedure described previously (28). Briefly, the homogenate prepared from the mammary tissue was centrifuged at low speed (600 x g for 10 min) and the pellet was suspended in 2.3M sucrose containing 3.3 mM CaCl$_2$. The suspension was filtered twice through 3 layers of cheesecloth. The resultant suspension was diluted 1:1 with 0.23M sucrose containing 0.33 mM CaCl$_2$ and centrifuged at 25,000 rpm for 1 hr at 0°C using a fixed angle rotor. The pellet containing purified nuclei was then washed twice in 0.23M sucrose and 0.33 mM CaCl$_2$ solution. DNA content was then measured in an aliquot of nuclear preparation using the diphenylamine procedure (29).

Nuclear Interaction of the Retinoid Binding Proteins

The nuclear suspension containing a known amount of DNA was pelleted using low speed centrifugation. The cytosol containing retinoic acid-bound RABP complexes was incubated with nuclei for 30 min at 0°C unless mentioned otherwise. The nuclei were separated, washed, and extracted with 1 ml of 0.4M KCl in Tris buffer. The KCl extract was analyzed for retinoic acid binding using 5-20% sucrose density gradients prepared in buffer containing 0.4M KCl. The procedure for determining the binding with this technique was as described above.

RESULTS

The selection of retinoids for a proposed study is usually based on relative biological activity, toxicity and tissue distribution. Structures of some natural and synthetic analogs of vitamin A are shown in Figure 1. It is apparent from several reports that the effectiveness of retinoids in suppression of cancers is organ specific. For example, 13-*cis*-retinoic acid inhibits N-butyl-N-(4-hydroxybutyl)nitrosamine-induced bladder cancers in rats and mice, but is relatively ineffective against MNU-induced mammary cancers in rats. Similarly, the trimethylmethoxyphenyl analog of retinoic acid ethyl ester can suppress the occurrence of mouse skin tumors but has no inhibitory effect on the induction of mammary or bladder cancers.

The effect of dietary supplementation with various retinoids on the incidence of MNU-induced mammary adenocarcinomas is shown in Figure 2. As indicated, retinyl acetate and 4-hydroxyphenyl retinamide significantly reduced the incidence of mammary cancer and increased the latency of the first palpable tumors. By contrast, 13-*cis*-retinoic acid has little effect on the appearance of mammary cancer, while retinyl methyl ether was of intermediate efficacy. These results demonstrate that a minor alteration in the basic retinoid structure can significantly alter the activity of the molecule with respect to prevention of MNU-induced mammary carcinogenesis.

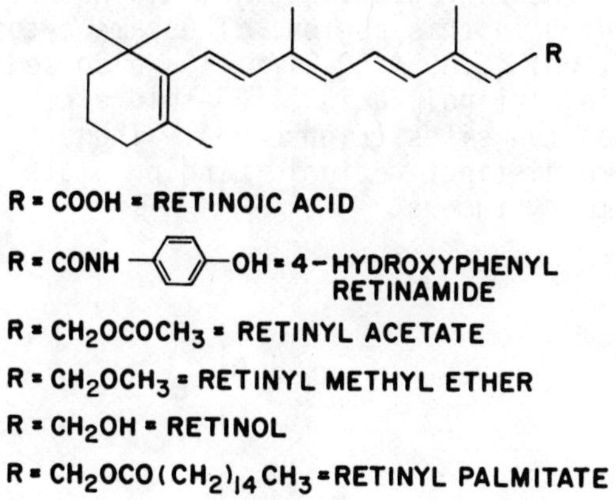

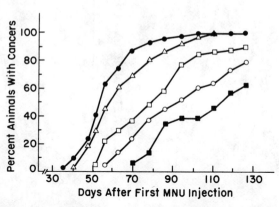

R = COOH = RETINOIC ACID

R = CONH ⟨phenyl⟩ OH = 4-HYDROXYPHENYL
                              RETINAMIDE

R = CH₂OCOCH₃ = RETINYL ACETATE

R = CH₂OCH₃ = RETINYL METHYL ETHER

R = CH₂OH = RETINOL

R = CH₂OCO(CH₂)₁₄CH₃ = RETINYL PALMITATE

Fig. 1.   Structures of retinoids.

Fig. 2.   Effect of retinoids on the incidence of MNU-induced
mammary carcinogenesis. ● - no retinoid; Δ - 13-*cis*-
retinoic acid; □ - retinyl methyl ether; O - retinyl
acetate; ■ - 4-hydroxyphenyl retinamide.

Retinoic acid binding proteins were detected in the cytosol of
MNU-induced adenocarcinomas by the use of sucrose density gradients.
The RABP-[3H]RA complex sedimented as a specific binding 2S component with nonspecific binding occurring as a 4S species (Figure 3A).
Unlabeled all-*trans*-retinoic acid at 25-fold excess inhibited the
binding only under the 2S region; retinol did not displace the [3H]-
retinoic acid binding in this region. The same cytosol, when incubated with [3H]retinol (S.A. 4.50 Ci/mmol), also sedimented as a 2S
component; unlabeled retinoic acid at 25-fold excess concentration
did not compete for the sites (Figure 3B). These results demonstrate
the presence of two distinct retinoid binding proteins in the cytosol
of MNU-induced mammary tumors.

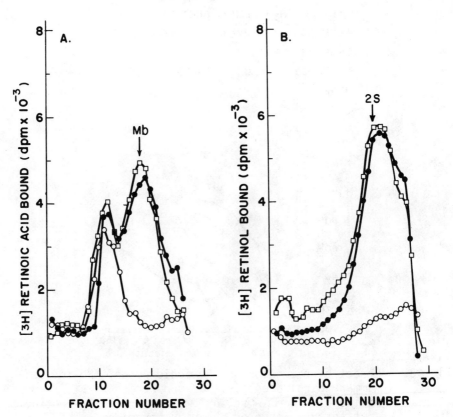

Fig. 3.   Sucrose density gradient profiles for retinoic acid (A)
           and retinol (B) binding proteins in the cytosol of MNU-
           induced mammary tumors. A. ● - [3H]retinoic acid; O -
           [3H]retinoic acid + 25 μM all-*trans*-retinoic acid; □ -
           [3H]retinoic acid + 25 μM unlabeled retinol. B. ● -
           [3H]retinol; O - [3H]retinol + unlabeled retinol; □ -
           [3H]retinol + 25 μM retinoic acid.

Further experiments were conducted to determine the ligand
specificity of the cRABP. Portions of mammary tumor cytosols were
incubated with 1 μM [3H]retinoic acid either alone or with several
concentrations of unlabeled retinoids ranging from 1 to 100-fold
excess. The results of this experiment are presented in Figure 4.
It was observed that only all-*trans*-retinoic acid and its isomer
13-*cis*-retinoic acid were competitive inhibitors for the binding
sites; other synthetic analogs, although effective against mammary
carcinogenesis, did not compete for retinoic acid binding sites.

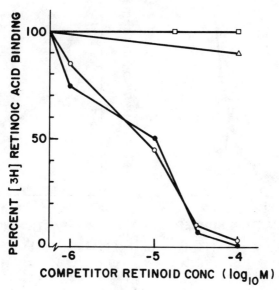

Fig. 4.   Retinoic specificity for retinoic acid binding proteins.
           A constant volume of tumor cytosol was incubated with [3H]-
           retinoic acid at 0°C for 16 hr. Competitors used for the
           study were: O - all-*trans*-retinoic acid; ● - 13-*cis*-
           retinoic acid; and Δ - retinyl acetate. Retinyl methyl
           ether, 4-hydroxyphenyl retinamide, retinyl butyl ether,
           retinylidene dimedone, axerophthene, retinol and retinyl
           palmitate did not compete and are represented by □.

Retinoid binding was further evaluated by reacting mammary tumor
cytosol with radioactive [3H]5,6-epoxyretinoic acid or [3H]4-hydroxy-
phenyl retinamide (S.A. 1.14 Ci/mmol) under identical conditions,
followed by analysis on sucrose density gradients. As shown in
Figure 5A, only the retinoic acid metabolite, 5,6-epoxyretinoic acid,
bound specifically to retinoic acid binding sites. Both unlabeled
all-*trans*- as well as 13-*cis*-retinoic acid were competitive inhibitors of 5,6-epoxyretinoic acid binding; 4-hydroxyphenyl retinamide

did not bind specifically to any cytosolic protein.

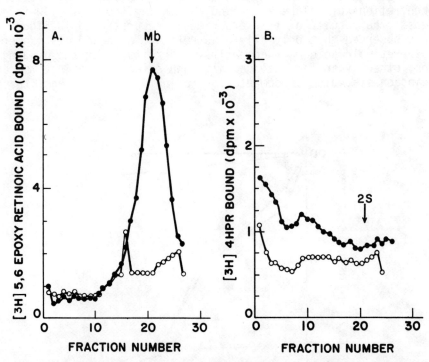

Fig. 5.   Retinoic specificity for retinoic acid binding sites.
A. ● - 1 μM [³H]5,6-epoxyretinoic acid; O - [³H]5,6-
epoxyretinoic acid + 25 μM all-*trans*-retinoic acid.
B. ● - 1 μM [³H]4-hydroxyphenyl retinamide, either alone
or O - in presence of unlabeled 4-hydroxyphenyl retinamide
(25 μM).

    Since the growth of many carcinogen-induced mammary tumors is
influenced by ovarian hormones, the levels of RABP in the cytosol
of ovarian hormone independent and responsive tumors were determined.
These results are summarized in Table 1. A considerable difference
was apparent in the cRABP levels between the tumors which grew and
those which regressed in the absence of ovaries.   The ovarian hormone
independent tumors contained 4.5 ± 0.7 pmol cRABP/mg protein whereas
binding of [³H]retinoic acid by dependent tumors was 0.65 ± 0.16
pmol/mg protein. Responsive tumors, those which grew in the ovariectomized host following daily injections of 5 μg estradiol and 5 mg
progesterone, showed a six-fold increase in the binding (3.90 ± 0.48
pmol/mg protein) when compared with the dependent tumors.

Table 1. Levels of cRABP on MNU-induced Mammary Tumors

Ovarian Hormone Dependence	Number of Tumors Examined	cRABP[a] (pmol/mgP)
Independent	19	4.57 ± 0.73^b
Regressing	5	0.65 ± 0.16^c
Responsive	18	3.90 ± 0.48^d

[a] The levels of cRABP were determined using sucrose density gradient procedure as described in Materials and Methods.

[b] Significantly different from c ($p < 0.025$)

[c] Significantly different from d ($p < 0.025$)

One implication of the results presented in Table 1 is that ovarian hormone independent tumors may be more responsive to retinoid treatment than are ovarian hormone dependent tumors. To test this possibility, an experiment was conducted which combined ovariectomy with retinoid feeding. These results, depicted in Figure 6, show a tumor incidence of 100% in intact, placebo-fed rats, while intact rats fed 328 mg retinyl acetate/kg diet had a tumor incidence of 77%. Presumably all tumors developing in the ovariectomized rat are ovarian hormone independent. Whereas a 28% incidence of mammary tumors was evident in animals ovariectomized two weeks post-carcinogen and fed placebo diet, the combined treatment of ovariectomy and retinyl acetate feeding reduced the tumor incidence to 3%. Tumor latency was also greatly increased by the combined treatment regimen.

Quantitative measurements for cRABP were also made in normal rat mammary gland during various stages of differentiation. The mammary gland from young virgin females contained very low levels of cRABP, ranging from nondetectable to 1 pmole per mg protein. Similar results were obtained from the lactating rat, while glands from pregnant animals had significantly elevated levels of cRABP (Table 2). It should be noted that this reflects an inverse relationship with the levels of estrogen receptors present during pregnancy and lactation. The experiments were extended further by measuring the levels of RABP in the mammary cytosol of lactating animals after increasing the levels of circulating estradiol by injecting 5 µg estradiol-17β every day for 7 days. Such treatment significantly elevated the levels of RABP, approaching the levels seen in preg-

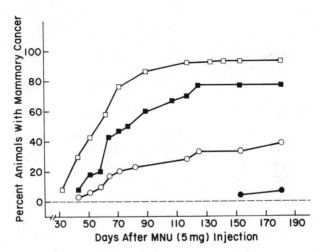

Fig. 6.   Effect of retinyl acetate and ovariectomy on latency of
           appearance of MNU-induced mammary cancer. □ - intact-
           placebo; ■ - intact-retinyl acetate (328 mg/kg diet);
           O - ovariectomized-placebo; ● - ovariectomized-retinyl
           acetate diet.

nancy. Similar results were obtained when young virgin female rats
were injected subcutaneously with 5 µg estradiol-17β for 7 days;
progesterone did not alter the RABP content of the mammary cells in
any animals tested.

The translocation of RABP to the nucleus was studied in MNU-
induced mammary cancers. As shown in Figure 7, the sedimentation of
nuclear RABP was as a 2S component. Thus, nuclear RABP sedimentation
was similar to that observed in the cytosol from the same tissue,
although no non-specific binding in the 4S region was found. To
insure that cRABP-retinoic acid complex is essential for the nuclear
translocation, both intact nuclei and KCl nuclear extracts were
incubated with [3H]retinoic acid. Intact nuclei were then extracted
with KCl, and both the pre- and post-incubation nuclear extracts were
subjected to sucrose gradient analysis as described earlier. Nuclear
binding of [3H]retinoic acid did not occur in the absence of cRABP-
retinoic acid complex (Table 3). Treatment of the cytosol with
dextran-coated charcoal prior to incubation with the nuclei had no

Table 2.   Influence of Ovarian Hormones on the Levels of
cRABP in Mammary Gland

Stage of Differentiation	Treatment	cRABP (pmol/mgP)
Virgin	None	0.42
Virgin	Estradiol[a]	1.97
Virgin	Progesterone[a]	0.73
Virgin	Estradiol + Progesterone	1.26
Pregnancy	None	3.04[b]
Lactation	None	0.62[c]
Lactation	Estradiol	2.43[d]

[a] Daily injection of 5 μg estradiol or 5 mg progesterone for 7 days were given subcutaneously.

[b] Significantly different from c ($p < 0.01$).

[d] Significantly different from c ($p < 0.025$).

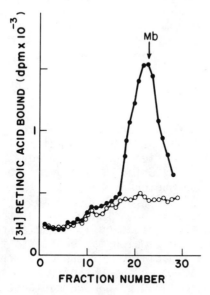

Fig. 7.   Retinoic acid binding proteins in the nuclear fraction of MNU-induced mammary tumors. ● - total binding; O - non-specific binding.   Procedures in detail are described in the text.

Table 3. Conditions for Nuclear Translocation

Reaction	Time and Temperature	nRABP[a] (pmol/100 µg DNA)
[^{3}H]RA + Nuclei	0°C 30 min	None
	25°C 30 min	None
[^{3}H]RA + KCl Extract of Nuclei	0°C 30 min	None
	25°C 30 min	None
[^{3}H]RA - cRABP 0°C + Nuclei	0°C 30 min	2.40
[^{3}H]RA - cRABP 25°C, 30 min + Nuclei	0°C 1 hr	2.50
[^{3}H]RA - cRABP 37°C, 30 min + Nuclei	0°C 1 hr	0.85

[a] Levels of nuclear retinoic acid binding proteins (nRABP) were estimated using sucrose density gradient procedure as described in Materials and Methods.

effect on the amount of nuclear RABP, indicating that the cRABP-retinoic acid complex and not unbound radioactive retinoic acid is interacting with the purified nuclei. Moreover, subjecting the [^{3}H]RA-RABP complex to 25°C for 30 min prior to the incubation with nuclei did not enhance the nRABP content. These results indicated that the activation of the [^{3}H]RA-RABP complex may not be required for the nuclear translocation. Incubation of the complex at 37°C for 30 min prior to the incubation with nuclei resulted in a reduction in the nRABP content, which may be due to thermal denaturation of the complex. The association of the cRABP-retinoic acid complex with nuclei is related to the amount of DNA present in the nuclear fraction, since [^{3}H]retinoic acid-RABP radioactivity from the nuclei increased linearly up to a concentration of 150 µg DNA. At a concentration of 150 µg DNA, binding of cRABP-retinoic acid plateaued (Figure 8); no further binding was evident with increasing DNA concentrations.

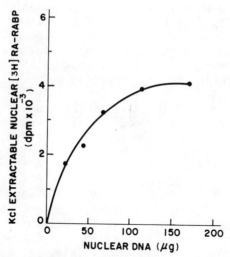

Fig. 8.   Effect of DNA concentration on nuclear binding of [3H]-
retinoic acid. A constant amount of [3H]RA-cRABP complex
was incubated with nuclei containing increasing amounts
of DNA. nRABP were separated on sucrose density gradients
as described in the text.

DISCUSSION

Early studies of cancer prevention by retinoids in animals
employed the natural retinoids retinyl acetate and retinyl palmitate.
A significant inhibition of chemically-induced lung cancer (30,31)
and mammary cancer (8,32) was achieved by these compounds. However,
a major problem of feeding high doses of the natural retinoids has
been toxicity; for this reason, a variety of synthetic retinoids
have been developed (33,34). These synthetic compounds have patterns
of metabolism and organ distribution which differ from the natural
retinoids, resulting in reduced toxicity. There are an increasing
number of reports indicating that the synthetic retinoids have a
better therapeutic index than natural retinoids for prevention of
cancer of the skin (35), urinary bladder (6,36) and mammary gland
(7-9,37).

Once ingested, the retinyl esters are hydrolyzed to free
retinol by pancreatic esterases and subsequently esterified with
long chain fatty acids and transported to the liver. The liver
synthesizes and stores a specific serum transport protein which
complexes with retinol and is then released to the blood, where

the retinol-RBP complex associates with prealbumin. The entire complex disassociates once the retinoid is delivered to the cell (38). Retinoic acid, on the other hand, is transported in the blood bound to serum albumin (39). The mechanism by which these natural retinoids enter the cell is unknown although membrane receptors for the retinoids have recently been implicated (40).

It is well documented that steroid hormones associate with specific cytosolic proteins (receptors) in the target cell and are subsequently translocated to the nucleus where regulation of gene expression occurs (19,41). However, the mechanism of retinoid action once it reaches the target cell is obscure. Although Prutkin and Bogart (42) showed specific uptake of retinoic acid by kerato-acanthoma cells *in vitro*, Basher, et al. (43) were the first to report the presence of specific retinol binding proteins sedimenting as a 2S component on the sucrose density gradients in the cytosols of retinol sensitive tissues. Since then, both retinol and retinoic acid binding protein with ligand specificity has been reported for a number of tissues in experimental animals (44,45) as well as in human tumors (46,47). Consistent with these studies, we have observed both retinol and retinoic acid binding proteins in mammary cancers induced in animals by chemical carcinogens (25) as well as in mammary cancers of human origin (26). Both retinoic acid and retinol bind to specific intracellular proteins; retinoic acid did not compete for retinol sites and retinol was unable to displace retinoic acid from its binding sites. Some of the retinoids which are effective against mammary carcinogenesis such as 4-hydroxyphenyl retinamide and retinyl acetate did not compete for the retinoic acid binding sites. These results suggest that the 4-hydroxyphenyl retinamide or other retinoid analogs may first require metabolism to a form which can bind to RABP. This is supported by the observation that [^{3}H]4-hydroxyphenyl retinamide did not bind to any cellular component. Moreover, high pressure ligand chromatographic analysis of mammary extracts from the animals which were chronically fed 4-hydroxyphenyl retinamide showed a number of retinoid metabolites, but very little, if any, of the parent compound (9). It has also been observed that treatment with very low nontoxic concentration of all-*trans*-retinoic acid significantly reduces the occurrence of mammary adenocarcinomas (48).

It is well known that DMBA-induced tumors are, at least, partially dependent upon the ovarian steroids for their growth. Approximately 60-70% of the tumors appear to be hormone dependent as indicated by regression following ovarian ablation (49); the remaining 30-40% do not regress after ovariectomy, and may cease growing (static) or continue to grow (independent). We have noted that 20-30% of the MNU-induced tumors are hormone independent. All chemically-induced mammary tumors appear to contain measurable levels of estradiol receptor; however, hormone dependent tumors contain greater numbers of estrogen receptors than do hormone independent

tumors (50,51). We have also observed variations in the levels of
retinoic acid binding proteins in these tumors. For our purpose,
we have classified these tumors one step further. The hormone
dependent tumors which regressed and responded to exogenous estradiol
by reinitiated growth were considered as ovarian hormone responsive.
To date all MNU-induced tumors which regressed after ovariectomy
responded to estradiol with renewed growth. A distinct difference
in the cRABP content of these tumors was evident; estrogen
treatment of ovariectomized animals significantly elevated the levels
of cRABP. A comparison of cRABP levels in hormone independent and
dependent tumors suggests that the ovarian hormone independent tumors
may be more susceptible to retinoid chemoprevention. Our preliminary *in vivo* experiments indicate that this may indeed be the case
since retinoid supplementation of the diet of ovariectomized, car-
cinogen-treated rats significantly reduces tumor incidence.

We have previously shown that both virgin mammary gland and
mammary tumors possess detectable levels of cRABP (25). Since the
role of retinoids in the normal differentiation of the mammary gland
is unknown, we extended our studies to determine mammary cRABP levels
during various stages of differentiation; we found that mammary
glands of pregnant animals contain significantly higher levels of
cRABP than that of lactating glands. Since it is well known that
the mammary gland of the pregnant rat contains either nondetectable
or a very low level of estrogen receptor which increases during
lactation, our results indicate an inverse relationship between
retinoid and estrogen receptors. Moreover, both hormone responsive
tumors and the glands of lactating animals treated with estrogen
exhibited increased cRABP levels. These observations appear to
indicate a possible induction of retinoid receptors by estradiol.

Little is known concerning the nuclear interaction of retinoids.
In an early report, Sani (52) indicated that when nuclei from lung
tumors and embryonic skin were incubated with radioactive retinoic
acid, a retinoic acid bound complex which sedimented as a 2S component on sucrose gradients was obtained. However, in our studies,
we found that the retinoic acid bound nRABP complex from the cytosol
is essential for such an interaction and that free [3H]retinoic acid
did not bind to any nuclear component. It is possible that the
dialysis technique used by Sani to separate cRABP from unbound retinoic acid compared to the dextran-coated charcoal procedure used in
the present study may account for this apparent discrepancy. In
support of our results, however, Takase et al. (23) reported that
retinol-cRABP complex was essential for the nuclear interaction of
retinol.

The results presented in this report indicate that the action
of retinoids may be mediated in a manner similar to that of the
steroid hormones, in that the complexing of retinoic acid with specific cytoplasmic binding proteins is a prerequisite for translocation

to the nucleus. However, it remains unclear whether cRABP simply delivers retinoic acid to the nucleus or if the complex itself enters the nucleus. Further information regarding the nuclear interaction of the retinoids will provide valuable insight into the molecular mechanism of these compounds and their effects on normal and neoplastic differentiation of mammary tissue.

ACKNOWLEDGEMENTS

This work was supported in part by Grant CA-26030 and Contracts NO1-CP-23292, NO1-CB-74207 and NO1-CP-75939 from the National Cancer Institute. We wish to thank Dr. David McCormick for valuable discussions and Ms. Cathy Fricks, Mrs. Wendy Cerny and the rest of our staff for expert technical assistance. Mrs. Margaret Collins provided excellent secretarial assistance in preparation of this manuscript. Radioactive retinoids were supplied by the Chemoprevention Program, Chemical and Physical Carcinogenesis Branch, National Cancer Institute, Bethesda, Maryland. Unlabeled retinoids were generously supplied by Dr. Michael Sporn, National Cancer Institute, Hoffmann-LaRoche, Inc., Nutley, NJ, BASF Aktiengesellschaft, Ludwigshafen, Germany and Johnson and Johnson, New Brunswick, NJ.

REFERENCES

1. D. P. Chopra and L. J. Wilkoff, Effect of retinoids and estrogens on testosterone-induced hyperplasia of mouse prostate explants in organ cultures, Proc. Exptl. Biol. and Med. 162:229 (1979).

2. I. Lasnitzki, Reversal of methylcholanthrene-induced changes in mouse prostates *in vitro* by retinoic acid and its analogues, Br. J. Cancer 34:239 (1976).

3. M. B. Sporn, G. H. Clamon, N. M. Dunlop, D. L. Newton, J. M. Smith, and U. Saffiotti, Activity of vitamin A analogues in cell cultures of mouse epidermis and organ cultures of hamster trachea, Nature 253:47 (1975).

4. D. L. Newton, C. A. Frolich, A. B. Roberts, J. M. Smith, M. B. Sporn, A. Nürrenbach and J. Paust, Biological activity and metabolism of the retinoid axerophthene (vitamin A hydrocarbon), Cancer Res. 38:1734 (1978).

5. M. S. Dickens, R. P. Custer, and S. Sorof, Retinoid prevents mammary gland transformation by carcinogenic hydrocarbon in whole gland culture, Proc. Natl. Acad. Sci. (U.S.A.) 76:589 (1979).

6. P. J. Becci, H. J. Thompson, C. J. Grubbs, R. A. Squire, C. C. Brown, M. B. Sporn and R. C. Moon, Inhibitory effect of 13-*cis*-retinoic acid on urinary bladder carcinogenesis induced in C57BL/6 mice by N-butyl-N-(4-hydroxybutyl)

7. C. J. Grubbs, R. C. Moon and M. B. Sporn, Inhibition of
    mammary cancer by retinyl methyl ether, Cancer Res.
    37:599 (1977).
8. R. C. Moon, C. J. Grubbs, and M. B. Sporn, Inhibition of 7,12-
    dimethylbenz(a)anthracene-induced mammary carcinogenesis
    by retinyl acetate, Cancer Res. 36:2626 (1976).
9. R. C. Moon, H. J. Thompson, P. J. Becci, C. J. Grubbs, R. J.
    Gander, D. L. Newton, J. M. Smith, S. L. Phillips, W. R.
    Henderson, L. T. Mullen, C. C. Brown and M. B. Sporn,
    N-(4-hydroxyphenyl)retinamide, a new retinoid for pre-
    vention of breast cancer in the rat, Cancer Res. 39:1339
    (1979).
10. J. E. Dowling and G. Wald, The biological function of vitamin
    A acid, Proc. Natl. Acad. Sci. (U.S.A.) 46:587 (1960).
11. G. Dennert, C. Crowley, J. Kouba, and R. Lotan, Retinoic acid
    stimulation of the induction of mouse killer T-cells in
    allogeneic and synergeneic mice, J. Natl. Cancer Inst.
    62:89 (1979).
12. L. M. DeLuca, P. V. Bhat, W. Sasak, and S. Adamo, Synthesis
    of phosphoryl and glycosyl phosphoryl derivatives of
    vitamin A in biological membranes, Fed. Proc. 38:2535
    (1979).
13. T. C. Kiorpes, Y. C. L. Kim, and G. Wolf, Stimulation of the
    synthesis of specific glycoproteins in corneal epithelium
    by vitamin A, Exp. Eye Res. 28:23 (1979).
14. C. H. Tsai, and F. Chytil, Effect of vitamin A deficiency on
    RNA synthesis in isolated rat liver nuclei, Life Sci.
    23:1416 (1978).
15. B. C. Johnson, M. Kennedy, and N. Chiba, Vitamin A and
    nuclear RNA synthesis, Am. J. Clin. Nutr. 22:1048 (1969).
16. T. W. Kensler, and G. C. Muller, Retinoic acid inhibition of
    comitogenic action mezerein and phorbol esters in bovine
    hepatocytes, Cancer Res. 38:771 (1978).
17. S. H. Yuspa, K. Eigjo, M. A. Morse, and F. J. Wiebel, Retinyl
    acetate modulation of cell growth kinetics and carcinogen-
    cellular interaction in mouse epidermal cell cultures,
    Chem.-Biol. Interact. 16:251 (1977).
18. R. G. Mehta, and R. C. Moon, Inhibition of DNA synthesis by
    retinyl acetate during chemically-induced mammary carcino-
    genesis, Cancer Res. 40:1109 (1980).
19. E. V. Jensen, T. Suzuki, T. Kawashima, W. E. Stumpf, P. W.
    Jungblut, and E. R. DeSombre, A two step mechanism for the
    induction of estradiol with rat uterus, Proc. Natl. Acad.
    Sci. (U.S.A.) 59:632 (1968).
20. J. Gorski, D. Williams, G. Giannopoulos, and G. Stancel, The
    continuous evolution of an estrogen-receptor model, Adv.
    in Exptl. Biol. and Med. 36:1 (1972).
21. D. E. Ong, F. Chytil, Cellular retinol binding proteins from
    rat liver: purification and characterization, J. Biol.

Chem. 253:828 (1978).

22. D. E. Ong and F. Chytil, Cellular retinoic acid binding pro-
     teins from rat testis: purification and characterization,
     J. Biol. Chem. 253:4551 (1978).

23. S. Takase, D. E. Ong and F. Chytil, Cellular retinol binding
     protein allows specific interaction of retinol with the
     nucleus *in vitro*, Proc. Natl. Acad. Sci. (U.S.A.) 76:2204
     (1979).

24. B. P. Sani, and M. K. Donovan, Localization of retinoic acid
     binding protein in nuclei and nuclear uptake of retinoic
     acid, Cancer Res. 39:2492 (1979).

25. R. G. Mehta, W. L. Cerny and R. C. Moon, Distribution of
     retinoic acid binding proteins in normal and neoplastic
     mammary tissues, Cancer Res. 40:47 (1980).

26. R. C. Moon and R. G. Mehta, Retinoid inhibition of mammary
     carcinogenesis: receptors, Cancer Treatment Report 63:
     1177 (1979).

27. W. J. Waddell, A simple ultraviolet spectrophotometric method
     for determination of protein, J. Lab. Clin. Med. 48:311
     (1956).

28. R. G. Mehta, Progestertone binding sites in nuclear fractions
     from mammary glands of lactating rats, Fed. Proc. 34:627
     (1975).

29. A. J. Shatkin, Colorimetric reactions for DNA, RNA and protein
     determinations, in: "Fundamental Techniques in Virology",
     K. Habel and N. Satzman, eds., Academic Press, N.Y. (1969).

30. U. Saffiotti, R. Montesano, R. Sellakumar and S. A. Borg,
     Experimental cancer of the lung. Inhibition by vitamin A
     of the induction of tracheobronchial squamous metaplasia
     and squamous cell tumors, Cancer 20:857 (1967).

31. P. Nettesheim and M. L. Williams, The influence of vitamin A
     on the susceptibility of the rat lung to 3-methylcholan-
     threne, Int. J. Cancer 17:351 (1976).

32. R. C. Moon, C. J. Grubbs, M. B. Sporn and D. G. Goodman,
     Retinyl acetate inhibits mammary carcinogenesis induced by
     N-methyl-N-nitrosourea, Nature 267:620 (1977).

33. M. B. Sporn, M. B. Dunlop, D. L. Newton, and J. M. Smith,
     Prevention of chemical carcinogenesis by vitamin A and its
     synthetic analogs, Fed. Proc. 35:1332 (1976).

34. M. B. Sporn and D. L. Newton, Chemoprevention of cancer with
     retinoids, Fed. Proc. 38:2528 (1979).

35. H. Mayer, W. Bollag, R. Hanni and R. Ruegg, Retinoids, a new
     class of compounds with prophylactic and therapeutic
     activities in oncology and dermatology, Experentia 34:1105
     (1978).

36. P. J. Becci, H. J. Thompson, C. J. Grubbs, C. C. Brown and R.
     C. Moon, Effect of delay of administration of 13-*cis*-
     retinoic acid on the inhibition of urinary bladder carcino-
     genesis in the rat, Cancer Res. 39:3141 (1979).

37. D. L. McCormick, F. J. Burns and R. E. Albert, Inhibition of rat mammary carcinogenesis by short dietary exposure to retinyl acetate, Cancer Res. 40:1140 (1980).

38. J. E. Smith and D. S. Goodman, Retinol binding protein and the regulation of vitamin A transport, Fed. Proc. 38:2504 (1979).

39. J. E. Smith, P. G. Milch, Y. Muto and D. S. Goodman, The plasma transport and metabolism of retinoic acid in the rat, Biochem. J. 132:821 (1973).

40. B. P. Sani, Retinoic acid binding protein: a plasma membrane component, Biochem. Biophys. Res. Comm. 91:502 (1979).

41. L. Chan and B. W. O'Malley, Mechanism of action of the sex steroid hormones, The New Eng. J. Med. 294:1322 (1976).

42. L. Prutkin and B. Bogart, The uptake of labeled vitamin A acid in keratoacanthoma, J. Invest. Dermatol. 55:249 (1970).

43. M. M. Bashor, D. O. Toft and F. Chytil, *In vitro* binding of retinol to rat tissue components, Proc. Natl. Acad. Sci. 70:3483 (1973).

44. B. P. Sani and T. H. Corbett, Retinoic acid binding proteins in normal tissues and experimental tumors, Cancer Res. 37:209 (1977).

45. P. W. Trown, A. V. Palleroni, O. Bohoslawec, B. N. Richelo, J. M. Halpern, N. Gizzi, R. Geiger, C. Lewinski, L. J. Machlin, A. Jetten, and M. E. R. Jetten, Relationship between binding affinities to cellular retinoic acid binding protein and *in vivo* and *in vitro* properties for 18 retinoids, Cancer Res. 40:212 (1979).

46. D. E. Ong, D. L. Page, and F. Chytil, Retinoic acid binding protein: occurrence in human tumors, Science 190:60 (1975).

47. R. Huber, E. Geyer, W. Kung, A. Matter, J. Torhorst, and U. Eppenberger, Retinoic acid binding protein in human breast cancer and dysplasia, J. Natl. Cancer Inst. 61:1375 (1978).

48. P. W. Trown. Personal communication.

49. C. Huggins, Two principles in endocrine therapy of cancers: Hormone deprival and hormone interference, Cancer Res. 25:1163, (1965).

50. J. L. Wittliff, R. G. Mehta, P. A. Boyd and J. E. Goral, Steroid binding proteins of the mammary gland and their clinical significance in breast cancer, J. Toxicol. Environ. Health (suppl.) 1:231 (1976).

51. W. L. McGuire and J. A. Julian, Comparison of molecular binding of estradiol in hormone dependent and hormone independent tumors, Cancer Res. 31:1440 (1971).

52. B. P. Sani, Localization of retinoic acid binding protein in nuclei, Biochem. Biophys. Res. Comm. 75:7 (1977).

FEEDBACK EFFECTS OF MAMMARY GLAND TUMORS

ON THE HOST PITUITARY PROLACTIN CELL

W. C. Hymer and Arthur Signorella

Biochemistry Program, Department of Microbiology
Cell Biology, Biochemistry & Biophysics
The Pennsylvania State University
University Park, PA 16802

SUMMARY

Prolactin (PRL) cells in pituitary glands of F-344 ♀ rats bearing transplantable mammary gland adenocarcionmas (13762, 3230) were smaller, contained less intracellular hormone, and released less hormone in culture relative to non tumor-bearing littermates. In some instances removal of the tumor by surgery or chemotherapy (PAM) resulted in restoration of function in vitro. On the other hand, PRL cells from pituitaries of breast cancer patients were often hypertrophied. Since these patients had mastectomies prior to hypophysectomy, the data are consistent with the hypothesis that the tumor exerts negative feedback at the pituitary or hypo- thalamic level. In support of this hypothesis we have discovered a potent PIF in rat serum. In addition, an experimental protocol involving a) encapsulation of pituitary cells in Amicon hollow fibers, b) their implantation in ectopic sites and c) their sub- seuqent in vitro culture yields data which suggest that the brain of the tumor bearing rat suppresses PRL release. It is suggested that decreased PRL cell function in animals bearing certain mammary tumors ultimately favors metastatic activity of the tumor cell.

INTRODUCTION

Evidence for the concept that prolactin (PRL) is a major hormone in controlling mammary tumor growth is almost over- whelming. Other polypeptide and steroid hormones also appear to be involved in tumor growth, but their roles are less well docu- mented. Precisely how these hormones interact in mammary tumorigenesis has occupied many investigators for the better part of 20 years.

The excellent and recent reviews by Welsch and Nagasawa (1) and Nagasawa (2) on PRL and mammary tumorigenesis in rodents and humans are recommended to the interested reader. As pointed out (1) most treatments that result in a hyperprolactinemia in female rats already bearing DMBA - or MCA - induced mammary tumors cause a striking increase in growth of these neoplasms. For example, adrenalectomy, pregnancy; pseudopregnancy, pituitary homografts, pituitary tumors, hypothalamic lesions, hypothalamic steroid implants, reserpine, perphenazine, haloperidol and high dietary fat all result in hyperprolactinemia and increased tumor growth (1). On the other hand, drugs which result in hypoprolactinemia, e.g., ergot alkaloids, ergolines, L-DOPA, pargyline and anti-rat PRL serum also cause marked decrease in tumor growth.

In every one of these studies, the young Sprague Dawley (SD) female rat was used as the tumor model of choice. Of course, it was recognized by Huggins some years ago (3,4) that a single intragastric feeding of 7,12-dimethylbenz(a)anthracene (DMBA) would readily induce multiple mammary adenocarcinomas in this animal. Hormone dependency by these induced tumors is documented by their regression after ovariectomy, hypophysectomy, certain steroids or anti-hormones. As emphasized by Bogden (5), the hormone dependent nature of this experimental tumor system "provides a useful model for the evaluation of the endocrine factors that are concerned in growth and maintenance of the mammary tumor." Bodgen has also pointed out some of the vagaries of this model system. They include, a) the innate variability between DMBA-induced tumor (in the same as well as among) bearing animals, b) the "subtotal, transient and sometimes biphasic response" of tumor growth or regression following certain protocols, c) the presence of hormone-independent cells within the hormone dependent tumor and d) changing responsiveness with tumor development.

Progression from hormone dependence to independence is a common feature for mammary tumors established in serial transplantation. That is to say, these tumors grow well in any syngeneic animal apparently independent of the endocrine status of the host (5). Of course, the MT-W9 and 13762 E carcinogen induced transplantable tumors (Wistar-Furth and Fisher 344 rats respectively) offer two well-documented examples of hormone dependency in transplantable tumor lines.

In addition, Bogden has emphasized the distinction between hormone dependent and hormone responsive tumors. Examples of tumor models in the latter category include stimulation of 13762

tumor growth after elevation of endogenous serum PRL by
perphenazine (6), and <u>retardation</u> of tumor growth in the R-35 (6)
and R3230AC (7) tumor after perphenazine-stimulated PRL release
in <u>vivo</u>.

That enhanced PRL levels may actually <u>retard</u> mammary tumor
growth in certain animal models is obviously of interest in light of
the opposite effects in the most often studied DMBA-induced mammary
tumor (MT) carried in the SD animal. Transplantable syngeneic
MT models, of which the R3230 and 13762 are examples, have certain
advantages. As Bogden (5) points out ..."In experimental breast
cancer, the need for tumors with well-defined growth and metastatic patterns as well as responsiveness to chemotherapy, to
ionizing radiation, and to immunotherapy is best met by the
syngeneic mammary tumor system that has been established and
stabilized in serial transplantation. The heterogeneity that one
encounters with autochthonous tumors, animal and human, is also
reflected in syngeneic tumor systems, except that the differences
are found among established tumor lines rather than among tumors
within a line. With careful monitoring, one finds that the characteristics peculiar to a particular tumor line are reproducible in
each of the tumors of that line, transplant generation after transplant generation, whether ten animals or a thousand animals are
implanted at any particular passage."

With particular regard to the use of inbred strains in transplantable MT's Bogden further points out "the purpose of inbred
strains, the members of which serve as recipients for syngeneic
tumor grafts, is to have available for experimentation a large
population of genetically identical animals in which the relationship of each animal to a neoplasm arising in one of its members
mimics the autochthonous tumor-host relationship. Thus, malignant
tumors should be 100% transplantable in syngeneic hosts, producing
progressive and eventually lethal growths."

Which MT model system is the best to use in the study of human
breast cancer? Is there a <u>best</u> model? Bogden, among others, has
attempted to get to the answer to such questions by using a block
of different MT's that reflect a spectrum of growth patterns and
reactivities (5). On the basis of Bogden's data, we chose the 13762
and R3230AC transplantable syngeneic rat mammary tumor models for
our studies. Both of these tumors a) are adenocarcinomas and
b) are carried in the young F-344 ♀ rat. Mean survival times are
48.7+8 and 49.8+16 days for the 13762 and 3230 respectively. Maximum growth rates (mm/day) are 1.85 for the 13762 and 1.35 for the
3230. Bogden has documented a key difference in % incidence of
metastases in these two MT's; 93% for the 13762 and 10% for the
3230. Metastases from subcutaneous grafts of the 13762 MT
apparently occur via blood and lymphatic systems to lungs and/or
other viscera about 20 days post-implantation. Finally, Bogden

et al. (8) were able to show the 13762 MT was among the most
responsive to chemotherapy. That is, phenylalanine mustard (PAM)
used alone, or in combination with 5-flurouracil and methotrexate,
was effective in inhibiting tumor growth. None of these treatments,
however, were effective on the 3230 tumor. According to Bogden
the 13762 MT, ..."best mimics the chemotherapy responsiveness and
acquired drug resistance of those human breast cancers that are
sensitive to the alkylating agents. It has also shown a degree of
selectivity for agents most active in breast cancer, and has been
used effectively in integrating immunotherapy with other therapeutic modalities." (5).

The specific aim of the studies described in this chapter was
to determine what differences, if any, existed in the pituitary
glands of animals bearing the 13762 and 3230 MT's. Special emphasis
was placed on in vitro characteristics of the PRL cell prepared from
these two model systems.

METHODS

Animals. Untreated 50-60 day old ♀ rats of the Fisher (F-344)
strain (Charles Rivers Corp., Wilmington, MA) were used. In a few
cases Sprague Dawley (SD) ♀'s of the same age were also used.
Animals were maintained in a temperature controlled (25° C) arti-
fically illuminated (14 hr. daily) animal room. In some experiments these rats were ovariectomized (5-14 days) or pretreated with
estrogen (E₂, estradiol benzoate, injected sc in sesame oil at
doses of 1, 5 or 20 μg/day/5-11 days) prior to kill.

Tumors. F-344 ♀ rats, 38-45 days of age, were implanted with either
a) the 13762B mammary ascites tumor (MAT), b) the 13762 solid
mammary adenocarcinoma or c) the R3230 mammary adenocarcinoma.
These transplantable tumor lines were obtained from the Animal and
Human Tumor Bank of the Mason Research Institute, Worcester, MA.
The MAT line was maintained by injecting 1x10⁶ cells, IP. Animals
bearing these ascites tumors survived for 11-13 days; the line was
maintained by routine transplantation at day 10. The 13762 solid
DMBA-induced mammary adenocarcinoma metastasizes regularly to
regional lymph nodes, lungs, abdominal organs, and occasionally the
brain and spinal column. The 3230 AC is a solid tumor of spontaneous
origin, metastasizes occasionally to regional lymph nodes and lungs,
and responds to exogenous estrogens by milk secretion. Both solid
tumors were transplanted with 1-2 mm³ pieces injected sc via trocar
midway between the axillary and inguinal areas.

Tumor Removal. Chemotherapy. Experimental protocols were similar
to those used in the studies detailed by Bogden (8). Phenylalanine
mustard (PAM) was formulated in a Klucel vehicle consisting of 0.39%
hydroxypropyl cellulose in physiological saline. Vehicle or PAM
was administered via intubation. In the case of animals bearing

ascites tumor cells, PAM (2 mg/kilo/day) was administered 24 hrs
after tumor cell innoculation and continued for 10 days. Obvious
signs of tumor development was seen in controls, but not experi-
mentals, 7 days post-treatment. Animals bearing 13762 or 3230 solid
tumors received PAM at a dose 2 mg/kilo/3x per week. Ten-12 days
after tumor innoculation, tumor sizes were estimated from calipers
$(\frac{L + W}{2}$ mm).

Surgery. Animals bearing 13762 tumors were anesthesized with
sodium pentobarbital followed by careful excision of the tumor.
Tumor bearing controls of the same age were sham operated (i.e.,
anethesized, an incision made at the site of the tumor, and the
incision closed with clips).

Preparation of Pituitary Cells. Pituitary glands from 6-9 tumor
bearing animals were usually required in each experiment. Equal
numbers of non tumor-bearing littermates of the same age served as
controls. Animals were killed with a guillotine, hypophyses removed asceptically within 60 seconds and posterior pituitary
discarded. Pooled tissues were minced into $\sim$ 1 mm^3 fragments
prior to dissociation into single cells. The dissociation medium
consisted of 0.1% trypsin (Difco 1:250), 0.1% bovine serum albumin
(BSA, Armour, Fraction V), prepared in minimum essential medium
(MEM) at pH 7.3. Dispersion was done in a siliconized 25 ml
Spinner flask (Bellco Glass Co.) equipped with a teflon impeller.
Cell yields averaged $1.5-2.0x10^6$/gland ($\sim$ 60-80% yield) with a
viability estimated to be 95% on the basis of trypan blue dye
exclusion. Further details of the dissociation procedures can be
found in references (9,10,11).

Separation of Pituitary Cells by Velocity Sedimentation at Unit
Gravity (IG). The sedimentation chamber and its operation have
been detailed in several previous reports (9,10,11). Basically the
method involves sedimentation of the cells through a shallow
(0.3-2.4%) BSA gradient prepared in Medium 199, pH 7.4. No more
than $10x10^6$ cells were separated in any given experiment. Sedimentation was routinely carried out for 1.25 hr. at room temperature, after which time successive 15-30 ml fractions were obtained
by pumping the gradient upward and out through the top of the
chamber. Cell recoveries ranged 75-85% and recoveries of prolactin (PRL) and other pituitary hormones ranged 78-90%.

Pituitary Cell Culture. In the usual experiment 25,000 pituitary
cells were seeded into 35 mm plastic dishes containing either 3 ml
of Medium 199 + 20% fetal calf serum or α-Modified Eagles Medium
(αMEM) + 20% horse serum fortified with antibiotics. Fresh medium
was sometimes added to the cells every 3-4 days and spent medium
stored at $-20°$ C for subsequent RIA. At the end of the experiment,

intracellular hormone was extracted with cold 0.01 N NaOH followed
by centrifugation and dilution in RIA buffer (9,10). Usually 4
dishes of cells were used for each experimental point.

RIA. Concentrations of pituitary hormones in culture media and cell
extracts were measured by double antibody RIA procedures using
materials kindly supplied by the NIAMDD, NIH. All samples were
assayed in duplicate according to procedures recommended by NIH.
Data were analyzed by logit transformation of response variable
vs $\log_{10}$ dose of standard using a PDP-11 computer.

RESULTS

A number of investigators have used the unit gravity velocity
sedimentation technique to separate different pituitary cell types
(reviewed in Hymer et al., 12). This method is particularly useful
for detecting size changes of the pituitary PRL producing cell.
As shown in Fig. 1, PRL cell hypertrophy induced by E_2-pretreatment
of SD rats or its decrease induced by ovariectomy are readily demonstrated by this separation technique.

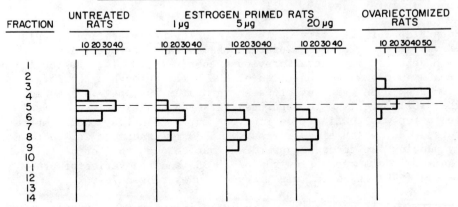

Fig. 1.   Separation of PRL cells from Sprague-Dawley ♀ rats by
          velocity sedimentation at unit gravity. Recovery of cell-
          associated PRL is represented by open bars; only the 4
          major fractions are shown. Cells in upper fractions are
          small, those in lower fractions are large. (Modified
          from Hymer et al. (10)).

A. Pituitary Cell Separation: Untreated F-344 Rat.

Since most of the work to be described in this report has been
done on the pituitary of the F-344 rat, we first studied glands of
untreated F-344 rats 47-145 days of age. As shown in the left
hand panel of Fig. 2, intracellular contents of PRL, GH, FSH, LH
and TSH in freshly trypsinized cell suspensions change with advancing age. Around 50 days of age, a time when animals receive
tumor implants, intracellular GH levels rise markedly, gonadotropins
fall, PRL levels rise slowly and TSH remains relatively constant.
The sedimentation profiles of these different cell types suggests
that size changes also take place during aging (Fig. 2, right panel).
The reader will recall that small cells are recovered from the
upper gradient fractions (e.g., #3) while large cells are recovered
from lower fractions (e.g., #8).

Pituitary glands of $\sim$ 50 day old rats contain PRL cells which
are widely dispersed throughout the gradient. This profile reflects
heterogeneity in size of this cell type. By 145 days of age, however, 50% of the recovered PRL is associated with cells sedimenting
to fraction 5 (i.e., smaller cells). GH cells also become smaller
as the animal ages. However, gonadotrophs and thyrotrophs show
little change in distribution profiles at each of the ages looked
at.

B. Pituitary Cell Separation: F-344 Rats Bearing Mammary Ascites Tumors (MAT).

Pituitary PRL cells from MAT bearing animals had significantly
less intracellular hormone than cells from non tumor-bearing littermates (Table 1). GH levels were also lower, while other pituitary
cell types were unaffected by the presence of the tumor.

Velocity sedimentation profiles of PRL and GH cells prepared
from MAT-bearing animals reflecting the changing intracellular
hormone levels of these two cell types. Thus, approximately 60%
of the recovered PRL ($\bar{x}$ of 4 experiments) was associated with cells
sedimenting to fraction 4 (Fig. 3). This sedimentation behavior is
in marked contrast to that of PRL cells prepared from non tumor-
bearing littermates (Fig. 3, top panel). Somatotrophs from pituitaries of the MAT animals also had slower sedimentation rates
relative to controls (cf Fig. 3, top 2 panels). The effects of
estrogen pretreatment, ovariectomy, and ovariectomy + estrogen
replacement therapy on subsequent sedimentation profiles of PRL
and GH cells from tumor bearing animals are given in the bottom 3
panels of Fig. 3. Ovariectomy had no effect on PRL or GH cell
size (panels 2 vs 3). However, E_2 administration resulted in
"reversion" of the PRL and GH cell from the tumorous state "back
to" the normal state.

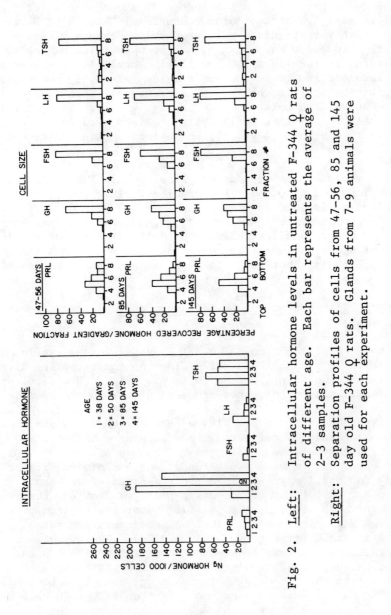

Fig. 2.   Left: Intracellular hormone levels in untreated F-344 ♀ rats
                  of different age. Each bar represents the average of
                  2-3 samples.

          Right: Separation profiles of cells from 47-56, 85 and 145
                  day old F-344 ♀ rats. Glands from 7-9 animals were
                  used for each experiment.

TABLE 1

Intracellular Hormone Contents of Dispersed Pituitary Cells
Prepared from Non-Tumor and Tumor-Bearing F-344 ♀ Rats.

Hormone	Nanograms Hormone/1000 Cells		
	No Tumor[+]	MAT[++]	MAT+E$_2$[+++]
PRL	5.7±0.6 (21)	3.0±0.3** (19)	13.3 (2)
GH	213.2 (2)	64.9 (2)	170 (1)
FSH	5.2±3.1 (3)	3.2±1.0 (3)	---
LH	14.6±6.4 (3)	15.6±5.4 (3)	---
TSH	64.7±5.9 (3)	50.8±9.1 (3)	---

[+]Untreated F-344 ♀'s, 48-57 days old. ( ) indicate #
of experiments. Usually 2 samples, each containing
300,000 cells, were extracted for hormone/exp.

[++]F-344 ♀ bearing 13762 mammary ascites tumor (MAT).
Tumor age 9-13 days; animals were littermates of controls.

[+++]F-344 ♀ bearing MAT (9-13 days). These animals were
injected sc with estradiol benzoate, 5 μg/day/11 days
prior to kill.

** = p < .01 vs control. FSH, LH and TSH not significant.

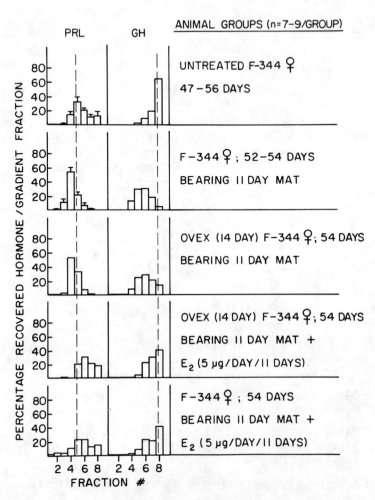

Fig. 3.   Velocity sedimentation profiles of PRL and GH cells from
F-344 ♀ rats bearing 13762 ascites tumors. Top 2 panels
represent the average of 4 experiments each (9 rats/experi-
ment). Although not shown, distribution profiles for
TSH, LH and FSH were unaffected by these treatments.

These results clearly document pituitary responsiveness to steroid administration in the tumor condition. Whether the E_2 acts directly at the pituitary level cannot, of course, be determined from these experimental designs. Although not shown in Fig. 3, we also assayed the various cell fractions of TSH, LH, and FSH. The sedimentation profiles of these cell types showed no difference between any treatment groups. The reader will recall that intra-cellular contents of the glycoprotein hormones were also not affected by the presence of the growing tumor (Table 1).

We were interested to find out when, during development of the 13762 MAT, we could begin to detect shifts in PRL cell size. In an extensive experimental series, animals bearing MAT were killed 4, 7, 10 and 11 days post-implantation. At each of these days, 7-9 animals were killed, their pituitaries pooled, dissociated, and separated by the IG technique. Results from 15 experiments (Fig. 4) are expressed as the percentage of PRL measured from cells sedimenting between fractions 1-4 (30-120 ml); i.e., permitting an estimation of the percentage of PRL cells in the total population which are "small." In 5 separate experiments, 8-27% of the PRL from cells of non tumor-bearing animals was recovered in fractions 1-4 (hatched area, Fig. 4). The frequency of small PRL cells in pituitaries of tumor-bearing animals increased linearly with tumor age (Fig. 4). As before (Fig. 3), E_2 administration (5µg/day/11 days) completely pre-vented the tumor-induced accumulation of cells in fractions 1-4.

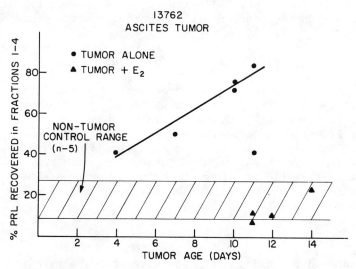

Fig. 4. Percentage of prolactin cells recovered in upper gradient regions after cell separation as a function of age of the tumor bearing host. Each point represents one experiment (7-9 animals).

The tumor-induced suppression of intracellular PRL (Table 1) was also examined as a function of tumor age. Animals bearing the tumor for 1-4 days had 3.3 ± 0.5 ng PRL/1000 cells vs 5.4 ± 0.8 ng PRL/1000 cells (N.S.) for controls of the same age. By 10-12 days, levels in the experimental groups were 2.2 ± 0.3 ng PRL/1000 cells vs 5.5 ± 0.7 for controls ($p<.02$). Taken together with the data in Fig. 4, it is obvious that tumor-induced suppression of PRL cell size and hormone content is related to tumor age.

C. Pituitary Cell Separation: F-344 Rats Bearing Solid Mammary Tumors.

PRL cells of rats bearing transplantable solid DMBA-induced 13762 and 3230 mammary tumors (MT) were also evaluated for intracellular hormone content and sedimentation behavior. Unlike the MAT animals, intracellular PRL levels in glands from animals bearing solid MT's were not significantly different from non tumor-bearing littermates.

Sedimentation profiles of PRL cells from animals bearing the 13762 or 3230 AC for 1, 2, 3 or 4 weeks are shown in Fig. 5. As before, glands from 7-9 tumor bearing animals were required for each experiment. In the 13762 model, significant shifts in PRL cell sedimentation were seen 2 weeks post implantation. One month post implantation, $\sim$ 60% of the cellular PRL was recovered from Fraction #4. The reader will recognize that this sedimentation profile was very similar to that of the 11 day MAT-bearing animal (cf. Figs. 5 to 3). On the other hand, cells from animals bearing the 3230 AC did not change in their sedimentation behavior until 1 month post implantation.

D. Pituitary Cytology of Tumor Bearing Rats.

Differential counts of cells from untreated F-344 rats gave the following distribution (Herlant's strain, $\bar{x}$ = 4 exps.): PRL cells 31.6 ± 1.5%; GH cells 31.6 ± 0.8%; TSH, FSH and LH cells (combined) 12.4 ± 1.0%; "chromophobes" 11.0 ± 1.4%; and "unknowns" 12.6 ± 2.4%. Similar counts on cells from glands of animals bearing the different tumor types discussed above failed to reveal any statistically significant change in this pattern. At the electron microscope level, cells from MAT animals were indistinguishable from untreated controls.

E. PRL Cell Culture.

It has been recognized for some time that the pituitary mammotroph is particularly well-suited to cell culture since it synthesizes and releases sizeable quantities of hormone over extended periods (13). We compared the capacity of PRL cells from tumor

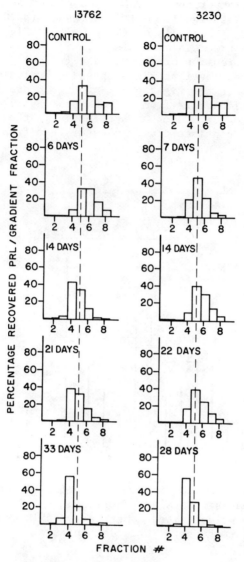

Fig. 5.   Velocity sedimentation profiles of PRL cells from animals
          bearing 13762 and 3230 solid MT.

bearing animals to release hormone during a 3 day period to controls.
Two medium formulations were used: a) TC 199 + 20% FCS and
b) αMEM + 20% HS.   In a recent study from our laboratory (13),
it was shown that the magnitude of PRL release was ∿ 5 fold higher
in the αMEM-HS system.   However, PRL synthesis takes place in both
since 2-8x as much PRL is recovered vs that originally seeded.

In each of 5 experiments, PRL release from cells of MAT bearing
rats (3-11 days) was significantly suppressed (p<.05) relative to
cells from non-tumor controls of the same age (Fig. 6). In another
5 exps., cells cultured in αMEM also consistently reflected the
tumor-related suppression of PRL release (p<.05). In none of these
experiments was the level of PRL suppression release related to
tumor age. Shown in the right panel of Fig. 6 are 6 additional
experiments in which cells from animals bearing 13762 or 3230 solid
MT's were cultured for 3 days. Suppression in the cells from the
13762 animals was consistently 2x greater than from 3230 tumor-
bearing animals.

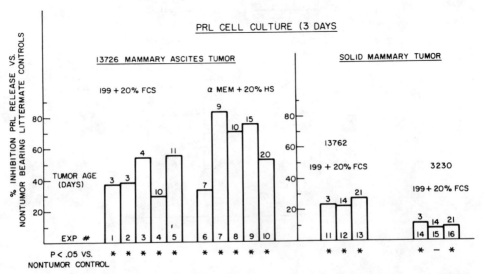

Fig. 6.   Culture of cells from tumor-bearing vs non tumor-bearing
          littermates. Data are expressed as 5 inhibition in PRL
          release vs untreated controls. 2.5x10^4 cells/dish; 4
          dishes/treatment. Three day culture.

F.   Tumor Removal.

Up to this point we have provided experimental evidence that
the PRL cell of tumor-bearing rats, relative to its counterpart in
non tumor-bearing littermates, contains significantly less intracellular hormone, b) is smaller and c) releases less PRL in vitro.
We reasoned that if PRL cell suppression was due directly to the
tumor, then its removal might result in restoration of function.

Surgery. Cell Culture. In 3 separate experiments, animals bearing
13762 solid mammary tumors for 1, 2 and 3 weeks were subjected to
surgery. One half of the animals (n = 10) had their tumors
surgically removed, while the other half were sham-operated. At
1, 3 or 7 days post-surgery the animals were killed and the dissociated pituitary cells cultured for 3 days. As shown in Fig. 7,
surgical removal of the 7 or 14 day tumor had no significant effect
on subsequent secretory capacity of the PRL cell in vitro relative
to PRL cells from the sham operated tumor-bearing controls. However, removal of the 3 week old tumor resulted in significantly
(p<.001) elevated PRL release 1 and 3 days post-surgery.

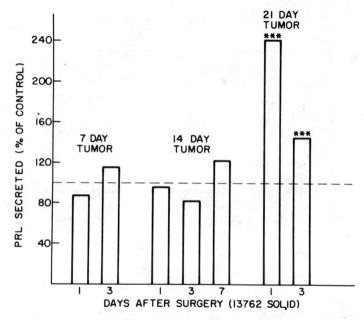

Fig. 7. Effect of surgical removal of the 13762 MT on subsequent
         PRL release from pituitary cells over a 3 day culture
         period vs that of cells prepared from sham-operated
         tumor-bearing controls.

Chemotherapy. Cell Culture. As an alternative method to tumor
removal we took advantage of Bodgen's observations (8) that
the 13762, but not 3230 MT is sensitive to PAM. In an extensive
series of experiments we tested effects of PAM treatment on
subsequent in vitro PRL cell function in normal F-344 animals

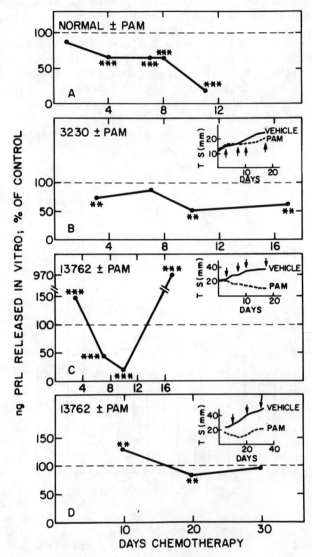

Fig. 8.   Effect of PAM administration in vivo on subsequent in vitro
PRL release (3 day culture) from nomal (panel A), 3230
(panel B) and 13762 (panels C and D) tumor bearing F-344
rats.   At times indicated, treated or vehicle-injected
littermates (5/group) were killed, pituitaries dissociated
and cells cultured for 3 days.   Inserts reflect PAM-induced
changes in tumor size.

subsequent in vitro PRL cell function in normal F-344 animals
(Fig. 8A), in 3230 MT bearing F-344 animals (Fig. 8B), and in
13762 MT bearing F-344 animals (Fig. 8C,D). Each point on the
figure represents data obtained from pooled pituitary cells of 5
animals/experimental point. Results from this experiment permit
the following conclusions: 1) PAM administration to untreated F-344
rats caused marked reductions in PRL release relative to vehicle-
injected controls. This reduction was apparent 1 day after PAM
treatment, and became progressively and significantly (p<.001)
lower with continued drug administration. 2) As expected, PAM
administration had little effect on the size of the 3230 tumor. In
vitro PRL release from these cells was also significantly lower
(p<.01) at 3 of 4 times tested. 3) PAM administration to animals
bearing 13762 tumors resulted in significant reduction in tumor
size during the first 2 weeks of therapy (Fig. 8C, D). Regrowth of
the tumor occurred ∿ 20 days into drug therapy (Fig. 8D).
4) Considering the data in panels C and D collectively, PRL release
from cells in the PAM treated groups were significantly (p<.001)
elevated, relative to vehicle in injected controls, 3 of 7 times
studied. However, this response was inconsistent, since significant suppressions were observed at 3 other times. The reader will
recall, however, that PAM treatment, by itself, suppressed in
vitro PRL release (Fig. 8, panel A).

In one other experiment involving PAM therapy, animals bearing
13762 MAT received the drug for 9 days. In vitro PRL release from
these cells was 1392+66 ng vs 1144+30 ng (p<.01) from vehicle
injected controls. Obvious signs of tumor development were seen in
controls, but not experimental animals, 7 days into treatment.

Chemotherapy. Intracellular PRL. We also tested the effects of PAM
treatment on intracellular pituitary PRL levels. As summarized in
Fig. 9, daily administration of PAM to the non-tumor bearing F-344
♀ rat resulted in the development of significant suppression of
intracellular PRL 7-11 days later. On the other hand, daily administration of PAM to animals bearing 13762 ascites tumors resulted
in decreased tumor growth (see Methods) and intracellular PRL
levels which were not suppressed relative to vehicle-injected tumor
bearing animals. Similarly, PAM administration to 13762-solid
tumor bearing rats sometimes resulted in signficantly elevated
levels of intracellular PRL. Taken together with the PRL release
data in Fig. 8, it appears that PAM treatment not only results in
tumor suppression, but in some instances, "recovery" of the PRL
cell as well.

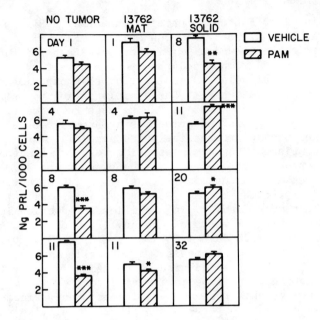

Fig. 9.   Effects of PAM treatment on intracellular PRL levels in
          tumor and non tumor-bearing F-344 littermates. PAM or
          vehicle was administered daily (see METHODS). Results
          represent average of 4 animals/group.

G.   Rat Serum Inhibition of PRL Release from Mammotrophs in Cell
     Culture.

     As discussed on pg. 13 (see Fig. 6), PRL cells in culture
synthesize and release considerable quantities of hormone. In a
recent study from our laboratory (13), we showed that the choice of
culture medium, pH and buffer composition all had significant effects
on PRL synthesis and release. For example, pituitary cells maintained in 20 different commercially available medium formulations
supplemented with 5% horse serum (HS) had vastly different secretory
capacities (Table 2). Thus, relative to the amount of cellular PRL
needed, mammotrophs cultured in αMEM for 9 days produced 25 times
their initial hormone content whereas those in Waymouth 752/1
medium produced only 1.2 times that amount. The high PRL levels
produced by cells in αMEM indicates that these cells renew their
complete hormone complement once every 9 hours.

TABLE 2

Effect of Medium Formulation and Serum Supplements
on PRL Production During a 9-Day Culture Period.

Medium[a]	PRL production index[b]	
	5% HS	5% CS
α-MEM	24.5 ± 2.9[c]	16.1 ± 1.7
DMEM	21.0 ± 2.7[c]	7.2 ± 1.4
RPMI 1640	17.4 ± 1.6	11.0 ± 1.9
MEMe	17.4 ± 3.2	13.5 ± 2.1
WE	16.9 ± 3.1	11.6 ± 2.1
Ham's F12	14.0 ± 1.6	11.1 ± 1.2
BMEe	13.4 ± 2.6	9.6 ± 1.5
Neuman, Tytell	13.4 ± 2.3	7.5 ± 1.1
McCoy's, 5A	13.2 ± 1.7	3.5 ± 0.4
BMEh	13.0 ± 2.3	11.3 ± 1.1
Leibovitz, L15	12.4 ± 0.9	10.8 ± 0.5
Ham's F10	10.8 ± 1.9	10.0 ± 1.1
MEMh	9.9 ± 1.6	8.5 ± 1.0
CGM	9.3 ± 1.3	6.1 ± 0.8
CMRL 1066	8.8 ± 1.1	1.5 ± 0.3
NCTC 135	8.7 ± 0.9	3.1 ± 0.6
Medium 199h	4.6 ± 0.7	2.2 ± 0.1
Swim's, S-77	1.8 ± 0.3	1.4 ± 0.2
Waymouth, 87/3	1.5 ± 0.3	1.0 ± 0.1
Waymouth, 752/1	1.2 ± 0.1	1.1 ± 0.1

Results represent average of 3 experiments.

a. BME, Basal Eagle's Medium; CGM, complete growth medium
(modified Puck's medium); e, with Earle's salts;
h, with Hanks' salts. Swim's S77 medium was supplemented
with $CaCl_2$ (200 mg/liter) and L-glutamine (280 mg/liter).

b. In vitro production of PRL and GH was evaluated by computing
a hormone production index based on the ratio of hormone
recovered from both medium and cells during culture to the
quantity of hormone originally seeded into the culture dish
[mean(± 1 SE) quantity of PRL and GH plated, 277±9 ng
PRL/dish and 1329±54 ng GH/dish, respectively]. Values
given are the mean ± 1 SE (n = 6).

c. Column treatment means with the same superscript are not
significantly different (p>0.05).

From Wilfinger, et al., 1979 (13).

In recent experiments, we have discovered that addition of small amounts of rat serum (RS) to cells maintained in this αMEM + 20% HS system dramatically inhibits PRL secretion in dose dependent fashion (Fig. 10).

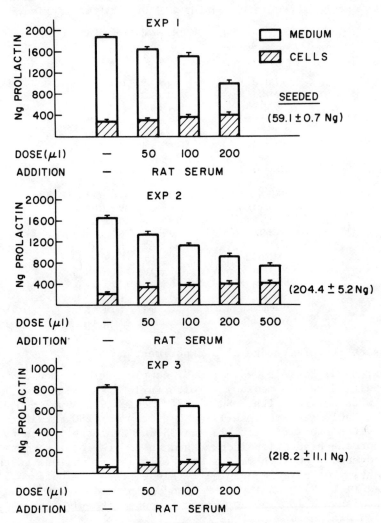

Fig. 10.   Effect of rat serum addition on subsequent PRL release from 2.5x10⁴ cells cultured for 3 days in αMEM+20% horse serum. Control plates (4/treatment) received an equivalent volume of αMEM. All experimental values are significantly different from each other (Duncan's multiple range).

In other experiments (not detailed here) we have determined
that a) cells can recover from RS induced inhibition, b) activity
is unaffected by addition of a wide range of protease inhibitors,
c) activity is non-dialyzable, heat labile and stable on freezing
and d) activity can be "generated" from whole clotted blood. Fractionation experiments of RS are currently underway. Results from
2 experiments involving gel chromatography on Sephacryl S-200 show
that PRL inhibitory activity is associated with molecules of
apparent MW $\sim$ 120,000 and $\sim$ 30,000 (Fig. 11).

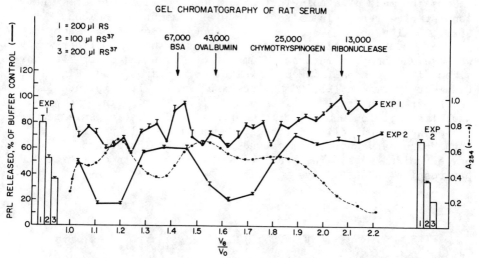

Fig. 11. Chromatography of rat serum on Sepharcyl S-200 columns.
Activity was determined by addition of eluant at indi-
cated fractions to 2.5×10^4 cells in culture αMEM+20% HS)
for 3 days. In both experiments the whole blood was
incubated at 37° C for 2 hours prior to preparation of
the serum. This procedure generates inhibitory activity.
Data are expressed as a percentage of PRL released
relative to column buffer-treated cells.

H. PRL Cell Function *In Vivo*.

The experimental results described thus far were generated
entirely from in vitro approaches. The direct approach of
measuring serum PRL levels in patients with breast cancer or in

animals bearing mammary tumors has been reported in many studies
over the last 5-10 years. Some investigators report a lack of
correlation between serum PRL levels and the presence or absence
of cancer, while others report a positive correlation (subject
reviewed in 1). In addition, estimations of serum PRL levels in
rats are of course also complicated by the well-documented phenomenon of stress-induced PRL release. Moreover, several studies
have appeared which suggest that clearance rates of PRL in mice
with mammary tumors may be altered, thereby rendering the value of
estimating serum PRL levels somewhat questionable (14).

A few years ago we began to study <u>in vivo</u> function of dispersed pituitary cells implanted in Amicon "hollow fibers." These
fibers are made of a polyvinyl chloride acrylic copolymer. They
consist of a very thin anisotropic Diaflo membrane (Amicon
Corp., Lexington, MA) and a thicker spongy layer of the same
polymer with increasingly larger openings. The XM-50 fiber which
we have used has an internal diameter of 500 μ and controlled pore
sizes with a nominal molecular weight cutoff at 50,000 (Fig. 12).
Pituitary hormones (22,500 MW) released from cells implanted into
the fiber lumen freely diffuse out of the fiber. Since immunoglobulins are 150,000 MW, molecular sieving by the capsule renders
the encapsulated cells, in theory, immunologically privileged.
Such "pituitary units," implanted into the brains of hypophysectomized rats, are capable of restoring growth over extended
periods (up to 40-60 days) (12,15).

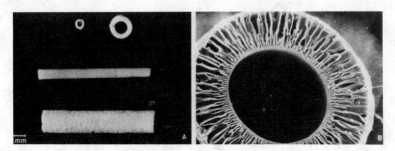

Fig. 12.   Amicon hollow fibers (left) and their appearance by
           scanning electron microscopy (right).

We have now begun, in preliminary studies, to study PRL
release from pituitary fiber units implanted ectopically in the rat.
In our particular experimental protocol it was important to first
show that encapsulated PRL cells could indeed release PRL from the
fiber. The results of two separate experiments (Fig. 13) indicate

that this is the case.   In these experiments, 25-400x10^3
pituitary cells prepared from 55 day old F-344 rats were either
plated directly into a culture dish (labeled "free") or encapsulated in 10 mm XM 50 hollow fibers prior to a 3 day culture.
Results showed a) that levels of PRL released from the encapsulated
cells into the medium (open bars, Fig. 13) were of the same order
of magnitude as that from the non encapsulated cells and b) that
the magnitude of hormone release was directly related to cell number.   These encouraging results prompted us to study PRL release
from encapsulated cells placed in various ectopic sites.   In one
recent experiment, pituitary cells from 53 day old untreated F-344
or 13762 ascites tumor bearing rats were encapsulated (150,000/
capsule) and placed either a) in culture, b) in brain parenchyma
or c) in the femur (marrow cavity) of normal or tumor bearing
(13762 ascites) recipients of the same age.   Animals bearing such

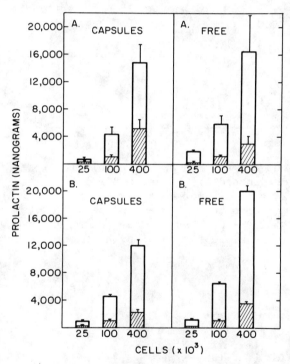

Fig. 13.   Release of PRL from dispersed pituitary cells in culture
          for 3 days.   In each of 2 experiments, indicated cell
          numbers were either encapsulated in Amicon hollow fibers
          prior to culture or otherwise added directly to the dish.
          Open bars indicate PRL in medium; hatched indicate intra-
          cellular hormone.

capsules appeared unaffected by the implant. After 4 days, the
capsules were removed (n = 5/group) and PRL release studied by a
perifusion technique. Briefly, this involved placement of capsules
in 1 cc glass columns maintained at 37° C in which buffer (Medium
199 + 0.1% BSA, pH 7.4) was pumped through the column at the rate
of 500 µl/min for a 2 hr. period). Results from this experiment
document the potential of this approach to the study of PRL cell
function in mammary cancer. Briefly they show (Fig. 14), a) that
cyclic patterns of hormone release occur, b) that encapsulated
pituitary cells from tumor bearing animals in general release less
PRL than pituitary cells from the non-tumor animals, c) that rather
different <u>patterns</u> of PRL release are seen from normal cells placed
in the head of the normal <u>vs</u> tumor-bearing recipient. The reader

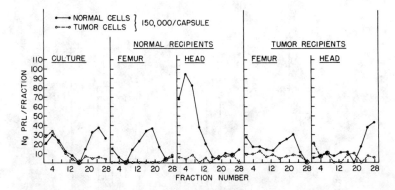

Fig. 14.   PRL release from encapsulated pituitary cells implanted
            in (or donated by) 53 day old F-344 ♀ rats (untreated or
            13762 ascites tumor-bearing littermates). After 4 days
            the capsules were removed and perifused for 2 hours in
            Medium 199 + 0.1% BSA. Capsules in culture were main-
            tained <u>in vitro</u> for the length of time the others were
            <u>in vivo</u>.

will recall that pituitary PRL cells from tumor bearing animals
release significantly less hormone <u>in vitro</u> relative to cells
from non-tumor littermates (Fig. 6). The data in Fig. 14 suggest
that the brain of the tumor bearing animal may be rich in prolactin
inhibitory material (dopamine?) relative to brains of normal
recipients (cf. normal cell PRL release kinetics in normal <u>vs</u>
tumor recipients). Such data offer the possibility of getting
at fundamental changes in the brain chemistry during mammary
tumorigenesis which, in turn, may eventually get at mechanisms
underlying PRL cell inhibition in these tumor-bearing rat models.

I. Human Pituitary PRL Cells from Breast Cancer Patients.

     A few years ago we had the opportunity to study pituitary PRL
cells from patients undergoing hypophysectomy for a variety of
diseases, including breast cancer. We were interested to find out
something about the human PRL cell in terms of a) its intracellular PRL levels, b) its sedimentation behavior at unit gravity
and c) its secretory characteristics in vitro. These studies were
published previously (16), and are therefore only summarized briefly
at this point.

     Intracellular PRL levels in dispersed cells of samples from 19
patients averaged 3.8 ng/1,000 cells (range 0.3-7.9). Ten of the
19 samples were derived from breast cancer patients, and these cells
averaged 4.6 ng/1,000 cells. The number of PRL cells, estimated by
immunocytochemistry, averaged ∿ 20% of the total population. None
of these parameters measured on glands of breast cancer patients
were strikingly different from the remainder of the patient population studied.

     Unit gravity velocity sedimentation profiles of dispersed
human pituitary cells in shallow BSA gradients are shown in Fig.
15. The cell distribution profiles serve as reference markers for
the distribution of recovered PRL. In all but one instance (chromo-
phobe adenoma), the major cell peak was recovered from fractions
3-6, i.e., a region encompassing 91-180 ml of the gradient. In each
of the three samples from "normal" tissue (2 post mortem , 1 diabetic)
the distribution of recovered PRL tended to follow that of the cells,
i.e., the PRL peak was associated with the major cell peak. With
cells prepared from breast cancer patients; however, 12-39% ($\bar{x}$ =
28%) of the PRL was associated with a minor population of cells that
sedimented further than fraction 6, whereas only 7-9% of the PRL
from normal tissue was recovered in this same gradient region.
These sedimentation profiles obviously suggest that the pituitary
gland of breast cancer patients contains some large PRL cells. In
support of this notion, an electron micrograph of a human pituitary
PRL cell (breast cancer) recovered from combined fractions 6-10
reveals a cell with hypertrophied golgi areas, abundant stacks of
ER, and irregular shaped secretory granules (Fig. 16). This
micrograph (and many others like it) offer morphological evidence
for actively secreting cells. In fact, these separated cells
were cultured for 21 days and were shown to be "active secretors"
(see (16) for further details).

     On the surface it would appear from our data that the pituitary
PRL cell of the breast cancer patient is rather different from its
counterpart in the DMBA-induced transplantable rat mammary adenocarcinoma. However, the pituitaries we studied were obtained from
patients with primary tumors removed surgically a good while before

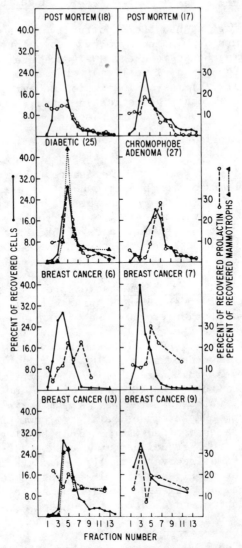

Fig. 15.   Percentage of recovered cells (●———●) and percentage
of recovered prolactin (O----------O) in 8 cell separation
gradients. Numbers in parentheses indicate patient information, see Hymer et al. (16) for further details.

hypophysectomy. This raises the possibility of feedback interaction between the tumor and pituitary, a notion which is considered
more fully in the following section.

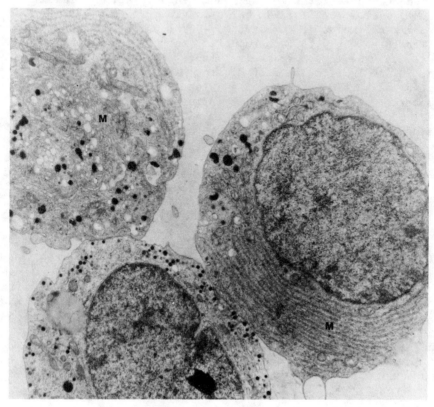

Fig. 16.   Electron microscopic appearance of two mammotrophs (M) recovered from lower gradient regions (fractions 6-10). These cells show morphologic signs of intense secretory activity, e.g., well-developed Golgi areas and endoplasmic reticulum.   X 13,000.

DISCUSSION

Our studies show that pituitary PRL cells prepared from animals
bearing the metastasizing, PAM sensitive, 13762 MT are different
from their counterparts in the non-metastasizing, PAM insensitive,
3230 MT model. That is, PRL cells in pituitaries of 13762 MT-
bearing rats, relative to non tumor-bearing littermates, are
smaller (Figs. 3, 4, 5), contain less intracellular hormone (Table
1), and release less hormone in culture (Fig. 6). On the other
hand, PRL cells from the 3230 MT show minimal cell size changes
(Fig. 5) and are only marginally affected in culture (Fig. 6). It
is interesting that age-associated changes in the sedimentation
profiles of the PRL and GH cells in glands of the untreated F-344
Q_+ rat are minced by the presence of the 13762 ascites or solid
tumor (cf. Fig. 2 vs 4 and 5). Whether it is correct to attribute
these pituitary changes of 13762 MT animals to activation of some
age-related process is, of course, a matter of conjecture. That
the tumor-induced suppression of PRL and GH function in the 13762
MT model is not merely due to a debilitating non-specific effect
of the tumor is suggested by the observations 1) that tumor-
bearing animals eat as much food as non tumor-bearing littermates
(Bogden, personal communication, 2) that FSH, LH and TSH cells
appear unaffected by the presence of the tumor, 3) that the in
situ PRL and GH cell in the tumor-bearing host can be stimulated
to return to "normal" by in vivo administration of estrogen (Fig.
3), and finally 4) that PRL cell function in the 3230 MT model is
only marginally affected by the presence of the tumor. Furthermore, the in vitro data (Figs. 7, 8) on PRL cells prepared from
glands of animals which had their tumors "removed" (at least
partially) by chemotherapy and/or surgery are also consistent with
the concept that the mammotrophs can recover from tumor-induced
suppression.

What is the mechanism(s) by which the tumor might suppress
pituitary PRL function? The model in Fig. 17 is not only intended
to provide an explanation for our results, but also to offer a
framework for future experimentation.

Path 1 - Metastasis (Fig. 17). In 1976 Kreider et al. (17)
demonstrated that the ascites form of the 13762 metastasizes at a
greater rate than the 13762 solid tumor and kills faster. Bogden
et al. (18) showed that by day 20 metastases from subcutaneous
grafts of the 13762 MT occurred to lungs and/or other viscera in
100% of the animals. In this same study it was shown that
excision of sc tumors on day 18-20 prolonged survival (mean
survival 48+7 days vs 66+8 days for the surgical group). Death
at 66+8 days was attributed to previous metastases in this
latter group. The reader will recall that surgical removal of
the 13762 MT lead to subsequent enhancement of PRL secretion only

after a time when metastases would have been firmly established
(i.e., 21 days). Furthermore, if path 1 in the model is correct,
then surgical removal of the primary at 7 and 14 days would not
be expected to affect PRL release since metastatic spread has
presumably not yet begun. The data in Fig. 7 are consistent with
this hypothesis.

MAMMARY TUMORS AND THE F-344 RAT: A MODEL

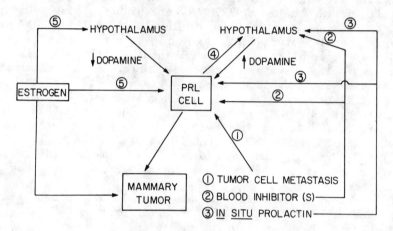

Fig. 17. A model to help explain PRL cell function in F-344 ♀
rats bearing the 13762 MT.

In 1975 Teears et al. (19) reviewed clinical details of 88
cases of carcinoma metastasizing to the human pituitary. Most
(70%) involved posterior lobe, 30% had anterior lobe involvement.
In these cases, breast and lung cancer were the most frequent
primary sites in women and men respectively. Teears et al. (19)
reviewed the literature on this apparently little-studied topic
and conclude that metastatic spread to the pituitary may be more
common than previously suspected. Since retrograde flow in the
pituitary-hypothalamus axis might very well involve vessels in the
neural capillary bed (20), micrometastases to this site could
conceivably alter PRL output.

Path 2 - Blood Borne Inhibitors (Fig. 17). The rat serum-
induced inhibition of PRL release in vitro is an entirely new and
somewhat provocative finding (e.g., Figs. 10, 11). This is a
repeatable result, but at this point it is not at all clear where

the inhibitory material comes from, nor whether it plays a physiological role in regulation of PRL release in vivo. If this
inhibitory material helps to explain the mechanism of tumor induced
suppression of PRL cell function, then RS from tumor bearing
animals might be expected to be more inhibitory than equivalent
amounts of normal rat serum. Studies which test this prediction
are currently in progress.

A particularly intriguing possibility for a blood-borne regulatory molecule affecting pituitary PRL comes from the studies by
Schlutz and Ebner in 1977 (21). They found, using a specific and
sensitive RIA, low but detectable levels of αlactalbumin in the
13762 solid MT. Their measured levels were 0.074 ng/ug protein.
Intracellular levels in the 3230 MT were higher, being 1.06 ng/ug
protein. In contrast, αlactalbumin levels in the 13762 MAT were
barely detectable, averaging 0.006 ng/10 ml packed cells. On the
other hand, serum αlactalbumin level in MAT bearing animals were
rather high. At 2 days after tumor implantation (a time at which
no ascites tumor is visible), levels were 40 ng/ml. By day 10,
these levels were 100 ng/ml. Thus PRL cell sizes get progressively
smaller in the 13762 MAT system at a time when αlactalbumin blood
levels are rising in approximately linear fashion. Serum from
rats bearing 3230 MT had less than 20 ng αlactalbumin/ml during
the first 20 days of tumor development. Recall that PRL cells of
the 3230 tumor bearing animal show minimal changes until day 28.

Qasba and Gullino (22) also measured αlactalbumin by RIA in the
3230 MT and reported a value of 0.86 ng/ug protein. They were unable to detect αlactalbumin in the 13762 MT. Based on the data
from both studies (21,22) it is obvious that tissue levels of α-
lactalbumin in the 13762 MT are extremely low but serum levels may
be high, implying rapid turnover of this protein. Horn and
Kano-Sueoha (23) have developed a transplantable MT in the AXC
rat which is dependent upon PRL for αlactalbumin activity.

It is becoming increasingly well established that agents which
affect PRL release do so by controlling turnover of hypothalamic
dopamine. It is therefore conceivable that blood borne factors
(rat serum, αlactalbumin, etc.) could act directly at the pituitary
level or else at a higher brain center to eventually modulate
(suppress) PRL cell function.

Path 3 - *In Situ* PRL (Fig. 17). The concept that PRL is
involved in controlling its own secretion (via the so-called
"short-loop" feedback system) enjoys considerable experimental
support. For example, host pituitary glands of animals bearing
PRL secreting pituitary tumors s.c. show suppressed PRL function
(24,25). Addition of ovine PRL to clonal 2B8 pituitary PRL cells
in culture will ↓ PRL release (26). Pathway 3 presupposes that

PRL produced from some ectopic site (mammary tumor?) could feed-back at the host pituitary directly, or via hypothalamic dopamine, to suppress PRL cell function. Ectopic PRL has been reported in lung and renal tumors (27) and in cells of the human gut (28). Ectopic hGH, in human mammary adenocarcinoma, has also reportedly been detected in breast cancer tissue as well as in ovaries of breast cancer patients (51 μg hGH/gm tissue (29). Others have detected hGH in lung tumors (30,31,32). Whether ectopic GH can inhibit release of PRL from tumor bearing rats is unknown.

Path 4 - Retrograde PRL Flow (Fig. 17). Within the last few years the notion that pituitary hormones, including PRL, might be delivered directly to the brain has met with some experimental support. Not only has the anatomical pathway been defined (20), but substantial quantities of PRL have been measured in the portal circulation (33) and observed by immunohistochemical techniques in hypothalamic nuclei (34). If future work substantiates this path-way, then the influence of tumor tissue on activity of this pathway would provide a mechanism for tumor-induced suppression of PRL cell function.

Path 5 - Estrogen (Fig. 17). That estrogen stimulates pituitary PRL cell function (synthesis, secretion and division) is axiomatic. The mechanism(s) by which this is accomplished is less clear, but many experimental results suggest direct action at the pituitary level. However, equally good evidence exists for site of action at the level of the hypothalamus (not reviewed here). Our data clearly support these E_2-mediated changes in PRL cell structure/function. The reader will recognize that the inhibitory effect of MT on PRL cells in the model (Fig. 17) are counter-balanced by the effects of estrogen.

The model in Fig. 17 was developed to help explain the results obtained with rats bearing 13762 and 3230 MT. How well does it apply to the human? Since our evidence shows some PRL cell hyper-trophy in the breast cancer patient, it would initially seem as if the model had little application to the human. However, hypo-physectomies were performed on these patients sometime after their primary tumor was removed. In this sense, then, results reflecting human PRL cell hypertrophy and increased hormone release in vitro (16) are somewhat analogous to those obtained with surgery and chemotherapy in the rat model.

Bogden has shown that administration of E_2 (140 μg/day/∿ 14 days) to 13762 MAT bearing animals prolongs average survival from 13.5+1.9 days to 15.6+3.5 days with some 20-30% of the animals surviving 23 days post-implantation (personal communication). It is of course tempting to attribute this kind of response to elevated PRL levels. In an extensive series of experiments in

the 13762 MAT cell system, we tested effects of hormone injection
on the tumor cell. We observed a) that E_2 treatment in vivo
resulted in reduction of tumor cell size, b) that E_2 treatment
increased protein synthesis in the tumor cells, c) that intracellular glycogen levels were lower after hormone treatment and
d) that in vivo administration of ovine PRL resulted in 3-5 fold
elevations of in vitro DNA synthesis as assessed by autoradiography. Finally, electronmicrographs of ascites tumor cells from
PRL vs saline injected animals (100 µg ovine PRL IP/day/10 days)
showed a large increase in the number of free polysomes and less
"fuzzy coat" material on the microvilli of the hormone-treated
cells (Fig. 18). Such data argue in favor of the hormone
responsiveness of the 13762 tumor cell. In light of the effects
of exogenous PRL/E_2 on size and membrane changes of the tumor
cell, we offer the suggestion that metastatic spread of tumor
cells is regulated, in part, by the activity of the pituitary PRL
cell.

Our studies have served to emphasize that changes in the
pituitary PRL and GH cells occur during mammary gland tumorigenesis.
They have also served to indicate that these changes may be correlated with tumor-specific characteristics (e.g., metastatic
incidence, chemotherapy sensitivity, and PRL responsiveness).
Furth et al. (35) have shown that pituitary PRL cells are first
detectable on day 15 in the developing rat; their number and intracellular content then increasing gradually throughout development.
On the other hand, plasma estrogen (probably of adrenal origin) are
first detectable on day 5, rise to a peak on day 19, and gradually
return to basal values by day 30. Furth suggests that it is
within this "window" that mammary tissue is particularly sensitive
and susceptible to events which eventually lead to tumor formation.
In this same vein, Kerdelhue et al. (36) have recently shown that
basal PRL and preovulatory gonadotropin surges are deranged in
the SD rat given DMBA, but not in the DMBA-resistant Wistar-Furth
rat. These exciting results implicate specific changes in the
hypothalamopituitary axis resulting from DMBA treatment.

Continued study of the PRL cell in these experimental animal
model systems will hopefully provide key clues to the initiation,
and therefore eventual control, of mammary gland tumorigenesis.

ACKNOWLEDGEMENTS

These studies were supported by grant CA23248 from the National
Cancer Institute, NIH. The able secretarial assistance of Mrs.
Linda Steyers is acknowledged.

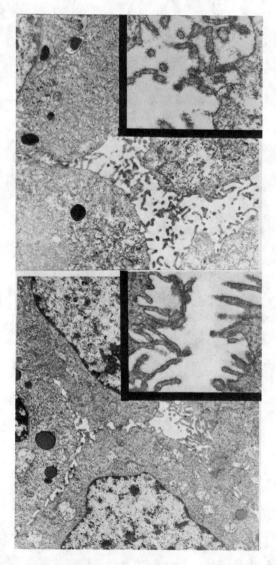

Fig. 18.   Electron micrographs of 13762 MAT cells taken from animals injected with either vehicle (top) or ovine PRL (100 µg IP/day/10 days) (bottom).

REFERENCES

1. C. W. Welsch and H. Nagasawa, Prolactin and Murine Mammary
    Tumorigenesis: A Review, Cancer Res. 37:951 (1977).
2. H. Nagasawa, Prolactin and Human Breast Cancer, Eur. J. Cancer
    15:267 (1979).
3. C. Huggins, G. Briziarelli, and H. Sutton, Jr., Rapid Induction
    of Mammary Carcinoma in the Rat and the Influence of Hormones
    on the Tumors, J. Exp. Med. 109:25 (1959).
4. C. Huggins, L. G. Grand, and F. P. Brillantes, Mammary Cancer
    Induced by a Single Feeding of Polynuclear Hydrocarbons
    and its Suppression, Nature (London) 189:204 (1961).
5. A. E. Bogden, Therapy in Experimental Breast Cancer Models, in
    "Breast Cancer," Vol. 2, W. L. McGuire, ed., Plenum
    Publishing Co. (1978).
6. A. E. Bogden, D. J. Taylor, Eric Y. H. Kuo, M. M. Mason, A.
    Speropoulos, The Effect of Perphenazine-Induced Serum Pro-
    Lactin Response on Estrogen-Primed Mammary Tumor-Host Systems,
    Cancer Res. 34:3018 (1974).
7. R. Hilf, C. Bell, H. Goldenberg, I. Michel, Effects of Fluphena-
    zine HCl on R3230 AC Mammary Carcinoma and Mammary Glands of
    the Rat, Cancer Res. 31:1111 (1971).
8. A. E. Bogden and D. J. Taylor, Predictive Mammary Tumor Test
    Systems for Experimental Chemotherapy, in "Breast Cancer:
    Trends in Research and Treatment," J. C. Heuson, W. H.
    Mattheiem, and M. Rozencweig, eds., Raven Press, New York
    (1976).
9. W. C. Hymer, W. H. Evans, J. Kraicer, A. Mastro, J. Davis, and
    E. Griswold, Enrichment of Cell Types from the Rat Adeno-
    hypophysis by Sedimentation at Unit Gravity, Endocrinol.
    92:275 (1973).
10. W. C. Hymer, J. Snyder, W. Wilfinger, N. Swanson, and J. A.
    Davis, Separation of Pituitary Mammotrophs from the Female Rat
    by Velocity Sedimentation at Unit Gravity, Endocrinol.
    94:107 (1974).
11. W. C. Hymer, Separation of Organelles and Cells from the
    Mammalian Adenohypophysis, in "The Anterior Pituitary,"
    Vol. 7, A. Tixier-Vidal and M. G. Farquhar, eds., Academic
    Press, New York (1975).
12. W. C. Hymer, R. Page, R. C. Kelsey, E. C. Augustine, W.
    Wilfinger, and M. Ciolkosz, Separated Somatotrophs: Their
    Use In Vitro and In Vivo, in Biochemical Endocrinology
    Series, K. W. McKerns and M. Jutisz, eds., Plenum
    Publishing Co., New York (1979).
13. W. W. Wilfinger, J. A. Davis, E. C. Augustine and W. C. Hymer,
    The Effects of Culture Conditions on Prolactin and Growth
    Hormone Production by Rat Anterior Pituitary Cells,
    Endocrinol. 105:530 (1979).

14. Y. N. Sinha, S. R. Baxter and W. P. Vanderlaan, Metabolic
     Clearance Rate of Prolactin During Various Physiological
     States in Mice with High and Low Incidences of Mammary
     Tumors, Endocrinol. 105:680 (1979).

15. W. C. Hymer, R. Page, R. C. Kelsey, E. C. Augustine and E.
     Hibbard, Implantable Artificial Pituitary Units Restores
     Growth of Hypophysectomized Rats. Abstract 229, The Endo-
     crine Society 61st Annual Meeting (1979).

16. W. C. Hymer, J. Snyder, W. W. Wilfinger, R. Bergland, B. Fisher
     and O. Pearsen, Characterization of Mammotrophs Separated
     from the Human Pituitary Gland, J. Natl. Cancer Inst. 57:995
     (1976).

17. J. W. Kreider, G. L. Bartlett and D. M. Purnell, Suitability of
     Rat Mammary Adenocarcinoma 13762 as a Model for BCG Immuno-
     therapy. J. Natl. Cancer Inst. 56:797 (1976).

18. A. E. Bogden, H. J. Esber, D. J. Taylor and J. H. Gray, Compara-
     tive Study on the Effects of Surgery, Chemotherapy and Immuno-
     therapy, Alone and in Combination, on Metastases of the 13762
     Mammary Adenocarcinoma, Cancer Res. 34:1627 (1974).

19. R. J. Teears and E. M. Silverman, Clinicopathologic Review of
     88 Cases of Carcinoma Metastatic to the Pituitary Gland,
     Cancer 36:216 (1975).

20. R. M. Bergland and R. B. Page, Can the Pituitary Secrete Directly
     to the Brain? Endocrinol. 102:1325 (1978).

21. G. S. Schlutz and K. E. Ebner, Measurement of α-Lactalbumin in
     Serum and Mammary Tumors of Rats by RIA, Cancer Res. 37:4539
     (1977).

22. P. K. Qasba and P. M. Gullino, α-Lactalbumin Content of Rat
     Mammary Carcinomas and the Effects of Pituitary Stimulation,
     Cancer Res. 37:3792 (1977).

23. T. M. Horn and T. Kano-Suevka, Effects of Hormones on Growth
     and α-Lactalbumin Activity in the Transplantable Rat Mammary
     Tumor MCCLX, Cancer Res. 39:5028 (1979).

24. R. MacLeod and J. E. Lehmeyer, Restoration of Prolactin
     Synthesis and Release by the Administration of Monoaminergic
     Blocking Agents to Pituitary Tumor-Bearing Rats, Cancer
     Res. 33:2903 (1973).

25. I. Nakayama and P. A. Nickerson, Suppression of Anterior
     Pituitary in Rats Bearing a Transplantable Growth Hormone
     and Prolactin-Secreting Tumor (MtT/W10). Endocrinology
     92:516 (1973).

26. D. C. Herbert, H. Ishikawa, and E. G. Rennels, Evidence for the
     Autoregulation of Hormone Secretion by Prolactin, Endocrinol.
     104:97 (1979).

27. L. H. Rees, Endocrine Manifestations of Cancer, S. Afr. Cancer
     Bull. 23:60 (1979).

28. F. W. Stevens and C. Shaw, Prolactin and the Human Gut, Ir.
     J. Med. Sci. 148:26 (1979).

29. A. Kaganowicz, N. H. Farkouh, A. G. Frantz and A. U. Blaustein,
     Ectopic Human Growth Hormone in Ovaries and Breast Cancer,
     J. Clin. Endocrinol. Metab. 48:5 (1979).

30. D. P. Camerson, H. G. Burger, D. M. DeKretger, K. J. Catt,
     and J. B. Best, On the Presence of Immunoreactive Growth
     Hormone in a Biochogenic Carcinoma, Aust. Ann. Med. 18:143
     (1969).

31. M. Sparagana, G. Phillips, C. Hoffman, and L. Kucera, Ectopic
     Growth Hormone Syndrome Associated with Lung Cancer,
     Metabolism 20:730 (1971).

32. C. Beck and H. G. Burger, Evidence for the Presence of Immuno-
     reactive Growth Hormone in Cancers of the Lung and Stomach,
     Cancer 30:75 (1972).

33. C. Oliver, R. S. Mical, and J. C. Porter, Hypothalami-
     pituitary Vasculature: Evidence for Retrograde Blood Flow
     in the Pituitary Stalk, Endocrinol. 101:598 (1977).

34. K. Fuxe, T. Hokfelt, P. Eneroth, J.A. Gustafsson, and P.
     Skett, Prolactin-like Immunoreactivity; Localiztion in
     Nerve Terminals of Rat Hypothalamus, Science 196:89 (1977)

35. J. Furth, H. J. Esber, A. E. Bogden and P. Moz, Evolution of
     Pituitary Tropic Cells and Estrogens in Relation to Differen-
     titation of the Mammary Gland and Mammary Tumorigenesis,
     Abstract 366.

MAMMALIAN CELL PROLIFERATION IS REGULATED BY THE SYNERGISTIC ACTIONS OF MULTIPLE GROWTH FACTORS

W. J. Pledger, C. A. Hart, and W. R. Wharton

Department of Pharmacology and Cancer Research Center
University of North Carolina Medical School
Chapel Hill, North Carolina 27514

Normal mammalian fibroblasts require serum for growth in culture. When serum is withdrawn from the culture medium or when a high cell density is reached, normal fibroblastic cells become growth arrested in a distinct region (Go) of the cell cycle with a G_1 content of DNA. When serum is added to quiescent growth-arrested fibroblasts, DNA synthesis begins after a 12 hour lag. Viral transformation of fibroblasts lessens their serum requirement and can alter the ability of the cells to enter the normal growth arrested state.

Serum provides hormones and growth factors that enable cells to sustain their growth and replication (1). It has now been recognized that some serum growth factors control distinct regulatory processes within the cell cycle (2). The identification of the serum factors required for growth will enable the investigation of the regulatory events that control the cell cycle. Such investigations can lead to an understanding of how transformation, by either viral or chemical means, alters normal regulatory processes.

Recently, it has been proposed that hormones and serum growth factors control an ordered sequence of events that result in the commitment of quiescent growth-arrested cells to undergo DNA synthesis and ultimately cell division (2). Commitment is defined as the point in the cell cycle when mitogenic stimuli can be removed and the cells will continue to undergo DNA synthesis. The point of commitment for normal fibroblasts is believed to immediately precede the S phase(3,4). In general, the events in the G_1 phase are thought to establish the rate of cellular replication within a population of cells (5). The aim of our work is to elucidate the regulatory events in the G_1 phase of the cell cycle and charac-

terize how serum factors regulate these putative events and define
the process by which transformation alters the normal regulation.

SERUM CONTROLS TWO DISTINCT STAGES OF CELL REPLICATION

Serum contains both platelet -derived growth factors and plasma-
derived growth factors (2). Platelet-derived growth factor (PDGF)
has been shown to be the serum mitogen required to stimulate fibroblast growth in culture medium supplemented with platelet-poor
plasma (PPP) (6,7,8). Plasma is the fluid portion of blood and
does not support the growth of fibroblasts. When serum is formed
from blood, platelet-derived growth factor is released from the
platelets into the fluid. Platelet-derived growth factor (PDGF)
has been recently purified to homogeneity (9,10) and is a cationic
peptide (pI 9.7) with a molecular weight of 30,000 daltons as determined with non-reducing polyacrylimide electrophoresis.

Even though the factors in platelet-poor plasma do not initiate cell replication or support growth, they do act synergistically with PDGF to stimulate DNA synthesis in quiescent density-
dependent growth inhibited Balb/c-3T3 cells (Figure 1). Various
concentrations of a heat treated (100° for 10 minutes) platelet extract were added to medium in several concentrations of PPP and
exposed to cultures of confluent Balb/c-3T3 cells. The percentage

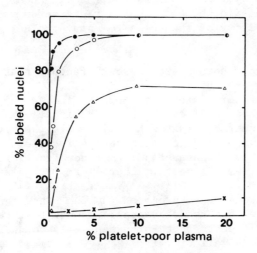

Figure 1: Effect of concentration of platelet-poor plasma on
platelet extract-induced DNA synthesis. Platelet extract (●, 100
ug; 0, 10 ug; △, 5 ug; or X, 0 ug) was added to cultures in 0.2 ml
of medium containing ^{3}H dThd and various concentrations of platelet-poor plasma. Cultures were fixed 36 hr later and processed for
autoradiography (2).

of cells synthesizing DNA within 36 hours was determined. The percentage of cells stimulated to synthesize DNA was a function of
both the amount of platelet extract and the platelet-poor plasma
(Figure 1).

Quiescent density-inhibited Balb/c-3T3 cells could be treated
transiently with platelet-derived growth factor and then exposed
to plasma after which the cells entered into DNA synthesis. Figure
2 illustrates that with increasing concentration of PDGF the cells
required a shorter time of exposure to the PDGF to become able to
respond to plasma-derived factors and enter S phase. Platelet-
derived growth factor makes cells "competent" to respond to plasma-
derived factors (2). Competence formation is temperature-dependent
in that the time necessary to render a population of cells competent
was shorter at 37°C than at 20°C, and at 4°C, treatment with PDGF
had almost no effect.

Once quiescent cells have been made competent by exposure to
PDGF, the competent cells are still 12 hours from entry into S
phase. Figure 3 shows that when cells are made competent, plasma

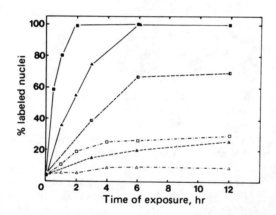

Figure 2: Temperature dependence of platelet extract-induced commitment to DNA synthesis. Cultures were incubated with the platelet extract in 0.2 ml of medium at 37° (■ , 100 ug; ▲, 50 ug), 25°
(▣, 100 ug; ▲ , 50 ug) or 4° (□ , 100 ug; △ , 50 ug). At the indicated times the platelet extract was removed and the cultures
were washed with 28 mM 2-mercaptoethanol followed by medium. The
cultures were placed in 0.2 ml of medium containing ^{3}H dThd and 5%
platelet-poor plasma. Cultures were fixed and processed for autoradiography at 36 hr (2).

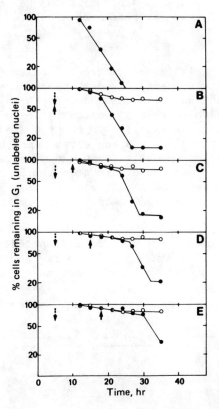

<u>Figure 3</u>: The stability of the platelet extract-induced committed
state. (A) Cultures were treated with 50 ug of platelet extract
at 37° in 0.2 ml of medium containing 5% platelet-poor plasma and
^{3}H dThd. At the indicated times, cultures were fixed and processed for autoradiography. (B-E) Cultures were treated with 50
ug of platelet extract in 0.2 ml of medium for 5 hr (↓) at 37°,
washed and returned to 0.2 ml of medium containing ^{3}H dThd but
lacking platelet-poor plasma. At the times indicated by (↑) the
medium was supplemented with platelet-poor plasma (●, 5%; 0, 0.25%).
The cultures were fixed and processed for autoradiography at time
intervals (2).

can be added after various times and the cells enter DNA synthesis
12 hours after the addition of plasma. These data indicate that
once cells were rendered competent, they remained in the competent
state for at least 13 hours.

Plasma derived factors promote the "progression" of competent
cells through the cell cycle. Only the cells rendered competent
undergo progression in plasma. The rate of entry of competent

cells into S phase, but not the 12 hour lag before DNA synthesis, was dependent on the concentration of platelet-poor plasma (2).

Two distinct plasma-dependent growth-arrest points were located in the 12 hour lag between competence formation and entry into DNA synthesis. PDGF-treated competent cells were exposed to 5% plasma for 10 hrs. Many of these cells (40%) synthesized DNA, but cell entry into the S phase ceased 5 hrs after the initial plasma was withdrawn. A second plasma treatment stimulated those cells that had not become committed to DNA synthesis by the first plasma exposure to synthesize DNA after a lag of only 6 hrs. (Figure 4C).

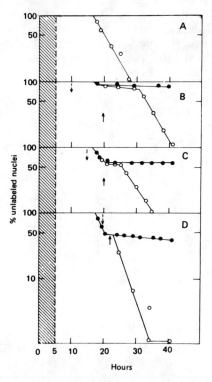

Figure 4: Sequential growth arrest points in the plasma-dependent progression of Balb/c-3T3 cells through G_0/G_1. Cultures were treated with 50 ug of the platelet extract for 5 hr at 37° (hatched bar) in 0.2 ml of medium. The platelet extract was then removed, and the cells were washed and returned to medium (0.2 ml) containing ^{3}H dThd and 5% plasma. (A) At the indicated times, cultures were fixed and processed for autoradiography. (B-D) At the indicated times (↓), the cultures were transferred to medium (0.2 ml) lacking plasma but containing ^{3}H dThd (●, no further additions; 0, at the times indicated (↑), the cultures were again transferred to medium (0.2 ml) containing 5% plasma and ^{3}H dThd). The cultures were fixed and processed for autoradiography at timed intervals (3).

Thus, in the absence of plasma some cells were arrested at a mid-
point in Go/G_1 6 hrs. from the S phase.

In similar experiments PDGF-treated cells were exposed to
plasma for 15 hrs. When the plasma was withdrawn, 56% of the cells
entered S phase; however, the remainder of the population became
growth arrested within 1-2 hrs. after the plasma was withdrawn.
This arrested population immediately began to enter S phase when
plasma was restored to the culture (Figure 4D). Therefore, a
growth-arrested point, dependent on plasma factors, was observed at
an apparent point between G_1 and S phase. The point 6 hrs. before S
phase was termed "V" and the point between G_1 and S phase was termed
"W". The "W" growth-arrest point requires protein synthesis to
allow cells to progress through G_1 and into S phase. The diagram
in Figure 5 illustrates the PDGF- and plasma-dependent growth-
arrest points in the Go/G_1 transition to S phase.

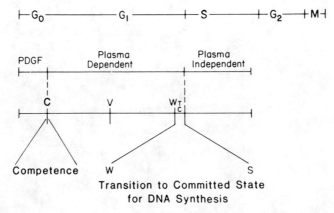

Figure 5: Model of several sequential events in Go/G_1 that precede
DNA synthesis (3).

These data indicate that serum contains two separate sets of
growth factors that regulate two distinct stages of Go/G_1 transition and commitment to DNA synthesis. The first stage is controlled
by platelet-derived growth factor. This stage is termed "competence"
and must occur before the second phase. The second phase is termed
"progression" and the events of regulation in this phase are regulated by plasma-derived factors. Because quiescent, density-arrested cells must become competent before they can undergo progression,
PDGF must initiate entry into the cell cycle.

COMPOUNDS THAT RENDER CELLS COMPETENT AND THE INVOLVEMENT OF PREF-
ERENTIAL SYNTHESIS

PDGF, as has been discussed, acts synergistically with plasma
to initiate DNA synthesis in quiescent cells. In fact, a transient
exposure of PDGF to quiescent cells allowed these cells when placed
in plasma-supplemented media to synthesize DNA. This has allowed
the development of a complementation test for various compounds
known to initiate growth by exposing such substances to quiescent
cells and then placing the treated cells into plasma supplemented
medium anddetermining the percent of cells that synthesize DNA.
Fibroblast growth factor, calcium phosphate, and wounding a confluent monolayer act synergistically with plasma factors to initiate
DNA synthesis in quiescent Balb/c-3T3 cells (4).

Treatment of quiescent Balb/c-3T3 cells with pure PDGF induced
the preferential synthesis of five cytoplasmic proteins (M.W. 20K,
29K, 42K, 60K and 72K detected by SDS-PAGE under reducing conditions)
as shown in Figure 6. Quiescent Balb/c-3T3 cells were treated with

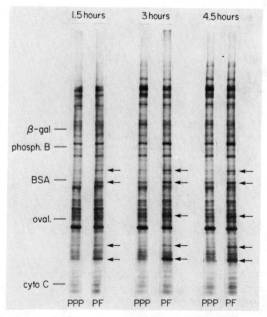

Figure 6: The incorporation of ^{35}S-methionine into NP40 soluble
Balb/c-3T3 cells after treatment with PDGF or PPP. Proteins were
analyzed on a 6-18% exponential acrylamide gel gradient. PF represents 25 ug partial purified PDGF activity and PPP was 5%. The
arrows indicate PF proteins that appear to be preferentially synthesized compared to 5% PPP.

PDGF or plasma supplemented media (2% normal methionine concentration) and at various times incubated with ^{35}S-methionine. After ^{35}S-methionine incorporation the cells were solubilized in 1% NP40 and this non-nuclear extract was boiled 3 minutes in SDS and mercaptoethanol. Exponential (6-18%) acrylamide gels were employed and after electrophoresis gels were processed through fluorography (11).

The 20K PDGF-induced proteins were observed within 40 minutes after PDGF addition. This protein was observed after treatment of quiescent cells with calf serum, pure PDGF, or FGF but were not observed observed after the addition of plasma, insulin, or epidermal growth factor to quiescent cells. The preferential synthesis of this protein (20K) is associated with competence formation.

PLASMA-DERIVED FACTORS REQUIRED FOR PROGRESSION

Quiescent 3T3 cells were exposed briefly to PDGF and trans-

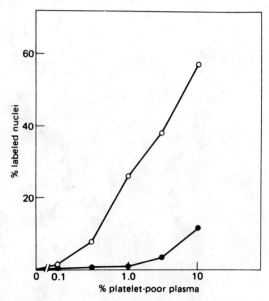

Figure 7: Plasma prepared from hypophysectomized rats is deficient in progression activity. Density-arrested 3T3 cells were treated with 57 ug of partially purified PDGF for 3 hrs. The culture medium was removed. Cell monolayers were washed once with saline containing 28 mM 2-mercaptoethanol and once with saline only. Fresh growth medium supplemented with ^{3}H dThd (5 uCi/ml; 1 Ci=3.7 x 10^{10} bequerels) was added to the cultures. Plasma from hypophysectomized (0) or normal (0) rats was added to the indicated concentration. After a 24 hr. incubation at 37°C, the monolayers were fixed and processed for autoradiography.

ferred to media containing plasma from a normal rat or plasma from
a hypophysectomized rat. Plasma from the hypophysectomized rat had
only 1/20th the progression activity as that found in normal rat
plasma (Figure 7).

These data indicate that a normal plasma-derived factor under
the control of the pituitary was required for progression through
G_1. When competent cells exposed to PDGF were placed in plasma
from a hypophysectomized rat, normal progression could be restored
by the addition of somatomedin C (Figure 8). These data indicate
that somatomedin C at a physiological dose (10^{-11}M) restored progression activity in the plasma from hypophysectomized rats. Insulin restored the progression activity when used at pharmacological
doses. It has recently been shown that when competent cells undergo progression in plasma from a hypophysectomized animal the cell
cycle becomes arrested at a point 6 hrs from S phase (V point)
(13). Insulin-like activity (ILA) and multiplication-stimulating
activity (MSA) are members of the somatomedin peptide family.
These peptides also restore progression activity to the plasma
from hypophysectomized rats (12).

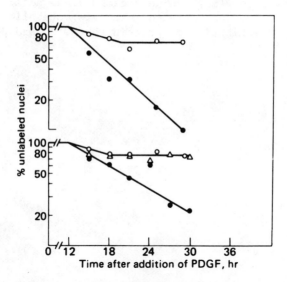

Figure 8: The addition of pure somatomedin C to hypophysectomized
rat plasma restores progression factor activity. Density arrested
3T3 cells were treated with PDGF, washed, and placed in ^{3}H dThd
medium as in Figure 1. The cells were fixed at intervals and processed for autoradiography. (Upper) The culture medium was supplemented with 3% plasma from control (●) or hypophysectomized (○) rats.
(Lower) Culture medium was supplemented with 3% plasma from hypophysectomized animals (○), 3% plasma from hypophysectomized
animals plus pure somatomedin C at 3 ng/ml ●), or pure somatomedin
C at 3 ng/ml only (△).

These experiments show that cells made competent by exposure
to PDGF not only required somatomedin C but also required other
factors in hypophysectomized rat plasma in order to progress
through the G_1 phase. Data from our laboratory and also from the
laboratory of Dr. C.D. Stiles indicates that epidermal growth factor,
transferrin, somatomedin C, and either bulk-non-specific protein
(such as ovalbumin) or an inhibitor of proteolytic activity can
provide the needed regulatory peptides to allow competent cells
to progress through G_1 and enter S phase. These factors are very
similar to the factors needed for several cell lines to grow in
serum-free medium as has been defined by Sato (14, 15).

Once cells are made competent, factors derived from plasma
allow progression until the cell has become committed to DNA synthesis. It has been suggested that commitment to DNA synthesis may
occur at a point in the cell cycle between the G_1 phase and S
phase (3, 4).

Recently, Wharton, et al., have demonstrated that methylgly-
oxal bis-(guanylhydrazone) (mGBG), a potent inhibitor of polyamine
synthesis, reversibly blocks cell cycle progression in G_1 (16).
mGBG inhibits S-adenosylmethionine decarboxylase activity and
Wharton, et al., have demonstrated that this metabolic block was
accompanied by an inhibition of protein synthesis and decreased

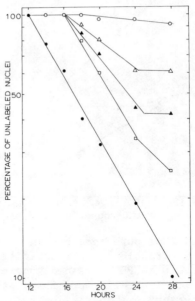

Figure 9: Quiescent cells were treated for 12 hrs. with PDGF, PPP
alone (●-●) or with 30 uM mGBG. The cultures treated with mGBG
were then washed and fresh media containing either media alone (0-0),
or 1.0% (△-△), 2.5% (▲-▲) or 5% (□-□) PPP was added. At the
times indicated the cells were fixed and processed for autoradiography.

stability of ribosomal-RNA (17). When quiescent cells that were
stimulated with serum to undergo cell replication in the presence
of mGBG are removed from the mGBG after 12 hrs. and placed in plasma
supplemented medium, they enter DNA synthesis after a lag of 4 hrs.
The rate of entry into the S phase, but not the lag time, was dependent on the plasma concentration (Figure 9).

It can also be seen in these data that once cells are removed
from the medium containing mGBG and placed in non-supplemented
medium, they do not progress through S phase. The addition of
somatomedin C to medium at physiological concentrations or insulin
at higher concentrations allows cells to commit to DNA synthesis
(Figure 10). We have tested epidermal growth factor, fibroblast
growth factor, PDGF, spermidine, and spermine and these compounds
did not allow cells after they were released from the mGBG block
to enter S phase. Clearly, somatomedin C alone allows progressing
cells to undergo commitment to DNA synthesis.

VIRAL TRANSFORMATION OF FIBROBLASTIC CELLS ABROGATES PDGF REQUIRE-
MENTS AND ALTERS DEPENDENCY ON PLASMA FACTORS

Multiple lines of evidence point to the conclusion that the
elucidation of the mechanism of action for the various growth factors demonstrated to be required for cell replication is important

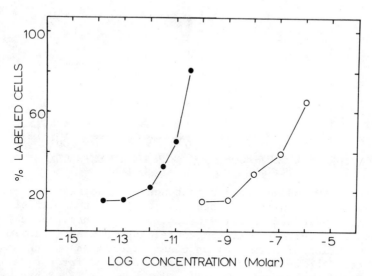

Figure 10: Cells were treated for 12 hrs. with PDGF, PPP and 30 uM
mGBG. The cultures were then washed and the indicated concentrations of either somatomedin C (●-●) or insulin (0-0) were added
and the number of cells which were labeled in the next 24 hrs.
was then determined.

in understanding neoplastic formation. Firstly, when normal fibroblastic cells are transformed with DNA or RNA tumorgenic virus the
transformants grow in platelet-poor plasma, whereas the normal
cells do not (18). Therefore, the transformation process abrogated
the requirement of the normal cells for platelet-derived growth
factor to initiate cell replication. This same observation can be
made a different way. When normal Balb/c-3T3 cells are plated at
low densities in plasma supplemented medium they do not grow. In
these conditions the cells undergo growth arrest and become quiescent. However, when plasma maintained quiescent cells were infected
with SV40 these quiescent cells initiated growth and were able to
undergo multiple rounds of cell division.

SV40 induces both competence and progression. Density arrested
3T3 cells replicate their DNA and divide after infection with SV40
(18). The mitogenic response of 3T3 cells to infection with SV40
is strictly a function of the virus multiplicity of infection since
increasing the concentration of plasma or exposing the cells to increasing concentrations of PDGF did not enhance DNA synthesis in the
SV40- infected cells (Figure 11).

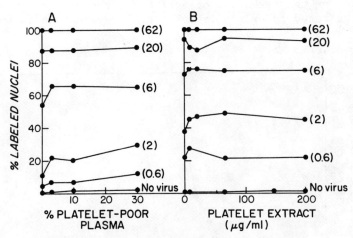

Figure 11: SV40 induces both competence and progression. (Left)
SV40 was added to density-arrested 3T3 cells at the multiplicity
of infection indicated in parentheses. After 3 hrs. the cells were
washed and transferred to medium containing ^{3}H dThd (5 uCi/ml) and
the concentration of normal human plasma indicated on the abscissa.
After 36 hrs. the cells were fixed and processed for autoradiography.
(Right) Density-arrested 3T3 cells were exposed for 3 hrs. to the
concentration of PDGF indicated on the abscissa. The medium was
removed and the cell monolayers were washed. Fresh medium containing ^{3}H dThd and 0.25% normal plasma was added to all cultures together with SV40 at the multiplicity of infection indicated in

parentheses. A supplement of 0.25% normal human plasma sustains cell attachment to the tissue culture dish but is not sufficient to cause progression of PDGF-treated cells into S phase. After 36 hrs, all cultures were fixed andprocessed for autoradiography.

DISCUSSION

The mechanism whereby cells that normally depend on serum growth factors for continued replication become independent of these factors is unknown. The temporal analysis of factors needed for the mitogenic response of fibroblasts may allow the normal biochemical processes needed for growth control to be documented. Once the growth factors and their ordered requirement in cell cycle traverse is learned, then their mechanisms of action can be investigated. Since transformation alters the normal requirement of serum factors for growth, a comparison of the normal cells to transformed cells can lead to the understanding of how transformed or neoplastic cells override growth dependency on mitogenic signals. These findings will enable us to determine how transformation mimicks the action of growth factors or overrides their requirement by a different mechanism other than the normal sequence of regulatory steps.

This research was supported by NIH grants CA 24193 and CA 16084. WRW is a recipient of an NIH fellowship GM 1477.

REFERENCES

1. Hormones and Cell Culture: Cold Spring Harbor Conferences on
       Cell Proliferation, Vol 6 1979. G. H. Sato and R. Ross.
       Cold Spring Harbor Laboratory, New York. pp. 982.
2. Pledger, W. J., C. D. Stiles, H. N. Antoniades, and C. D. Scher.
       1977 Induction of DNA synthesis in Balb/c-3T3 cells by serum
       components: Reevaluation of the commitment process. Proc.
       Natl. Acad. Sci. 74:4481.
3. _____ 1978. An ordered sequence of events is required before
       Balb/c-3T3 cells become committed to DNA synthesis. Proc.
       Natl. Acad. Sci. 75:2839.
4. Brooks, R. Regulation of the fibroblast cell cycle by serum.1976
       Nature 260.248
5. Pardee, A.B., R. Dubrow, J. L. Hamlin, R. E. Kletzien. (1978)
       Animal Cell Cycle. Ann. Rev. Biochem. 47:715.
6. Balk, S. 1971. Calcium as a regulator of normal but not of
       transformed chicken fibroblasts in a plasma-containing
       medium. Proc. Natl. Acad. Sci. 68:271
7. Kohler, N. and A. Lipton. 1974 Platelets as a source of a
       fibroblast growth-promoting activity. Exp. Cell Res. 87:297
8. Ross. R.,J. Glomset, B. Kariya, and L. Harker. 1974. A platelet-
       dependent serum factor that stimulates the proliferation of
       arterial smooth muscle cells in vitro. Proc. Natl. Acad. Sci.

arterial smooth muscel cells in vitro. Proc. Natl. Acad. Sci. 71:1207.

9. Antoniades, H. N., C. D. Scher, C. D. Stiles 1979. Purification of human platelet-derived growth factor. Proc. Natl Acad Sci. 76:1809

10. Heldin, C. H., B. Westermark, A. Wasteson 1979. Platelet-derived growth factor: Purification and partial characterization. Proc. Natl. Acad. Sci. 76:3722

11. Bonner, W. M., R. A. Laskey 1974. A Film Detection method for tritium-labelled proteins and nucleic acids in polyacrylamide gels. Eur. J. Biochem. 46:83.

12. Stiles, C.D. G.T. Capone, C. D. Scher, H. N. Antoniades, J. J. Van Wyk, and W. J. Pledger 1979b. Dual control of cell growth by somatomedins and platelet-derived growth factor. Proc. Natl. Acad. Sci. 76:1279

13. Stiles, C. D., W. J. Pledger, J. J. Van Wyk, H. N. Antoniades, C. D. Scher 1979. Hormonal control of early events in the Balb/c-3T3 cell cycle; commitment to DNA synthesis. Hormones and Cell Culture. Cold Spring Harbor Laboratory, New York, p. 425.

14. Serrero, G. R., D. B. McClure, G. H. Sato 1979. Growth of mouse 3T3 fibroblast in serum-free, hormone-supplemented media. Hormones and Cell Culture. Cold Spring Harbor Laboratory, New York, p. 523.

15. Bottenstein, J. E., G. H. Sato, J. P. Mather 1979. Growth of neuroepethelial-derived cell lines in serum-free hormone-supplemented media. Hormones and Cell Culture. Cold Spring Harbor Laboratory, New York, p. 531.

16. Wharton, W. R., J. Van Wyk, W. J. Pledger 1980. Inhibition of polyamine synthesis leads to a block of Balb/c-3T3 cells in late G_1. Submitted.

17. Wharton, W. R., J. Van Wyk, W. J. Pledger, 1980. Effects of methyglyoxal bis-(guanylhydrazone) on macromolecular synthesis and stability in Balb/c-3T3 cells. Submitted.

18. Scher, C. D., W. J. Pledger, P. Martin, H. N. Antoniades, and C. D. Stiles 1978. Transforming viruses directly reduce the cellular growth requirement for a platelet derived growth factor. J. Cell. Physiol. 97:371

DEFECTIVE STEROID RECEPTORS IN A GLUCOCORTICOID RESISTANT

CLONE OF A HUMAN LEUKEMIC CELL LINE

J. M. Harmon, T. J. Schmidt,* and E. B. Thompson

Laboratory of Biochemistry
Division of Cancer Biology and Diagnosis
National Cancer Institute
National Institutes of Health
Bethesda, MD 20205

INTRODUCTION

The ability of steroid hormones to elicit changes in cell physiology, metabolism and differentiation, and their role in both developmental and homeostatic regulation has prompted extensive study of the mechanism of action of these hormones. These studies have defined a general pathway for the action of steroid hormones whose first step is the binding of the steroid to a specific receptor localized in the cell cytoplasm. This steroid receptor complex then undergoes a conformational alteration ("activation") and enters the nucleus where either through direct interaction with chromatin, or through an acceptor mediated interaction with chromatin, specific changes in gene transcription are produced. The specific transcripts of these genes when expressed as proteins produce the ultimate observed cellular responses.

While specific receptors have been identified for each class of steroid hormone, the manner in which they regulate gene expression is basically unknown. In large measure this is due to the difficulties encountered in obtaining these receptors in pure form in sufficient quantity for adequate study of their molecular properties. Thus while significant progress has been made in defining the

---

* Present address: Fels Research Institute
                     Temple University Medical School
                     Philadelphia, PA   19140

structure and organization of specific, steroid regulated genes, comparatively little progress has been made in identifying how steroid receptor complexes influence the expression of these genes.

One approach we have recently pursued to gain insight into receptor function is to isolate mutant cell lines containing altered or defective receptors[1,2] and to thus correlate specific alterations in receptor properties with specific loss of function. To do this requires a specific steroid response whose expression or lack thereof provides a basis for detection of responding or non-responding cells. Such a response is glucocorticoid-induced lymphocytolysis. It has been shown for the mouse S49 and WEH1-7 lymphoma tissue culture cell lines that steroid resistant mutants can be isolated which are completely resistant to the cytolytic effects of glucocorticoids.[3,4] These mutants either lack receptor entirely (r^-) or contain receptors with a reduced capacity for nuclear transfer in the cell and a reduced affinity for DNA-cellulose in vitro (r^+,nt^-).[5-7] An additional class of receptor defects ($r^+,nt^{\overline{1}}$) involves receptors with an unusually high capacity for nuclear translocation and a greater than normal affinity for DNA cellulose.[6] Thus receptor defects in the mouse cell line seem to define the end-points of receptor action; either no binding of steroid or defective interaction with the nucleus. Clearly, additional receptor defects would serve to further characterize the mechanism of action of steroid receptors and define their intrinsic properties. Based on our present knowledge of glucocorticoid receptors such mutations might affect the interconversion of the steroid binding and non-binding forms of the receptor,[8,9] the ability of the receptor to undergo "activation" or the affinity of the receptor for steroid. Intrinsic to any discussion of altered receptor function is the assumption that there may be modulators or regulatory components of the receptor, as yet unidentified, mutations in which could lead to defective receptor function, and that isolation of steroid resistant mutants could indirectly identify such regulatory components.

ISOLATION OF GLUCOCORTICOID-RESISTANT HUMAN LYMPHOBLASTS

When the human T-cell-derived lymphoblastoid cell line CEM-7 is exposed to 10^{-6} M dexamethasone a classic lympholytic response is observed.[10,11] Cell growth is slowed and cell death is observed 18-24 hours after exposure, with cells becoming irreversibly arrested in G_1 at the same time.[11] The extent of the lympholytic response is essentially total. Microscopic examination of steroid treated cultures reveals no viable cells. However, if sufficient (>10^5) cells are plated in semisolid medium in the presence of 10^{-6} M dexamethasone a limited number of colonies are formed.[12] When these colonies are isolated and returned to culture they are found to be completely resistant to steroid. In addition, their plating efficiencies in

the presence of steroid are identical to those for untreated controls, suggesting that steroid resistance is a stable phenotype. As
was the case for the steroid-resistant mutants isolated from the
mouse cell lines S49 and WEH1-7, Luria Dulbrück fluctuation analysis[13] established that resistance is acquired randomly in the absence of selective pressure. Analysis of the data from several such
experiments has placed the rate of acquisition of this phenotype
between $2\text{-}3 \times 10^{-5}$/cell/generation, a rate consistent with spontaneous mutation in a haploid or functionally heterozygous locus.[12]

    Using this information we were able to isolate 54 steroid re-
sistant subclones of CEM-C7 whose independent origin could be guar-
anteed. The scheme for the isolation of these clones is shown in
Figure 1. A culture of CEM-C7 is diluted to a concentration of
0.2 cells/ml and distributed in 0.2 ml aliquots into microtiter
wells. Ten days later a small, presumably steroid sensitive,
colony ($\sim 10^3$ cells) was picked and redistributed to several flasks.
Each of these flasks is then grown to $\sim 2 \times 10^5$ cells/ml and then
cells from each flask are plated in semisolid medium in the presence
of 10^{-6} M dexamethasone. One resistant colony from each set of
plates corresponding to each flask inoculated was selected for further study. The steroid sensitivity of the initial subclone of
CEM-C7 was determined by its growth inhibition in medium containing
steroid. Since the spontaneous rate of acquisition of the resistant
phenotype is $\sim 2\text{-}3 \times 10^{-5}$ per cell per generation and since only 50
cells were inoculated into each flask when the sensitive subclone
was divided it is certain that no steroid resistant cells were present in the initial inoculations. Thus, any steroid resistant cell
which gives rise to colony in the presence of steroid must have
arisen during cell proliferation to 2×10^6 cells/flasks. Therefore, by choosing only one colony from each set of plates corresponding to a single flask no two colonies can contain resistant
cells from a common resistant precursor.

CHARACTERIZATION OF STEROID RESISTANT MUTANTS

Steroid Receptor Content

The preponderance of the steroid resistant mutants isolated from S49
and WEH1-7 contain no steroid binding activity.[5-7] In contrast,
each of the 54 steroid resistant subclones of the CEM-C7 cell line
contains at least some residual binding activity. Table 1 shows the
relative receptor content of the 54 steroid subclones. All but five
of these clones contain significantly less receptor than the sensitive parent with the majority (28/54) having between 10 and 30% of
wild-type levels. Since these assays were performed at a single
(5×10^{-8} M) concentration of steroid, one possibility for the reduced binding observed is that these resistant clones contain receptors with decreased affinity for steroid.

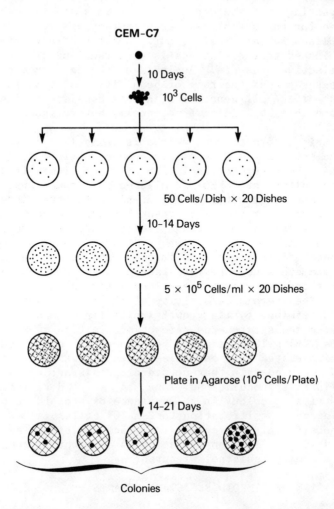

Fig. 1. Schematic representation of the isolation of independent steroid resistant subclones of CEM-C7. A single cell of CEM-C7 was grown to a small colony of about 1000 cells. This colony was divided into 20 separate cultures, and each culture was grown to a density of 5 x 10^5 cells/ml. Cells were plated in semisolid medium (indicated by cross hatches) and in the presence of 10^{-6} M dexamethasone and colonies appearing after 14-21 days were isolated.

Table 1. Receptor Content of Spontaneous Steroid Resistant Mutants

% of Wild-Type[1]	Number of Clones
0	0
1-10	1
10-20	13
20-30	15
30-40	5
40-50	7
50-60	4
60-70	2
70-80	1
80-90	1
90-100	3
>100	2

[1]Receptor content was measured using a whole cell binding assay. Cells were incubated for 1 h at 37°C with 5 x 10^{-8} M ^{3}H-dexamethasone in tricine buffered RPMI 1640 with 10% fetal calf serum. Free steroid was removed by washing cells in Hanks Balanced Salt Solution and competable binding was determined as the difference between incubations containing either no or a 200-fold excess of unlabeled steroid. Results are expressed as a percent of the steroid sensitive parent cell line.

Measurements of affinity of receptor for dexamethasone in both whole cell, and cell-free binding assays for three steroid resistant mutants 3R7, 3R43, and 4R4 are shown in Table 2. Although some differences in affinity may exist between the receptors from the resistant mutants and those from CEM-C7 these differences are not enough to explain the lower receptor content of the mutants measured in the whole cell assay at 5 x 10^{-8} M dexamethasone. Indeed calculations of the number of receptors per cell based on Scatchard plots[14] of concentration dependent binding curves show the mutants to have considerably less receptor than the wild-type. More importantly, these data demonstrate that at 10^{-6} M dexamethasone, the concentration used to select resistant clones, receptors of the mutants would have been completely occupied, thus eliminating the possibility that simple differences in affinity for steroid can account for steroid resistance.

Table 2. Affinity of Receptors from Steroid Resistant Mutants for
Dexamethasone

Clone	Sites/Cell[1]	K_D Whole Cell	K_D Cytosol
C7	20,000	1.2×10^{-8}	3.3×10^{-8}
3R7	10,000	1.4×10^{-8}	6.2×10^{-8}
3R43	3,500	3.4×10^{-8}	5.0×10^{-8}
4R4	5,900	7.3×10^{-8}	4.2×10^{-8}

[1]Sites per cell and equilibrium dissociation constants (K_D's)
were calculated from equilibrium binding assays performed on
whole cells and cell cytosols in the presence of various concentrations of ^{3}H-dexamethasone from 10^{-9} to 10^{-7} M by the
method of Scatchard.[14] Competable binding was determined as
the difference between assays containing either no, or a
200-fold excess of unlabeled steroid.

Nuclear Transfer of Steroid Receptor Complexes

Given that receptors capable of binding steroid do exist in the
steroid resistant clones, the ability of these complexes to enter
the nucleus under physiological conditions was examined. Cells
incubated with ^{3}H-dexamethasone for 1 h at 37°C were fractionated
into nuclear and cytoplasmic compartments and the proportion of
competable binding in each fraction was determined. The results of
these experiments are presented in Table 3.

In the three resistant clones examined the proportion of steroid receptor complex found in the nucleus was much less than in the
sensitive parent CEM-C7. These results suggest that nuclear translocation, an obligatory step in the effective action of steroid
hormones, is either inhibited or defective in these clones.

In Vitro Activation of Steroid Receptor Complexes

It has been suggested that the conformational change preceding
nuclear translocation of steroid-receptor complexes can be induced
in vitro.[16-19] This change, generally termed "activation," has
been reported to be accelerated by heat, high salt, gel filtration,
dilution, or various combinations of these.[16,17,19-21] Methods of
measurement of activation include binding of steroid-receptor
complexes to DNA,[16,20-22] DEAE-sephadex,[23] and DEAE-cellulose.[24] In

Table 3. Nuclear Transfer of Steroid-Receptor Complexes

Clone	% Nuclear Transfer[1]
CEM-C7	40
3R7	15
3R43	1
4R4	0

Nuclear transfer was measured by a minor modification of the technique of Munck and Wira.[15] Cells were incubated with ^{3}H-dexamethasone as in Table 1, washed and nuclei separated from cell cytoplasm by centrifugation after hypotonic lysis in 15 mM $MgCl_2$. Competable binding in the nuclear and cytoplasmic fractions was then determined.

the case of glucocorticoid receptor, activated steroid-receptor complexes can be resolved from unactivated complexes by DEAE-cellulose chromatography.[24]   Activated steroid-receptor complexes bind less tightly to DEAE-cellulose and can be eluted with approximately 50 mM potassium phosphate (PKI) whereas unactivated complexes bind more tightly and require 0.22 M potassium phosphate for elutions (PKII). Recently Munck and Foley[25] have shown in intact thymocytes that steroid-receptor complexes from cells labeled with ^{3}H-dexamethasone contain steroid-receptor complexes which progressively shift from the high to the low salt eluting DEAE binding forms under physiologic conditions providing strong evidence that these two forms do indeed represent the two forms of the steroid-receptor complex.

The observation that the steroid resistant mutants contain receptors defective in nuclear translocation suggested a possible defect in the activation process. Such a defect could involve an inability of complexes to undergo transformation to the activated form. Alternatively, such complexes could be labile under activating conditions and thereby fail to maintain sufficient steroid-receptor complexes for effective function. These possibilities can be tested and differentiated by chromatography of steroid-receptor complexes from both mutant and wild-type on DEAE-cellulose after activation. Abortive activation would result in the lack of

conversion of the high salt to the low salt eluting form, while
loss of complexes upon activation would indicate lability.

Figure 2 shows the results of experiments in which steroid-
receptor complexes from CEM-C7 and the steroid resistant mutant 4R4
were labeled with ^{3}H-triamcinolone acetonide and then were chromatographed either prior to (Fig. 2A) or after (Fig. 2B) activation
for 30 min at 20°C in the presence of 0.2 M KCl. Receptors from
the wild-type sensitive parent are eluted in the high salt (unactivated) form if applied to DEAE-cellulose prior to activation and
predominantly in the low salt (activated) form if applied after
activation. If during the initial incubation an excess of
unlabeled steroid is included there is no binding of labeled complexes to DEAE-cellulose (data not shown). In contrast, steroid-
receptor complexes from the mutant 4R4 can only be chromatographed
prior to activation. While unactivated complexes elute at the
same salt concentration as do the unactivated complexes of the
sensitive parent (Fig. 2C), chromatography of cytosol which had
been subjected to activating conditions shows the loss of the
unactivated form without any concommitant increase in the activated
form (Fig. 2D). Since all of the competable binding present after
activated charcoal adsorbtion of the steroid or G-25 chromatography
of labeled cytosols is retained on DEAE, the results in Figure 2D
represent a net loss of total receptor, and not a failure of activated complexes from the mutant to bind to DEAE. Therefore,
steroid receptor complexes from the steroid resistant mutants are
significantly more labile during in vitro activation than complexes
of the steroid sensitive parent. This instability could account
for both the lower number of receptors measured in the mutants in
whole cell binding assays and for the decreased proportion of
nuclear localization since these assays were performed under conditions favoring receptor activation, and suggest a possible mechanism
for the steroid resistance observed, namely, the failure to generate
stable, functional activated complexes. This phenotype termed
"receptor positive, activator labile" (r^+, act[l]) has also been found
in three other steroid resistant clones tested, and therefore
appears to be a significant mechanism for the acquisition of steroid
resistance in this cultured cell line.

Sodium molybdate ($NaMoO_4$) has been shown to both inhibit the
conversion of unbound glucocorticoid receptor to a form unable to
bind steroid,[8,9] and to inhibit the activation of glucocorticoid
and other steroid hormone receptors.[26-28] We have used this latter
property to determine if it is the unactivated form of the steroid
receptor complex which is excessively labile under activating conditions or whether the increased lability of such complexes is a
property of their activated forms. Steroid receptor complexes from
both mutant and wild-type were activated in the presence and absence
of 50 mm $NaMoO_4$ and then analyzed by DEAE-cellulose chromatography

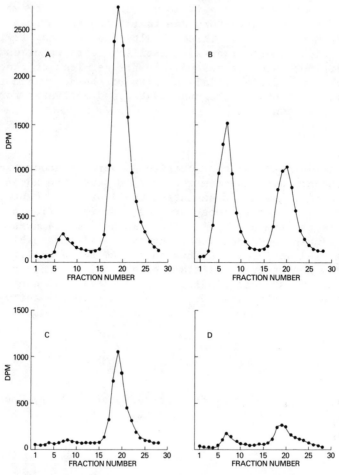

Fig. 2. Cytosols (100,000 x g supernatants) in 5 mM potassium buffer, pH 7.4, prepared from CEM-C7 (A,B) and the steroid resistant subclone 4R4 (C,D) were labeled with ^{3}H-dexamethasone acetonide for 2 h at 0-2°C. Samples of the labeled cytosols were applied to DEAE-cellulose either before (A,C) or after (B,D) activation at 20°C in 0.2 M KCl for 30 min. Prior to application on DEAE-cellulose unbound steroid was removed by gel filtration and G-25. Columns were eluted with linear gradients of 5 mM-0.4 M potassium phosphate and 1.0 ml fractions were collected and assayed for radioactivity.

for the presence of the high (unactivated) and low (activated) salt
eluting forms. The results, Table 4, indicate that when activation
is blocked by molybdate there is no conversion of wild-type
complexes to the activated form and that there is no loss of
complexes from the mutant. These results suggest that it is not a
simple case of a general increased lability of receptor under activating conditions which is responsible for net loss of receptor but
a more complicated differential lability of the activated form or
some intermediate between the unactivated and activated form of the
steroid-receptor complex.

SUMMARY

We have isolated and characterized several glucocorticoid
resistant mutants derived from the steroid sensitive human leukemic
cell line CEM-C7. Among these mutants, all of which contain residual high affinity steroid receptors, we have identified a class of
receptor defects termed r^+act^1. These mutants contain receptor
capable of binding glucocorticoid but apparently incapable of undergoing successful activation. Thus they seem to be qualitatively
distinct from the steroid resistant mouse cell line mutants which
either contain no steroid binding capacity,[4,5,7] or contain receptors with aberrant affinity for DNA cellulose in the activated
form.[6,7]

Table 4. Effect of Molybdate on Receptor Lability Under
              "Activation" Conditions[1]

Condition	CEM-C7		4R4	
	PKI	PKII	PKI	PKII
Unactivated	1586	5196	1557	8319
Activated no molybdate	3258	1868	1128	3088
Activated plus molybdate	942	6001	1169	8071

[1]Cytosols of the sensitive parent (CEM-C7) and the resistant mutant
(4R4) were labeled with ^{3}H-triamcinolone acetonide and then chromatographed on DEAE-cellulose as in Figure 2. Fractions of the
gradient elution were collected and the radioactivity in each peak
was determined. Results are expressed as the total eluted dpm in
each peak.

The significance of this new class of receptor defect with respect to mechanism of steroid response in tissues and animals remains to be determined. However, our results underscore the fact that mere presence of steroid binding activity, even in cells or tissues which generally express steroid regulated functions, does not guarantee the existence of a functional, steroid responsive, pathway. It is not enough to establish the presence of steroid receptors to conclude that cells will or even should respond to steroids.

Chemotherapeutic treatment of acute lymphoblastic leukemia (ALL) relies heavily on the use of corticosteroids. Several studies have attempted to identify whether a correlation between glucocorticoid receptor concentration and degree of response to therapy exists.[29,30] While some correlation seems to exist if ALL is subdivided into Null and T cell leukemias, it is obvious that there are patients containing comparatively high levels of gluco-corticoid receptors who respond less well than those with lower receptor levels. Our preliminary characterization of human leukemic cells which spontaneously become steroid resistant in culture would suggest that more detailed analyses of glucocorticoid receptors from clinical material may be required to establish a relationship between receptors and clinical response.

We gratefully acknowledge editorial assistance of Mrs. Jean Regan in preparing the manuscript. T. J. S. was supported by an NIH postdoctoral fellowship (1F32 CA05447-02) awarded by the National Cancer Institute.

REFERENCES

1. J. M. Harmon, M. R. Norman, and E. B. Thompson, Human leukemic cells in culture—A model system for the study of glucocorti-coid-induced lymphocytolysis, in: "Steroid Receptors and the Management of Cancer," E. B. Thompson and M. L. Lippman, eds., CRC Press, Boca Raton, FL (1979).
2. J. M. Harmon and E. B. Thompson, Acquisition of steroid resis-tance in human leukemic cells through alterations in steroid receptors (abstract), J. Cell Biol. 83:274 (1979).
3. C. H. Sibley and G. M. Tomkins, Isolation of lymphoma cell variants resistant to killing by glucocorticoids, Cell 2:213 (1974).
4. S. Bourgeois and R. F. Newby, Diploid and haploid states of the glucocorticoid receptor gene of mouse lymphoid cell lines, Cell 11:423 (1977).
5. C. H. Sibley and G. M. Tomkins, Mechanism of steroid resistance, Cell 2:221 (1974).

6. K. R. Yamamoto, M. R. Stampfer, and G. M. Tomkins, Receptors from glucocorticoid-sensitive lymphoma cells and two classes of insensitive clones: Physical and DNA-binding properties, Proc. Natl. Acad. Sci. USA 71:3901 (1974).

7. M. Pfahl, T. Sandros, and S. Bourgeois, Interaction of glucocorticoid receptors from lymphoid cell lines with their nuclear acceptor sites, Mol. Cell. Endocrinol. 10:175 (1978).

8. J. J. Sando, A. C. LaForest, and W. B. Pratt, ATP-dependent activation of L cell glucocorticoid receptors to the steroid binding form, J. Biol. Chem. 254:4772 (1979).

9. J. J. Sando, N. D. Hammond, C. A. Stratford, and W. B. Pratt, Activation of thymocyte receptors to the steroid binding form: The roles of reducing agents, ATP and heat-stable factors, J. Biol. Chem. 254:4779 (1979).

10. M. R. Norman and E. B. Thompson, Characterization of a glucocorticoid-sensitive human lymphoblastoid cell line, Cancer Res. 37:3785 (1977).

11. J. M. Harmon, M. R. Norman, B. J. Fowlkes, and E. B. Thompson, Dexamethasone induces irreversible G_1 arrest and death of a human lymphoid cell line, J. Cell. Physiol. 98:267 (1979).

12. J. M. Harmon and E. B. Thompson, Isolation and characterization of glucocorticoid resistant mutants of the human leukemic cell line CEM-C7 (Submitted for publication).

13. S. E. Luria and M. Delbrück, Mutations of bacteria from virus sensitivity to virus resistance, Genetics 28:491 (1943).

14. G. Scatchard, The attractions of proteins for small molecules and ions, Ann. N. Y. Acad. Sci. 51:669 (1949).

15. A. Munck and C. Wira, Methods for assessing hormone-receptor kinetics with cells in suspension: Receptor-bound and non-specifically bound hormone; cytoplasmic-nuclear translocation, in: "Methods in Enzymology, Vol. XXXVI, Hormone Action," B. W. O'Malley and J. G. Handman, eds., Academic Press, New York (1975).

16. J. D. Baxter, G. G. Rousseau, M. C. Benson, R. L. Garcea, J. Ito, and G. M. Tomkins, Role of DNA and specific cytoplasmic receptors in glucocorticoid action, Proc. Natl. Acad. Sci. USA 69:1892 (1972).

17. M. Kalimi, M. Beato, and P. Feigelson, Interaction of glucocorticoids with rat liver nuclei. I. Role of the cytosol proteins, Biochemistry 12:3365 (1973).

18. M. Beato, M. Kalimi, M. Konstam, and P. Feigelson, Interaction of glucocorticoids with rat liver nuclei: II. Studies on the nature of cytosol transfer factor and the nuclear acceptor site, Biochemistry 12:3372 (1973).

19. S. J. Higgins, G. G. Rousseau, J. D. Baxter, and G. M. Tomkins, Early events in glucocorticoid action activation of the steroid receptor and its subsequent specific nuclear binding studied in a cell free system, J. Biol. Chem. 248:5866(1973).

20. E. Milgrom, M. Atger, and E.-E. Baulieu, Acidophilic activation of steroid hormone receptors, Biochemistry 12:5198 (1973).

21. J. A. Goidl, M. H. Cake, K. P. Dolan, G. L. Parchman, and G. Litwack, Activation of the rat liver glucocorticoid-receptor complex, Biochemistry 16:2125 (1977).

22. J. A. Cidlowski and A. Munck, Comparison of glucocorticoid-receptor complex binding to nuclei and DNA cellulose: Evidence for different forms of interaction, Biochem. Biophys. Acta 543:545 (1978).

23. L. G. Parchman and G. Litwack, Resolution of activated and unactivated forms of the glucocorticoid receptor from rat liver, Arch. Biochem. Biophys. 183:374 (1977).

24. Y. Sakaue and E. B. Thompson, Characterization of two forms of glucocorticoid hormone-receptor complex separated by DEAE-cellulose chromotography, Biochem. Biophys. Res. Commun. 77: 533 (1977).

25. A. Munck and R. Foley, Activation of steroid hormone-receptor complexes in intact target cells in physiological conditions, Nature 278:752 (1979).

26. K. L. Leach, M. K. Dahmer, N. D. Hammond, J. J. Sando, and W. B. Pratt, Molybdate inhibition of glucocorticoid receptor inactivation and transformation, J. Biol. Chem. 254: 11884 (1979).

27. D. Toft and H. Nishigori, Stabilization of the avian progesterone receptor by inhibitors, J. Steroid Biochem. 11:413 (1979).

28. T. J. Schmidt, J. M. Harmon, and E. B. Thompson, submitted for publication.

29. M. E. Lippman, G. Konior Yarbro, B. G. Leventhal, and E. B. Thompson, Clinical correlations of glucocorticoid receptors in human acute lymphoblastic leukemia, in: "Steroid Receptors and the Management of Cancer," E. B. Thompson and M. E. Lippman, eds., CRC Press, Boca Raton, FL (1979).

30. P. A. Bell and U. M. Bothwick, eds., "Glucocorticoid Action and Leukemia," Proc. 7th Tenovus Workshop, Alpha Omega Publishing, Cardiff, Wales (1979).

DEACYLCORTIVAZOL, A POTENT GLUCOCORTICOID WITH UNUSUAL

STRUCTURE AND UNUSUAL ANTI-LEUKEMIC CELL ACTIVITY

E. B. Thompson, S. S. Simons, Jr.,* and J. M. Harmon

Laboratory of Biochemistry
Division of Cancer Biology and Diagnosis
National Cancer Institute
and
*Laboratory of Chemistry
National Institute of Arthritis, Metabolism
  and Digestive Diseases
National Institutes of Health
Bethesda, MD 20205

INTRODUCTION

The currently accepted dogma of steroid action states that the structure required for potent glucocorticoid action must at least contain the pregna-4-ene-11β-ol-3,20-dione skeleton. This struc.re presumably is necessary for the steroid to fit in its binding site on specific glucocorticoid receptors.[1,2] This steroid-receptor interaction is widely accepted as the first of a series of molecular events which determine specific steroid-induced cellular responses.[3,4] Bulky substituents on the A-ring have been reported to decrease this activity.[1,2,5] We were therefore intrigued to find brief mention in the literature of a group of pyrazolo-steroids with extremely high anti-inflammatory activity despite the presence of bulky A-ring substituents and the absence of the 3-keto group.[6-8] Because of this interesting structure we decided to examine this type of steroid for its interaction with glucocorticoid receptors and for its potency as a glucocorticoid. We were able to take advantage of two well-studied tissue culture cell systems available in our laboratory. These have permitted examination of two phenotypically different aspects of glucocorticoid action: a classic hepatic glucocorticoid response, the induction of tyrosine

315

aminotransferase (TAT); and the lympholysis of T-derived leukemic
lymphoblasts. Our findings show that these pyrazolo-steroids are
extremely potent glucocorticoids and that they bind tightly to
glucocorticoid receptors. Our studies also point up the occasional
inadequacy of standard cell-free competitive receptor binding assays
for demonstrating the proper affinity relationships between steroids. Such assays do not reflect the high potency of the pyrazolo-steroids. However, whole cell binding assays carried out at
37°C more nearly do so, as the data below will show.

An unexpected and interesting additional finding has been that
these compounds also kill leukemic lymphoblasts selected from an
originally steroid-sensitive population for resistance to high
concentrations of the potent glucocorticoid dexamethasone. Our
results suggest, therefore, that these pyrazolo-steroids have two
types of toxic effects on the lymphoblasts. One effect appears to
be that of extremely high potency glucocorticoids acting by the
classic glucocorticoid receptor mechanism; the other seems to be
independent of glucocorticoid receptor. These compounds therefore
have potential as chemotherapeutic agents, especially in glucocorticoid resistant leukemia in relapse. In this report we will review
our data concerning the action of one such steroid, deacylcortivazol
(DAC), whose structure is that of compound IIa), below.

$$\underline{II} \quad a)\ X = H$$
$$b)\ X = F$$

Deacylcortivazol in HTC Cells

HTC cells are a line of rat hepatoma cells[9] in which a
limited number of responses to glucocorticoids have been defined.[10]
These cells contain glucocorticoid receptors, and these have been
well characterized.[11] The most studied response of the HTC cells
to steroids is that of TAT induction, for which it has been shown
that glucocorticoids indeed increase enzyme synthesis[12] and the
quantity of translatable TAT mRNA.[13] The extent of induction of
TAT corresponds to the extent of receptor occupancy by the inducing
steroid, and various steroids' potency as agonists or antagonists

correspond to their affinity for receptor sites in these cells.[11]
The effect of DAC on TAT induction in HTC cells was therefore
examined.[14] The half maximal concentrations for induction of
TAT activity by DAC and dexamethasone in HTC cells show that DAC
is an optimal inducer and is about 35 times more potent than dexamethasone (Fig. 1.) Based on other experiments in HTC cells comparing the relative potency of dexamethasone and cortisol, DAC is
calculated to be about 400 times more potent than cortisol.

When DAC and other glucocorticoids were compared with respect
to their affinities for glucocorticoid receptors from HTC cells,
different results were obtained in each of two different assays.
A standard cell-free assay carried out at 0-4° C, in which varying
concentrations of DAC, dexamethasone, or cortisol were used to
compete for a constant concentration of tritiated dexamethasone
binding to the receptor sites, indicated that DAC bound more
tightly than cortisol but less tightly than dexamethasone (Fig. 2a).
This, of course, is in sharp contradistinction to its biological
behavior. However, when whole cell binding assays were carried
out, as shown in Figure 2b, DAC displayed greater binding affinity
than dexamethasone for the corticosteroid receptor sites of whole

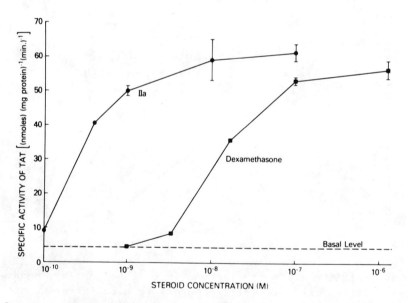

Fig. 1. Dose-response curves for DAC (here labeled IIa) vs Dexamethasone. TAT was induced overnight in monolayer cultures of HTC
cells, the cells harvested and assayed for the activity of the
enzyme. From reference 14, with permission.

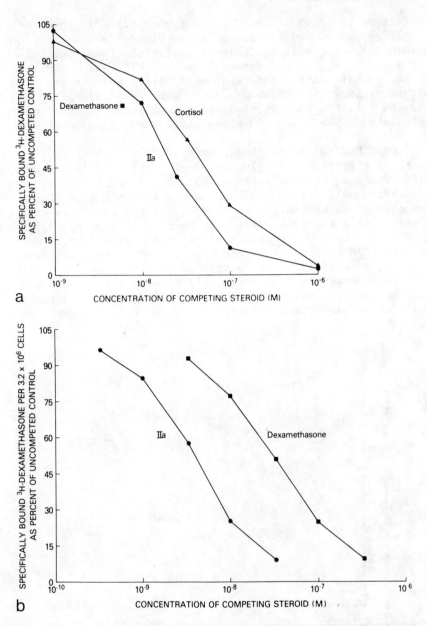

Fig. 2a.   Relative affinities of DAC (here labeled IIa), dexamethasone and cortisol for HTC cell receptors in a cell-free competition
assay.   Incubation for 2 h at 0°C.

2b.   Relative affinities of DAC (IIa) and dexamethasone for HTC
cell receptors in a whole cell competition assay.   Incubation for 30
min at 37°C.   For experimental details, see reference 14, from which
the above has been reproduced, with permission.

cells. The degree of affinity did not correlate precisely with the
biological activity, being only nine-fold greater than that of dexamethasone, but was certainly in closer agreement than that estimated by the cell-free binding assay. The explanation for this discrepancy in the different affinity determinations which we favor is
that the affinities of potent glucocorticoids are largely determined
by differences in their off-rate.[15,16] Thus with a very long $T_{1/2}$
for dissociation, (that of dexamethasone being approximately 100 h
at 0°C), competition assays such as those shown in Figure 1a usually
do not achieve equilibrium. If the off-rate of DAC is even slower
than that of dexamethasone, then the time required to reach equilibrium conditions would be so long that the system would not survive
the experiment. However, in the whole-cell assay carried out at
37°C for 30 min the approximation of the competitive binding to
equilibrium conditions would be greater. Thus, we believe, the 37°C
whole-cell assay better reflects the functional affinity of the compound for its receptor sites and is more appropriate in explaining
the whole cell glucocrticoid potency of DAC. Additional evidence
that DAC acts as a glucocorticoid through the standard mechanism is
provided by HTC cell variants. Clones of HTC cells have been isolated which possess basal levels of TAT and glucocorticoid receptors, but in which TAT is not inducible by glucocorticoids.[17]
When these cells were tested for their ability to be induced by DAC
the compound failed to raise the basal level of the enzyme. This
provides some slight additional evidence that DAC is not acting to
induce TAT through some mechanism other than that of standard glucocorticoids. At concentrations up to 10^{-6} M, HTC cells show no
significant growth inhibition by potent glucocorticoids such as dexamethasone, cortisol, triamcinolone, or by DAC. In this sense they
differ from the cells which will be discussed in the next section.

Deacylcortivasol in CEM Cells

One of the earliest observations concerning adrenalcorticoste-
roids was that they cause the lysis of thymocytes.[18] This property
has been put to wide pharmacological use and in particular has
formed the theoretical basis for employing glucocorticoids in the
treatment of certain leukemias. As the preceding paper by Harmon
et al. explains in detail, CEM-C7 cells are a clonal, steroid-sensitive, glucocorticoid receptor-containing line of human acute leukemic lymphoblasts.[19] This line of cells also contains glutamine
synthetase activity which is induced by glucocorticoids and which
seems to provide a marker for functional glucocorticoid receptors.[20,21] This line of lymphoblasts therefore provided us with an
excellent opportunity to test the potency of DAC in an entirely
different system, one which we feel represents a useful model for
steroid-sensitive human leukemia.

As in the case of tyrosine aminotransferase induction in HTC cells, we found DAC to be many times more potent than dexamethasone with respect to both glutamine synthetase induction and its ability to compete for glucocorticoid sites in a 37°C whole-cell assay. When examined for its ability to kill CEM-C7 cells, DAC was found to have even greater relative potency (Table 1). This greater potency for cell killing as compared to enzyme induction and/or receptor occupancy seemed of special interest and accordingly additional experiments were performed. The ability of the pyrazolo-steroid to induce glutamine synthetase clearly established the fact that this steroid analog was acting as a glucocorticoid in the CEM cells, but the imbalance between its potency as enzyme inducer and cell lytic agent suggested that the compound might be acting through an additional pathway for cell lysis.

Exposure of CEM-C7 cells to 10^{-6} M dexamethasone allows one to isolate the resistant clones arising spontaneously in the wild-type population at a rate of about 10^{-5} per cell per generation. The concentration of dexamethasone used to isolate these clones was more than sufficient to fully saturate glucocorticoid receptors, and therefore presumably was sufficient to have been exerting maximal steroid effect. However, when we attempted to isolate resistant clones from CEM-C7 with 10^{-6} M DAC, we were unable to find any resistant clones arising from a total number of 2 x 10^7 cells exposed. Thus, the frequency at which resistant cells were arising to DAC was significantly lower than that at which dexamethasone resistant cells arose. This, along with the dose response data, further suggested that either the principles of glucocorticoid receptor

Table 1. Comparison of Dexamethasone (Dex) amd Deacylcortivazol (DAC) for their Effects on CEM Human Leukemic Lymphoblasts

	Molar Concentration (x 10^{10}) Required for 50% Maximum Effect		
Steroid	Induction of Glutamine Synthetase	Competition with ^{3}H-Dexamethasone for Receptor Sites	Reduction in Cloning Efficiency
Dex	360	680	300
DAC	10	30	5.5

Glutamine synthetase was assayed as described in Schmidt and Thompson.[21] Whole-cell competitive binding assays and the method and rationale for estimation of effects on cell viability by reduction in cloning efficiency have been described.[19,22]

occupancy/cellular response had to be reconsidered, at least with
respect to cell killing, or that DAC was acting differently from
standard glucocorticoids.

The existence of more than 100 resistant clones which we had
previously derived from C-7 allowed us to examine these possibilities. These clones were of two types. The first group, derived
by selection in dexamethasone without mutagenesis, all had residual
glucocorticoid binding sites with decreased ability to undergo
nuclear transfer. Glutamine synthetase could not be induced in any
of these clones. Biochemical examination of these receptors in
several clones showed them to display increased lability compared to
that of wild-type receptors. Specifically, they appear to be unable
to form a stable, activated steroid receptor complex. The other
group of resistant clones was derived by first treating the C-7
cells with mutagenic agents (ICR 191, nitrosoguanidine) and then
selecting for dexamethasone resistance. The great majority of these
clones had no, or very few, receptor sites left, and, of course,
were noninducible with respect to glutamine synthetase. We tested
representative clones of each type for their sensitivity to DAC.
All of several clones representative of the first group showed cessation of growth and cell lysis when exposed to μM DAC. As we have
pointed out before, the lethal effect of dexamethasone on wild-type
CEM-C7 cells only begins after an exposure of approximately 18-24 h.
The DAC effect in the Dex-resistant clones took even longer to manifest itself. However, after several days exposure, cell growth
ceased and the cells died. It seemed possible to us that the DAC, by
virtue of its greater affinity for receptor sites, might be able to
stabilize and somehow utilize the poor receptors which remained in
the spontaneous-resistant clones and thereby kill the cells.
Accordingly, we also examined the effect of the compound on clones
of mutated dexamethasone-resistant receptorless cells, and we found
that in these as well 10^{-6} M DAC killed the cells. In fact it did
so even more promptly than in some of the spontaneous Dex-resistant
clones.

Since we had been unable to isolate DAC-resistant clones by
exposing wild-type CEM-C7 cells to μM DAC, we pursued the idea
that DAC might be acting through two different mechanisms, involving separate, event-limiting steps. If each key site were undergoing spontaneous change to resistant phenotype at a rate of 10^{-5}
or 10^{-6}, and if DAC were acting both as a glucocorticoid and in some
other fashion to kill the cells, then utilizing cells which had been
preselected for glucocorticoid resistance might allow us to see the
appearance of DAC-resistant cells. These might arise by virtue of
alteration occurring in the second putative event-limiting site of
DAC action. Accordingly, we placed both classes of dexamethasone-
resistant cells in μM DAC and indeed found that resistant clones

grew out at a frequency of approximately 5×10^{-5}. Furthermore we noted that in the instance of Dex-resistant spontaneous clones which still maintained a measurable level of residual glucocorticoid receptors, selection for DAC resistance did not do away with these steroid binding sites. Examples of these results are shown in Table 2. We conclude from these data that indeed DAC has dual effects on these leukemic lymphoblasts. One of its effects is that of a classic glucocorticoid with high potency. This effect accounts

Table 2.   Resistance of Various Subclones of Leukemic Lymphoblasts to Dexamethasone (Dex) and Deacylcortivazol (DAC)

		Response to	
Cell Line	Receptor Sites/Cell	Dex	DAC
Parental wild-type CEM-C7	20,000	S[a]	S
Spontaneously resistant subclones			
3R7[b]	12,000	R	S
3R7R1)			
R2)	8400–9600	R	R
R3)			
R4)			
3R43	3500	R	S
4R4	5900	R	S
4R4R1)			
R2)			
R3)	4200–6860	R	R
R4)			
R5)			
Mutagenized resistant subclones			
ICR19[d]	300	R	S
ICR27	0	R	S

a. S indicates sensitive, i.e. killed by the steroid. R indicates resistant, i.e. able to grow and form colonies in 10^{-5} M Dex or 10^{-6} M DAC.

b. 3R7, 3R43, and 4R4 arose spontaneously from CEM-C7, and were picked as colonies growing in 10^{-6} M Dex.

c. 3R7R1-R4 and 4R4R1-R5 are subclones of 3R7 and 4R4, respectively. They arose spontaneously and were picked for their ability to grow in 10^{-6} M DAC.

d. ICR19 and ICR191 grew as colonies in 10^{-6} M Dex after their parent clone, CEM-C7 had been treated with the mutagen ICR191.

for its ability to induce glutamine synthetase, to occupy glucocorticoid receptors, and to kill the cells at appropriate concentrations. The other effect, at some unknown site, is demonstrated by the ability of the compound to kill completely glucocorticoid-resistant clones irrespective of their residual receptor content. This second effect, coupled with the observation that steroid-sensitive cells give rise to DAC-resistant clones at a very low rate, make this compound and others of its class of interest for their potential as chemotherapeutic agents in certain blood dyscrasias. Important questions of possible general cellular toxicity to normal cells and therefore therapeutic ratio in vivo remain. The compound is now being tested on a standard tumor panel at the National Cancer Institute, and if these tests bear out the promise the compound shows in our tissue culture systems, we hope to bring it to Phase I trials in the future.

REFERENCES

1. A. Goldstein, L. Aronow, and S. M. Kalman, "Principles of Drug Action: The Basis of Pharmacology," 2nd Edition, John Wiley and Sons, New York, pp. 36-39 (1974).
2. M. E. Wolff, Structure activity relationships in glucocorticoids, in "Glucocorticoid Action," J. D. Baxter and G. G. Rousseau, eds., Springer-Verlag, New York, pp. 97-107 (1979).
3. E. B. Thompson and M. E. Lippman, Mechanism of action of glucocorticoids, Metabolism 23:159 (1974).
4. R. J. B. King and W. I. P. Mainwaring, "Steroid-cell Interactions," Univ. Park Press, Baltimore (1974).
5. G. G. Rousseau and J.-P. Schmit, Structure-activity relationships for glucocorticoids--I: Determination of receptor binding and biological activity. J. Steroid Biochem. 8:911 (1977).
6. J. H. Fried, H. Mrozik, G. E. Arth, T. S. Bry, N. G. Steinberg, M. Tishler, R. Hirschmann, and S. L. Steelman, 16-methylated steroids IV. $6,16\alpha$ dimethyl-Δ^6-hydrocortisone and related compounds, J. Amer. Chem. Soc. 85:236, (1963).
7. S. L. Steelman, E. R. Morgan, and M. S. Glitzer, Heterocyclic corticosteroids I. Biological properties of the 6,16α-dimethyl-4,6-prenadiene-11β,17,21-triol-20-one(3,2c)-2'-phenylpyrazole-21-acetate and its 21-desoxy derivative, Steroids 18: 129 (1971).
8. J. P. Dausee, D. Duval, P. Meyer, J. C. Gaignault, C. Marchandeau, and J. P. Raynaud, The relationship between glucocorticoid structure and effects upon thymocytes, Mol. Pharmacol. 13:948 (1977).
9. E. B. Thompson, G. M. Tomkins, and J. C. Curran, Induction of tyrosine α-ketoglutarate transaminase by steroid hormones in a newly established tissue culture cell line, Proc. Natl. Acad. Sci. USA 56:296 (1966).

10. R. D. Ivarie and P. H. O'Farrell, The glucocorticoid domain: Steroid-mediated changes in the rate of synthesis of rat hepatoma proteins, Cell 13:41 (1978).

11. G. G. Rousseau, J. D. Baxter, and G. M. Tomkins, Glucocorticoid receptors: relations between steroid binding and biological effects, J. Mol. Biol. 67:99 (1972).

12. D. K. Granner, E. B. Thompson, and G. M. Tomkins, Dexamethasone phosphate-induced synthesis of tyrosine aminotransferase in hepatoma tissue culture cells. Studies of the early phases of induction and of the steroid requirement for maintenance of the induced rate of synthesis, J. Biol. Chem. 245:1472 (1970).

13. P. Olsen, E. B. Thompson, and D. K. Granner, Regulation of HTC cell tyrosine aminotransferase mRNA by dexamethasone, Biochemistry, in press.

14. S. S. Simons, Jr., E. B. Thompson, and D. F. Johnson, Antiinflammatory pyrazolo-steroids: Potent glucocorticoids containing bulky A-ring substituents and no C_3-carbonyl, Biochem. Biophys. Res. Commun. 86:793 (1979).

15. W. B. Pratt, J. L. Kaine and D. V. Pratt, The kinetics of glucocorticoid binding to the soluble specific binding protein of mouse fibroblasts, J. Biol. Chem. 250:4584 (1975).

16. G. G. Rousseau and J. D. Baxter, Glucocorticoid receptors, in: "Glucocorticoid Action," J. D. Baxter and G. G. Rousseau, eds., Springer-Verlag, New York, pp. 50-77 (1979).

17. E. B. Thompson, D. K. Granner, T. D. Gelehrter, and G. L. Hager, Unlinked control of multiple glucocorticoid-sensitive processes in spontaneous cell variants, in: "Hormones and Cell Culture," eds. R. Ross and G. Sato, Cold Spring Harbor Conferences on Cell Proliferation, Vol. 6, pp. 339-360 (1979).

18. T. Dougherty and A. White, Functional alterations in lymphoid tissue induced by adrenal cortical secretion, Am. J. Anat. 77: 81 (1945).

19. M. R. Norman and E. B. Thompson, Characterization of a glucocorticoid-sensitive human lymphoid cell line, Cancer Res. 37: 3785 (1977).

20. J. M. Harmon, T. J. Schmidt, and E. B. Thompson, Loss of glutamine synthetase induction in human leukemic T cells selected for resistance to dexamethasone, J. Cell Biol. 79(2,2):200a (1978).

21. T. J. Schmidt and E. B. Thompson, Glucocorticoid receptors and glutamine synthetase in leukemic Sezary cells, Cancer Res. 39: 376 (1979).

22. J. M. Harmon, M. R. Norman, B. J. Fowlkes, and E. B. Thompson, Dexamethasone induces irreversible G_1 arrest and death of a human lymphoid cell line, J. Cell. Physiol. 98:267 (1979).

NEW OBSERVATION ON ANDROGEN ACTION: ANDROGEN RECEPTOR

STABILIZATION AND ANTISTEROID EFFECTS OF LHRH AGONISTS.

W. Wright, K. Chan, K. Sundaram, and C.W. Bardin

The Population Council, The Rockefeller University

New York, New York 10021

The androgenic activity of testosterone and its 5α-metabolites is classically defined as the growth promoting effect on the male reproductive tract. By contrast, the stimulatory effect of these hormones on nitrogen balance and body weight is referred to as their anabolic action (1). This latter effect results from androgen stimulation of protein synthesis in tissues, such as liver, kidney, bone and muscle, which compromise a major portion of body mass. Even though the anabolic and androgenic actions of testosterone were once thought to be distinct effects of a hormone, it is now clear that these are organ-specific responses. In most tissues, the effects of androgens are mediated via androgen receptors (2-4) and are inhibited by antiandrogens (5). In addition, the post-receptor actions of androgens are mediated via common intracellular events regardless of the tissue (6).

An understanding of the action of testosterone and other androgens depends on the accuracy and precision of assays for their receptors. Insights into androgen action are also provided by drugs which antagonize or modify the response of this class of steroids. The purpose of this report is to review new observations on improved assay conditions for androgen receptors and to report the antiandrogenic and antiestrogenic effects of LHRH agonists on reproductive tissues.

MATERIALS AND METHODS

Animals

For the receptor studies, mature male and female Balb/c mice were purchased from the Charles River Breeding Laboratories. Male animals were castrated one day before the experiment. For studies with LHRH agonists, 25- to 28-day old rats (Charles River) were castrated and used one week later in experiments in which either testosterone propionate or estradiol was administered in oil with or without 10 µg of an LHRH agonist.

Reagents

[17-methyl-^{3}H]-methyltrienolone (87 Ci/mmol) ([^{3}H]-R-1881), [1,2-^{3}H]-testosterone (52 Ci/mmol) ([^{3}H]-T) and methyltrienolone (R-1881) were purchased from New England Nuclear. Other steroids were purchased from Steraloids. All steroids were stored in absolute ethanol at 4C, under an atmosphere of nitrogen. The LHRH agonists [D-Trp^6,Pro^9-NEt]-LHRH and [(imBzl)D-His^6,Pro^9-NEt]-LHRH were prepared by J. Rivier and W. Vale of the Salk Institute and used in studies previously described (7).

Preparation of the Cytosol

Animals were killed by cervical dislocation and the kidneys placed in ice-cold phosphate buffered saline. All subsequent steps were carried out in a cold room (4C) with the tissue packed on ice. The kidneys were cleaned of adhering fat, placed in 2 volumes of 50mM Tris, 0.1 mM EDTA, 10% glycerol, 5mM dithiothreotol, pH=7.4, (TEGD) or TEGD with 20 mM Na$_2$MoO$_4$, pH=7.4 (TEGDMo) and homogenized with two or three 10 sec bursts of a Brinkman Polytron with a rheostat setting of 7. The cytosol fraction was isolated by centrifugation of the homogenate at 10,000 rpm for 20 min in a JA-20 rotor (Beckman) followed by centrifugation at 50,000 rpm in a Ti-50 rotor (Beckman). Aliquots of the cytosol were stored at -20C for subsequent analysis of protein concentration by the method of Lowrey et al. (8), using bovine serum albumin as standard. Cytosolic protein concentration was 1.6-2.2 mg/ml.

Assay of Receptor-Bound Steroid

The amount of radiolabeled steroid specifically bound to the androgen receptor was determined essentially as described before (9). Varying amounts of radiolabeled and radioinert steroids were added to 10x 75 mm glass culture tubes and dried under purified nitrogen (see specific studies for details). Two hundred twenty or 250 µl of cytosol were added to the tubes and incubated at 0-4C for 8 hr. Duplicate 100 µl aliquots of cytosol were transferred to DEAE filters (DE-81, Whatman) and incubated for 90 sec. The filters were then washed six times with 50mM Tris, 0.1mM EDTA, 0.25% Triton X-100, pH=7.4. During this washing procedure, negative pressure was applied to the filters on a filter box (Hoefer). It was critical that the pressure was constant from one batch of filters to the next in order to minimize intra-assay variability.

FACTORS AFFECTING ANDROGEN RECEPTOR STABILIZATION

The Use of [^{3}H]-Methyltrienolone (R-1881) for Assay of Androgen Receptor

Several investigators indicated that [^{3}H]-R-1881 is useful for measuring androgen receptors in a variety of tissues (10-12). In the present study, R-1881 was compared with testosterone as a ligand for androgen receptor measurement in mouse kidney. Kidneys from castrated male mice were homogenized in TEGD buffer and the cytosol incubated with varying amounts of [^{3}H]-R-1881 or [^{3}H]-T with and without a 1,000 molar excess of radioinert testosterone. Incubations were carried out on ice for 22 hr since preliminary studies indicated that at least 18 hr were required for steroid and receptor to reach equilibrium. In addition, there was no metabolism of R-1881 during this incubation period as determined by thin layer chromatography. Scatchard analysis of androgen receptor binding to [^{3}H]-R-1881 and [^{3}H]-T are shown in Figure 1. The apparent Kds of the androgen receptor for R-1881 and T were 0.6 x 10^{-9} M and 3.0 x 10^{-9} M, respectively. Both ligands detected the same number of binding sites (44 fmoles/mg protein).

The relative binding affinity of R-1881 and other steroids which are known to bind to the androgen receptor are shown in Figure 2. In this study, cytosol was incubated on ice for 3 hr with R-1881 (5nM) and varying amounts of the indicated steroids. The relative binding affinities, calculated from the concentration of competitor required to compete 50% of the specifically bound [^{3}H]-R-1881, were 100, 25, 2, and 0.4 for R-1881, T, estradiol, and progesterone, respectively. This study confirms the previous observations that R-1881 has a higher affinity for the androgen receptor than testosterone. These and other experiments suggested that this ligand would be superior to testosterone for receptor measurements. Accordingly, R-1881 was used in all further studies.

Optimal Sodium Molybdate (Na$_2$MoO$_4$) and pH for Androgen Receptor Measurement

The studies of Pratt and his colleagues (13-15) have demonstrated the stabilizing effect of Na$_2$MoO$_4$ on the glucocorticoid receptor. These investigators believed that this receptor was

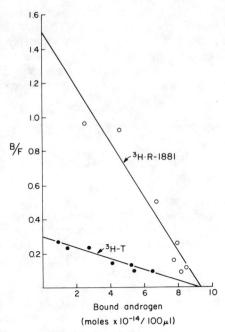

Figure 1:   Scatchard analysis of the androgen receptor binding to [^{3}H]-methyl-trienolone   ([^{3}H]-R-1881)   and   [^{3}H]-testosterone ([^{3}H]-T). Kidney cytosol was incubated on ice for 22 hr with varying concentrations of the two steroids + a 1000-fold excess of T.

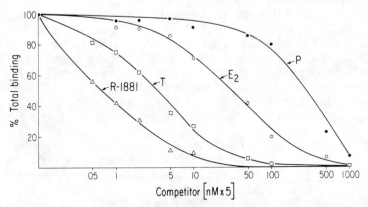

Figure 2:   Relative binding affinities of R-1881, testosterone (T), estradiol (E$_2$), and progesterone (P) for the androgen receptor. Cytosol in TEGD buffer was incubated for three hr on ice with 5 nM [^{3}H]-R-1881 and varying concentrations of the indicated steroids.

phosphorylated and that the effects of molybdate related to its known action as a phosphatase inhibitor. Recent studies of progesterone receptors have suggested, however, that molybdate has a direct stabilizing effect upon the receptor per se (16). Since a major problem of measuring androgen receptor relates to the instability of its binding site, we thought it pertinent to investigate the effects of Na_2MoO_4 on androgen receptor stability in mouse kidney and in other tissues.

The optimal concentration of Na_2MoO_4 required for stabilizing unoccupied androgen receptor binding sites was first determined. Cytosol from kidneys of female mice was prepared in TEGD buffer and aliquoted into tubes containing TEGD buffer with various concentrations of Na_2MoO_4 (0-100mM). The final pH of each tube was 7.4. The samples were incubated at 20C for 4 hr, and the residual binding activity was determined by a second incubation at 4C with 6nM [³H]-R-1881. In the absence of molybdate only 10% of the receptor activity remained after a 4 hr incubation at 20C. In the presence of 5-20nM Na_2MoO_4 there was no loss of steroid binding activity. Higher concentrations of molybdate (40-100mM) were slightly inhibitory.

The stability of the unoccupied and occupied androgen receptor at various pHs was next investigated. Two cytosol samples were prepared in phosphate or Tris buffer with 20mM Na_2MoO_4, 0.1mM EDTA, 10% glycerol and 5mM dithiothreotol. One of the samples was then incubated at 4C with 6nM [³H]-R-1881 for 2 hr (occupied receptor). Aliquots from both cytosol samples were then mixed with buffers of pH ranges from 6.0 to 8.25. All tubes were incubated at 20C for 4 hr, and the residual receptor measured with the R-1881 assay described above. A pH optimum for stability of the occupied receptor was noted between pH 6.6 and 7.6. By contrast, a more narrow pH optimum for stability was noted for the unoccupied receptor between 6.8 and 7.4. The results of these studies suggest that the androgen receptor is more easily degraded following a pH change in the absence than in the presence of ligand. These observations are particularly important since the addition of various ingredients to buffers, such as Na_2MoO_4, may shift pH. It is, therefore, important to maintain the androgen receptor at its pH optimum throughout every experiment.

Effects of Na_2MoO_4 on Stability of the Unoccupied Androgen Receptor

Cytosol from kidneys of female mice was prepared in TEGD or TEGDMo buffer. Aliquots of cytosol were incubated at seven different temperatures (4C-41.5C) and, after various times, samples were removed and incubated a second time with 6nM [³H]-R-1881 to measure residual binding activity. The presence of Na_2MoO_4 significantly stabilized unoccupied androgen receptors at all

temperatures examined. Representative inactivation curves from
this study are shown in Figure 3. The half times ($t_{1/2}$) of receptor inactivation at 4C were 7.4 hr and 204 hr in the absence and
presence of molybdate, respectively. The stability of the receptor in the presence of molybdate at 27.5C was comparable to that
of the unprotected receptor at 4C (Fig. 3). Arrhenius analysis of
the rates of degradation indicate that in the presence of molybdate, androgen receptors have a ΔH of inactivation 21% greater
than in the absence of this ion (ΔH_{mo} =31.87 Kcal/mole versus
ΔH=26.35 Kcal/mole). It is not possible to ascertain from these
observations why the receptor is thermodynamically more stable in
the presence of molybdate. However, from these and other studies
we believe that Na_2MoO_4 is not interacting with receptors to block
proteolytic degradation. If this were the case, no difference in
ΔH inactivation would be expected.

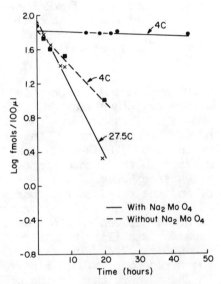

Figure 3:   Inactivation of the unoccupied androgen receptor in the
            presence and absence of sodium molybdate (Na_2MoO_4).
            Cytosol from female mouse kidneys was prepared in TEGD
            buffer with or without Na_2MoO_4. Cytosol was incubated
            without steroid for various times at the indicated tem-
            peratures and then residual binding activity was
            assayed at 4C.

Effects of Molybdate on Binding Kinetics

Association and dissociation binding kinetics of [³H]-R-1881
with the androgen receptor were determined using pools of kidney
cytosol prepared in the presence and absence of Na_2MoO_4. To measure the association of the steroid to the androgen receptor,

[^{3}H]–R–1881 was added to aliquots of cytosol to produce final concentration of 6nM. At various times after additions, samples were
applied to DEAE filters and the amount of bound steroid determined. The k_1 of the androgen receptor for R–1881 in the presence
of Na$_2$MoO$_4$ (2.9 x 10^8 M^{-1} hr^{-1}) was comparable to that in the
absence of molybdate (3.1 x 10^8 M^{-1} hr^{-1}). Similarly, the dissociation rate (k_{-1}) of R–1881 from the androgen receptor was measured in pools of cytosol which were first equilibrated with 6nM
[^{3}H]–R–1881 for 2 hr at 4C. Testosterone was added to an aliquot
of this cytosol (final concentration, 6μM) to determine the rate
of apparent dissociation of [^{3}H]–R–1881 from receptor. In another
aliquot of cytosol to which no testosterone was added, receptor
degradation was measured. These latter measurements were used to
correct the apparent dissociation rate measured in the absence of
molybdate. The results of these experiments indicate that the
dissociation rate constants were comparable in the presence and
absence of Na$_2$MoO$_4$ (Table 1). The results of these studies suggest that Na$_2$MoO$_4$ has no detectable effect on the kinetics of R–
1881 binding to the androgen receptor.

Table 1: Binding Parameters of the Androgen Receptor in the Presence and Absence of 20mM Sodium Molybdate (Na$_2$MoO$_4$).

Incubation Condition	Apparent Receptor Concentration (fmol/mg ptn.)	K_d (Mx10^{-9})	k_1 (M^{-1}hr^{-1})	k_{-1} (hr^{-1})
Without Na$_2$MoO$_4$	30	1.90	2.9x10^8	0.026
With Na$_2$MoO$_4$	45	0.86	3.1x10^8	0.034

The effect of molybdate on the equilibrium binding kinetics
of androgen receptor was studied next.   Kidney cytosols were
prepared in the presence and absence of Na$_2$MoO$_4$ and were mixed
with various concentrations of [^{3}H]–R–1881. The samples were
incubated at 4C for 24 hr and specific binding was measured using
DEAE filtration. The results of a typical experiment are shown in
Figure 4. In the absence of molybdate the receptor concentration
was reduced and the apparent equilibrium dissociation constant
(Kd) was increased (Table 1). This experiment was repeated on
several occasions.   In each instance the receptor concentration
was reduced in the absence of molybdate as in Table 1.   In some
experiments, however, the apparent Kds were similar in the presence and absence of this ion (not shown). The results of these
studies indicate that receptor degradation occurs during prolonged
incubation (greater than 18 hr) required to equilibrate R–1881
with receptor.   In all instances, this results in a decreased

number of binding sites detected and, in some instances, the
degradation in the samples containing the low concentrations of
ligand may be sufficient to alter the slope of the Scatchard plot
and thus change the apparent Kd.

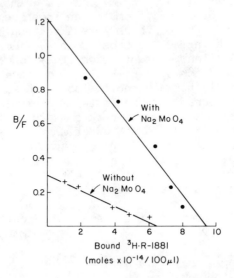

Bound ^{3}H·R-1881
(moles x 10^{-14}/ 100μl)

Figure 4: The effect of sodium molybdate (Na_2MoO_4) on equilibrium
binding kinetics of the androgen receptor for [^{3}H]–R-
1881. Cytosol samples from female mouse kidneys were
prepared in TEGD with and without Na_2MoO_4 and were
incubated at 4C for 24 hr with varying concentrations
of [^{3}H]–R-1881 ± a 1000-fold excess of radioinert testosterone.

     In conclusion, the use of [^{3}H]–R-1881 and DEAE filters has
eliminated many of the undesirable features of previous androgen
receptor assays (9,17). R-1881 is a steroid that binds to the
androgen receptor with high affinity, and is not metabolized during the prolonged incubation periods required to reach equilibrium. The androgen receptor assay described in this report was
also improved by the addition of Na_2MoO_4. This ion stabilized the
unoccupied androgen receptor for greater than 200 hr, permitting
its study under a variety of situations. As a consequence,
equilibrium binding constants have been measured under conditions
where degradation of unoccupied sites did not occur. The ability
to stabilize unoccupied androgen receptors will contribute to the
development of an androgen receptor exchange assay which will
markedly facilitate studies of hormone action on a variety of tissues. In addition, purification of stabilized androgen receptors
is now possible.

ANTIANDROGENIC AND ANTIESTROGENIC EFFECTS OF LHRH AGONIST

In addition to their action on the pituitary, LHRH agonists are known to have a direct effect both upon the testis and the ovary (18-20). Preliminary studies from our laboratory suggested that LHRH agonists could also be antiandrogenic when administered with testosterone propionate in hypophysectomized castrate animals. To further investigate this possibility, castrate immature male rats were treated with testosterone propionate (25 or 100 μg/day) with and without 10 μg of the LHRH agonist - [D-Trp^6,Pro^9-NEt] LHRH. The animals were treated for 5 days, killed on the sixth day and the organs of the reproductive tract examined (Table 2). The LHRH agonist produced an antiandrogenic effect on both prostate and seminal vesicles. To assure that the observed results were not a unique effect of one LHRH agonist, the studies were repeated with [(imBzl)D-His^6,Pro^9-NEt] LHRH. A similar antiandrogenic effect of this agonist was also observed (7). This was an unexpected observation and, to our knowledge, is the first time that a hypothalamic peptide such as LHRH had been shown to have antisteroid activity.

Table 2: Antiandrogenic Effects of [D-Trp^6-Pro^9-NEt]-LHRH on Ventral Prostate and Seminal Vesicles of Testosterone Propionate (TP)-Treated Rats.

Group #	Testosterone Propionate (μg/day)	LHRH agonist (μg/day)	Ventral Prostate (mg)	Seminal Vesicles (mg)
1	0	0	7.9+1.0[a]	8.3+0.4
2	25	0	31.8+2.5	75.3+2.6
3	25	10	26.1+1.4[b]	47.5+2.0[c]
4	100	0	54.2+2.2	81.3+3.6
5	100	10	38.9+2.7[d]	63.4+1.9[d]

[a] Mean + SEM
[b] Significantly different from TP-treated rats (P <0.05).
[c] Significantly different from TP-treated rats (P <0.01).
[d] Significantly different from TP-treated rats (P <0.005).

In view of the surprising effect of LHRH agonists on the male reproductive tract, we next investigated whether this peptide influenced the actions of estrogen on the uterus. Immature female rats, castrated for one week, were treated with estradiol (0.01

and 0.1 μg/day) with and without 10 μg of LHRH agonist per day (Table 3). The agonist completely inhibited the increase in uterine weight induced by 0.01 μg of estradiol. The agonist partially inhibited the effect of the higher dose of estradiol (0.1 μg per day) (7).

Table 3: Antiestrogenic Effects of [D-Trp^6,Pro^9-NEt]-LHRH on Uterine Weight of Estradiol-Treated Rats.

Group #	Estradiol (μg/day)	LHRH agonist (μg/day)	Uterine weight (mg)
1	0	0	37.4+1.8[a]
2	0.01	0	63.3+5.4
3	0.01	10	34.6+1.6[b]
4	0.1	0	134.3+9.2
5	0.1	10	113.7+5.2

[a] Mean + SEM
[b] Significantly different from estradiol treated-rats ($P < 0.005$).

In conclusion, a new effect of LHRH agonist on steroid sensitive tissues has been demonstrated. The results of studies in castrate and castrate-hypophysectomized animals indicate that these peptides can have a direct action on both the prostate and uterus. At the doses tested, two LHRH agonists demonstrated antiandrogenic and antiestrogenic activities. These observations suggest that LHRH agonists could be used to treat a variety of androgen and estrogen responsive tumors (7).

ACKNOWLEDGEMENTS

This research was supported by NIH Grant No. HD-13541. The technical assistance of Ms. Kathryn Connell is gratefully acknowledged. We also thank Jean Schweis for preparing this manuscript.

REFERENCES

1. Kochakian, C.D. Definition of androgens and protein anabolic steroids. Pharmac. Therap. B.1:149-177, 1975.
2. Bardin, C.W., Bullock, L.P., Mills, N.C., Lin, Y.-C. and Jacob, S.T. The role of receptors in the anabolic action of

androgens. In: Receptors and Hormone Action, Vol. II, Chap. 4 (B.W. O'Malley, ed.), Academic Press, New York. pp. 83-103, 1978.

3. Bardin, C.W., Bullock, L.P., Sherins, R.J., Mowszowicz, I. and Blackburn, W.R. Androgen metabolism and mechanism of action in male pseudohermaphroditism: A study of testicular feminization. Rec. Prog. Horm. Res. 29:65-109, 1973.

4. Bardin, C.W., Janne, O., Bullock, L.P. and Jacob, S.T. Physiochemical and biological properties of androgen receptors. In: Hormonal Regulation of Spermatogenesis (F.S. French, V. Hansson, E.M. Ritzen and S.N. Nayfeh, eds.), Plenum Press, New York. pp. 237-255, 1975.

5. Mainwaring, W.I.P. Monographs on Endocrinology. The Mechanism of Action of Androgens, Vol. 10, Springer-Verlag, New York. 1977.

6. Bardin, C.W., Brown, T.R., Mills, N.C., Gupta, C. and Bullock, L.P. The regulation of the β-glucuronidase gene by androgens and progestins. Biol. Reprod. 18:74-83, 1978.

7. Sundaram, K., Cao, Y.-Q., Rivier, J., Vale, W. and Bardin, C.W. Antisteroidal activity of LHRH agonists: A new biological effect. Nature(in press), 1980.

8. Lowry, O.H., Rosebrough, N.J., Farr, A.L. and Randall, R.J. Protein measurement with the Folin phenol reagent. J. Biol. Chem. 193:265- 1951.

9. Bullock, L.P., Bardin, C.W. and Sherman, M.R. Androgenic, antiandrogenic, and synandrogenic actions of progestins: Role of steric and allosteric interactions with androgen receptors. Endocrinology 103:1768-1782, 1978.

10. Bonne, C. and Raynaud, J.-P. Methyltrienolone, a specific ligand for cellular androgen receptors. Steroids 26:227-232, 1975.

11. Bonne, C. and Raynaud, J.-P. Assay of androgen binding sites by exchange with methyltrienolone (R-1881). Steroids 27:497-507, 1976.

12. Zava, D.T., Landrum, B., Horowitz, K.B. and McGuire, W.L. Androgen receptor assay with [^{3}H]-methyltrienolone (R-1881) in the presence of progesterone receptors. Endocrinology 104:1007-1012, 1979.

13. Nielsen, C.J., Sando, J.J., Vogel, W.M. and Pratt, W.B. Glucocorticoid receptor inactivation under cell-free conditions. J. Biol. Chem. 252:7568-7578, 1977.

14. Nielsen, C.J., Vogel, W.M. and Pratt, W.B. Inactivation of glucocorticoid receptors in cell-free preparations of rat liver. Cancer Res. 37:3420-3426, 1977.

15. Sando, J.J., Hammond, N.D., Stratford, C.A. and Pratt, W.B. Activation of thymocyte glucocorticoid receptors to the steroid binding form. J. Biol. Chem. 254:4779-4789, 1979.

16. Toft, D. and Nishigori, H. Stabilization of the avian progesterone receptor by inhibitors. J. Steroid Biochem. 11:413-416, 1979.

17. Bullock, L.P. and Bardin, C.W. Androgen receptors in mouse
     kidney: A study of male, female and androgen-insensitive
     (Tfm/Y) mice. Endocrinology 94:746-756, 1974.

AXC RAT PROSTATIC ADENOCARCINOMA:

CHARACTERIZATION OF CELLS IN CULTURE

Sydney A. Shain, Robert W. Boesel, S. S. Kalter,
and Richard L. Heberling

Southwest Foundation for Research and Education
San Antonio, Texas 78284

INTRODUCTION

Characterization of hormonal regulation of prostatic cancer cell growth has been limited. Although a number of human prostate cancer cell lines have been described (1-3) and at least one spontaneously derived rat prostate cancer cell line has also been described (4), these cells were not useful for studies of hormonal regulation of prostate cancer because they were unresponsive to changes in hormonal milieu (1-4). Transplantable prostatic adenocarcinomas have been described in four breeds of rats (5-9). Androgen responsiveness has been established for certain of the Copenhagen and Nb rat tumors (8-10), is indicated for the AXC rat tumors (7), and apparently is absent in Lobund Wistar rat tumors (4,6). Initial biochemical characterization of the AXC and Copenhagen rat transplantable tumors has been reported (7,10,11).

We have derived transplantable prostatic adenocarcinomas (7) from spontaneous adenocarcinomas of the AXC rat ventral prostate (11,12). Moderately well to well differentiated prostatic adenocarcinomas have been established as either rapidly growing (palpable within 3 to 4 weeks post-inoculation) or more slowly growing (palpable within 2 to 3 months post-inoculation) transplantable tumor lines. Transplantable prostatic adenocarcinoma tissue from an AXC rat bearing a second passage tumor was used to establish rat prostatic cancer in cell culture.

AXC rat prostatic cancer cells have now been maintained in continuous culture for one year without any apparent change in the properties of these cells. The rat prostatic cancer cell line, LSC-AXC, yields well to moderately well differentiated prostatic

337

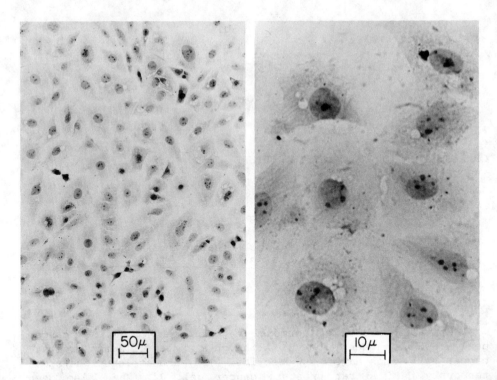

Figure 1. LSC-AXC rat prostate cancer cells in culture. Left.
The culture consists of polygonal epithelial cells which contain
enlarged, pleomorphic nuclei. Infrequent, multinucleated cells
are seen. Right. Most nuclei contain multiple, prominent
nucleoli and are surrounded by well defined granular cytoplasm.
H & E.

adenocarcinomas when inoculated subcutaneously into inbred AXC
rats. In this report we describe some of the biochemical properties of the LSC-AXC prostate cancer cell line which suggest these
cells are highly androgen responsive.

ESTABLISHMENT OF LSC-AXC CELL CULTURES

     Primary AXC rat prostatic adenocarcinoma was obtained from
the ventral prostate of a 38-month-old male. A testosterone containing silastic capsule had been subcutaneously implanted 4
months prior to sacrificing the rat. Subcutaneous inoculation of
small pieces of the primary tumor into 60-day-old male AXC rats
yielded palpable tumors at 5 to 6 months. One of the prostatic
adenocarcinomas was minced (1 mm^3) and inoculated into 22 AXC
male rats which were 80 to 90 days old. Palpable tumors were

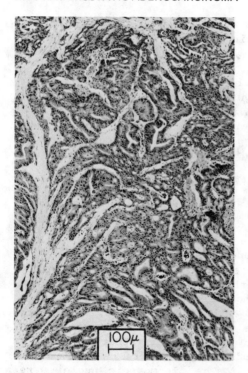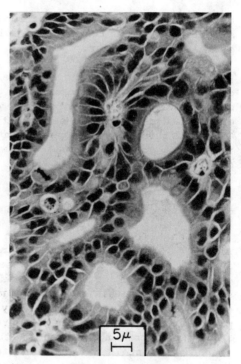

Figure 2.   LSC-AXC rat prostatic adenocarcinoma derived by s.c.
inoculation of AXC rats with LSC-AXC cells.   Left.   The
proliferating neoplastic epithelium are arranged in cribriform
patterns.   Numerous luminal spaces contain secretion products.
Hemorrhage and necrotic debris are present.   Right.   Luminal
spaces are surrounded by tall columnar neoplastic epithelium
containing basally polar, pleomorphic nuclei.   Numerous glands
contain epithelium which show a uniform supranuclear region
suggestive of active Golgi function.   Abundant secretions are
present in luminal spaces.   One gland contains a mitotic figure at
the luminal margin.   H & E.

detectable in all recipients within 60 to 80 days post-inoculation.

    Tumor was aseptically removed from one recipient at 130 days
post-inoculation and minced into 1 mm^3 pieces which were
dispersed into plastic tissue culture flasks containing modified
Eagles minimal essential medium, 10% fetal bovine serum, 100 U/ml
penicillin and 100 µg/ml streptomycin. After overnight incubation
at 37°C in 5% CO_2 in air, additional medium was added.   Medium
was routinely changed thrice weekly.   Initial confluency was
obtained in approximately 5 weeks and cultures were passaged after

harvesting by brief incubation at 37°C with a trypsin-EDTA solution (13). Cultures were split 1:2 until passage 6 and then split 1:10 thereafter.

LSC-AXC prostate cancer cells grow as typical epithelial cells in monolayer culture (Figure 1). The polygonal cells contain large, granular nuclei with prominent nucleoli. These epithelial cells have been maintained in continuous culture for 1 year without any apparent change in appearance, growth characteristics, or other properties which are described in following sections.

LSC-AXC TUMORS IN AXC RATS

When 60- to 80-day-old male AXC rats were inoculated (s.c.) with 10^7 LSC-AXC rat prostate cancer cells, palpable tumor was detectable within 25 days. These established tumors subsequently grew to 1 cm in most animals within 20 days. The tumors were solid masses containing varying amounts of hemorrhage. Histologically the tumors were moderately well differentiated, cribriform prostatic adenocarcinomas (Figure 2). Proliferating neoplastic cells were commonly arranged to form acinar structures which frequently contained secretion products. Chords of cells or cells in sheets were not commonly seen. The pleomorphic nuclei were enlarged, granular, and usually contained prominent nucleoli. Mitotic figures were numerous and often located at luminal margins (Figure 2). The morphologic characteristics of these LSC-AXC tumors are comparable to those of primary and transplantable AXC rat prostatic adenocarcinomas previously described by us (7,11,12).

BIOCHEMICAL CHARACTERIZATION OF LSC-AXC PROSTATE CANCER CELLS AND TUMORS

A.   Characterization of Androphiles

Exchange saturation analysis protocols which were developed in these laboratories for measurement of total androgen receptors in rodent (14), canine (15), and human (16) prostate were used to characterize androphiles in LSC-AXC prostate cancer cells and tumors. Single concentration inhibition studies of steroid specificity showed that only androgens which did not require metabolic conversion in order to be effective in prostate were potent inhibitors of R1881 (17β-hydroxy-17α-methyl-estra-4,9,11-trien-3-one) binding to cytoplasmic androphiles or of 5α-dihydrotestosterone (5α-DHT) binding to nuclear androphiles (Tables 1 and 2). Progesterone, estradiol-17β, and cortisol were either ineffective or

Table 1. Relative Steroid Specificity of Total Cytoplasmic
          Androgen Receptors in AXC Rat Prostatic Tissues

| | Specific Binding (% Control) | | |
Competitor	Ventral Prostate	LSC-AXC Cells	LSC-AXC Tumors
None	100	100	100
R1881	4 + 2	7 + 5	4 + 3
5α-Dihydrotestosterone	4 + 4	10 + 2	11 + 4
19-Nortestosterone	4 + 4	14 + 2	2 + 2
5α-Androstane-3α,17β-diol	48 + 20	78 + 3	42 + 10
4-Androstenedione	86 + 14	106 + 4	41 + 11
Estradiol	83 + 13	94 + 3	62 + 5
Progesterone	88 + 8	99 + 6	84 + 9
Cortisol	95 + 9	116 + 6	92 + 3

Probe, R1881, concentration was 10 nM. Competitor concentration
was 500 nM. Incubation was at 15°C for 20 to 24 hr. Data are the
mean $\pm$ SEM, n = 3-5.

Table 2. Relative Steroid Specificity of Nuclear Androgen
          Receptors in AXC Rat Prostatic Tissues

| | Specific Binding (% Control) | | |
Competitor	Ventral Prostate	LSC-AXC Cells	LSC-AXC Tumors
None	100	100	100
5α-Dihydrotestosterone	6 + 4	0	0
R1881	7 + 3	4 + 2	23 + 6
19-Nortestosterone	12 + 6	10 + 6	16 + 4
5α-Androstane-3α,17β-diol	78 + 8	83 + 2	74 + 7
4-Androstenedione	97 + 3	93 + 3	91 + 7
Estradiol	59 + 7	69 + 1	63 + 5
Progesterone	83 + 6	83 + 2	88 + 5
Cortisol	97 + 6	100 + 3	102 + 8

Probe, 5α-DHT, concentration was 10 nM. Competitor concentration
was 500 nM. Incubation was at 2°C for 20 to 24 hr. Data are the
mean $\pm$ SEM, n = 3-5.

poor inhibitors of androgen binding to cytoplasmic or nuclear androphiles in LSC-AXC prostatic cancer cells and prostate tumors. Notably, steroid specificity of R1881 binding to cytoplasmic androphiles or 5α-DHT binding to nuclear androphiles in LSC-AXC prostatic cancer cells or tumors was indistinguishable from that characteristic of R1881 binding to cytoplasmic or 5α-DHT binding to nuclear androgen receptors of rat ventral prostate (Tables 1 and 2).

Cytoplasmic androphiles measured by exchange saturation analysis (incubation with R1881 at 15°C) presented heterogeneous patterns when analyzed by sedimentation on low ionic strength sucrose density gradients (Figure 3). Some analyses showed a single broad peak of specific binding activity which sedimented at 8-10S, whereas other analyses showed two well defined peaks of specific binding activity, one of which sedimented at 8-10S and another which sedimented at 3-4S. Both gradient patterns were obtained with different specimens of either LSC-AXC prostatic cancer cells or tumors. Steroid unoccupied cytoplasmic androphiles of LSC-AXC prostatic cancer cells or tumors, measured by incubation at 2°C, showed a single peak of specific binding activity which sedimented at 9S on low ionic strength linear sucrose density gradients (Figure 3). Nuclear androphiles measured by incubation with 5α-DHT at 2°C showed a single peak of specific binding activity which sedimented at 3-4S on high ionic strength (0.6 M KCl) linear sucrose density gradients (Figure 3). Based upon analyses of relative steroid specificity (Tables 1 and 2), sedimentation properties on linear sucrose gradients (Figure 3), and apparent steroid dissociation constants (data not shown), the cytoplasmic and nuclear androphiles of LSC-AXC prostatic cancer cells and tumors are prostatic androgen receptors.

B.   Androgen Regulation of Androgen Receptor Distribution in
      LSC-AXC Cancer Cells and Tumors

At 24 hr post-orchiectomy, cytoplasmic androgen receptor content of ventral prostate of young or aged AXC rats is indistinguishable from that of intact AXC rats (Figure 4). The predominant effect of orchiectomy upon AXC rat ventral prostate cytoplasmic androgen receptors is depletion of steroid from androgen-occupied cytoplasmic receptors (14). Cytoplasmic androgen receptor content of LSC-AXC tumors is comparable to that of ventral prostate of aged AXC rats. At 48-hr post-orchiectomy, cytoplasmic androgen receptor content of LSC-AXC tumors is somewhat enhanced when compared to that of intact AXC rats bearing LSC-AXC tumors (Figure 4). Cytoplasmic androgen receptor content of LSC-AXC cells grown in either the absence or presence of added androgen is significantly less than that of LSC-AXC tumors or ventral prostate of young or aged AXC rats (Figure 4). As was the case for LSC-AXC

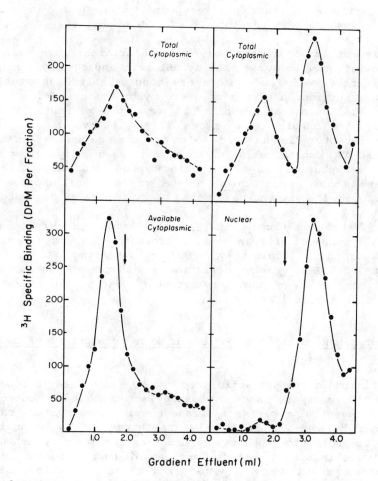

Figure 3. Sucrose density gradient analysis of LSC-AXC prostatic cancer cells or prostatic tumor androgen receptors. Total cytoplasmic (R_C plus $R_C A$) receptors were labeled with R1881 by incubation at 15°C for 20 to 24 hr and analyzed by centrifugation through 10-30% buffered sucrose. Available cytoplasmic receptors (R_C) were labeled with R1881 by incubation at 2°C for 2 hr and analyzed by centrifugation through 10-30% buffered sucrose. Total nuclear receptors were labeled by incubation with 5α-DHT at 2°C for 20 to 24 hr and analyzed by centrifugation through 5-20% buffered sucrose containing 0.6 M KCl. All gradients were developed by centrifugation for 2 hr at 2°C at 65 K rpm (VTi 65 rotor). The arrow indicates the position of sedimentation of human γ-globulin.

tumors, cytoplasmic androgen receptor content was greatest in LSC-AXC cells grown in the absence of added androgen.

This effect of androgen may be more apparent than real. We have consistently observed that cytoplasmic androgen receptors of LSC-AXC cancer cells and tumors are considerably less stable to exchange saturation analysis than are cytoplasmic androgen receptors of AXC rat ventral prostate (14) or canine prostate (15). We currently are unable to overcome this problem of cytoplasmic androgen receptor "inactivation" during exchange saturation analysis of LSC-AXC cancer cells and tumors. Consequently, cytoplasmic androgen receptor values reported in Figure 4 for LSC-AXC cancer cells and tumors maintained in the presence of androgen may represent significant underestimates of actual receptor content.

At 24-hr post-orchiectomy, nuclear androgen receptors are essentially undetectable in ventral prostate of young or aged AXC rats (Figure 5). Orchiectomy of AXC rats bearing LSC-AXC tumors or growth of LSC-AXC cancer cells in the absence of added androgen also reduced nuclear androgen receptor content to essentially undetectable levels (Figure 5).

C.   Androgen Regulation of Prolactin Receptor Content of LSC-AXC Tumors

Iodinated ovine prolactin prepared by a modified lactoperoxidase procedure may be used to measure lactogen binding components in AXC rat ventral prostate membrane preparations. Since rat FSH and growth hormone are ineffective inhibitors of ovine prolactin binding to prostatic membranes, whereas rat prolactin does inhibit ovine prolactin binding, these lactogen binding components of AXC rat ventral prostate may be considered to be prostatic prolactin receptors. Orchiectomy profoundly diminishes prolactin receptor content of ventral prostate of young mature or aged AXC rats (Figure 6). This effect of orchiectomy upon ventral prostate prolactin receptor content in young mature rats has been reported by others (17,18). Prolactin receptor content of LSC-AXC tumors in intact AXC rats is nearly fourfold greater than that of ventral prostate of aged AXC rats and is only modestly less than that of ventral prostate of young mature AXC rats. Notably, orchiectomy of AXC rats bearing LSC-AXC rat tumors results in a nearly complete loss of LSC-AXC tumor prolactin receptors (Figure 6).

D.   Androgen Regulation of Enzymes of Polyamine Synthesis in LSC-AXC Tumors

At 48 hr post-orchiectomy S-adenosyl-L-methionine decarboxylase (AMDC) content of ventral prostate of young mature or aged AXC

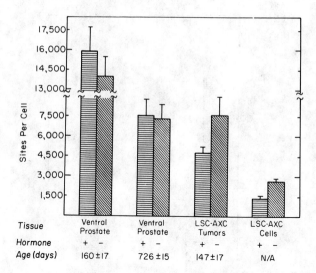

Figure 4. Effect of androgen upon total cytoplasmic androgen receptor content of AXC rat prostatic tissues. Normal AXC rats or LSC-AXC prostatic tumor bearing rats were intact (+) or orchiectomized (-) 24 (normal rats) to 48 (tumor bearing rats) hr prior to sacrifice. LSC-AXC prostate cancer cells were either grown in the presence (+) or absence (-) of added androgen (10^{-7}M). Quantitation of total and available androgen receptors was performed as described in Figure 3.

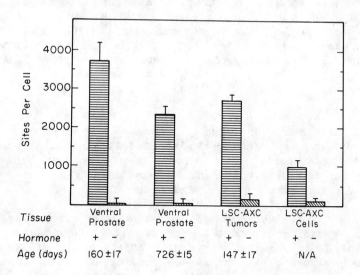

Figure 5. Effect of androgen upon total nuclear androgen receptor content of AXC rat prostatic tissues. All conditions are as described in Figure 4.

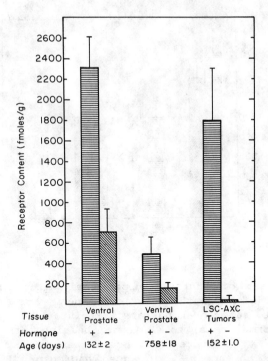

Figure 6. Effect of androgen upon prolactin receptor content of
AXC rat prostatic tissues. Washed plasma membranes were prepared
from homogenized tissue by centrifugation at 27 K x g. Receptor
content was quantitated by saturation analysis performed in 300 µl
of pH 7.6 buffer containing 25 mM Tris, 10 mM CaCl₂, 0.067% BSA,
200 U/ml penicillin, 200 µg/ml streptomycin and 200 µg/ml kanamy-
cin. Incubation was for 48 hr at 25°C and was terminated by
adding 2 ml buffer followed by centrifugation for 5 min at
1 K x g. The washed pellet was counted for ^{125}I content.
Orchiectomy was at 48 hr prior to sacrifice.

rats is significantly diminished (Figure 7). AMDC content of
LSC-AXC prostatic tumors is not altered following orchiectomy of
AXC rats bearing these tumors. Notably AMDC content of LSC-AXC
prostatic tumors is significantly less than that of ventral
prostate of young mature or aged AXC rats (Figure 7).

At 48 hr post-orchiectomy, L-ornithine decarboxylase (ODC)
content of ventral prostate of young mature or aged AXC rats is
significantly diminished (Figure 8). Orchiectomy of AXC rats
bearing LSC-AXC prostatic tumors also causes a diminution in ODC
content. As was the case for AMDC content of LSC-AXC prostatic
tumors, ODC content of these tumors is significantly less than
that of either young mature or aged AXC rats (Figure 8).

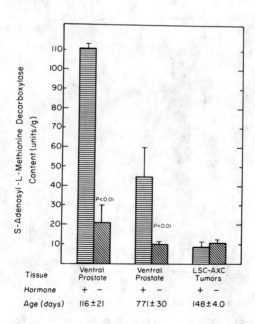

Figure 7. Effect of androgen upon S-adenosyl-L-methionine decar-boxylase content of AXC rat prostatic tissues. Enzyme activity was assayed by a micromodification of the procedure originally described by Pegg et al. (21). One unit of enzyme activity produces one nmole CO_2/30 min. Orchiectomy was at 48 hr prior to sacrifice.

That AMDC and ODC content are transiently elevated in both normal and neoplastic tissue following an acute growth stimulus is well documented (19). It is also established that AMDC or ODC content is not necessarily elevated in some neoplastic tissues (19,20). The decrease in ODC content of LSC-AXC prostatic tumors is in contrast to the generally observed two- to eightfold eleva-tion of hepatoma ODC content as opposed to normal liver ODC content (20). The decrease in AMDC content of LSC-AXC tumors is characteristic of the change in AMDC content of hepatomas (20).

E.   Acid Phosphatases of LSC-AXC Tumors

Both secretory, androgen dependent, and lysosomal, androgen independent acid phosphatases of ventral prostate of aged AXC rats are significantly diminished compared to ventral prostate of young mature AXC rats (Figure 9). Secretory acid phosphatase content of LSC-AXC prostatic tumors is comparable to that of ventral prostate of aged AXC rats, whereas lysosomal acid phosphatase content of LSC-AXC prostatic tumors is greater than that of ventral prostate

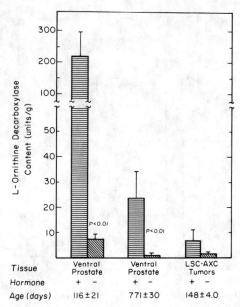

Figure 8. Effect of androgen upon L-ornithine decarboxylase content of AXC rat prostatic tissues. All definitions and conditions are as described in Figure 7.

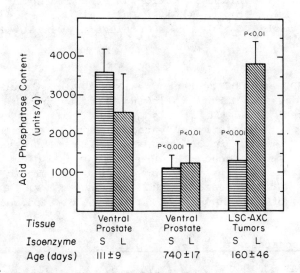

Figure 9. Secretory (S) and lysosomal (L) acid phosphatase content of AXC rat prostatic tissues. Enzyme activity was assayed by a minor modification of the procedure of Helminen et al. (22) and used α-naphthol phosphate as substrate. One unit of enzyme activity hydrolyzes one nmole α-naphthol phosphate/60 min. Other definitions and conditions are as described in Figure 7.

of young mature AXC rats (Figure 9).   The presence of secretory acid phosphatase in LSC-AXC tumors at a level identical to that of ventral   prostate   of   aged   AXC   rats   suggests   maintenance   of significant androgen responsive differentiated function in LSC-AXC prostatic tumors.

SUMMARY

We   have   described   the   establishment   of   AXC   rat   prostatic cancer cells in continuous culture.   When injected into isogeneic male   rats,   these   cells   produce   prostatic   adenocarcinomas.   The response of androgen and prolactin receptors and ODC in LSC-AXC prostatic cancer cells and tumors to androgen ablation is indistinguishable from that of ventral prostate.   In addition, LSC-AXC prostatic   tumors   retain   levels   of   secretory   acid   phosphatase comparable to those of ventral prostate of aged AXC rats.   These data demonstrate that LSC-AXC prostatic cancer cells and tumors retain a high degree of differentiated, androgen regulated function.   The LSC-AXC prostatic cancer cells and tumors appear to represent a unique model system for combined in vivo and in vitro studies of androgen regulation of prostate cancer cell function.

ACKNOWLEDGEMENTS

These studies were supported in part by the National Cancer Institute CA 21864 and CP 33379, the National Institutes of Health RR 00361, and the World Health Organization V4/181/38.   We are grateful to Nancy Dawson, Robert Klipper, Judi Koger, and Anita Moss for their expert assistance.

REFERENCES

1.   Kaighn, M. E., Narayan, K. S., Ohnuki, Y., Lechner, J. F., and Jones, L. W.:   Establishment and characterization of a human prostatic carcinoma cell line (PC-3).   Invest. Urol. 17:16-23, 1979.

2.   Stone, K. R., Mickey, D. D., Wunderli, H., Mickey, G. H., and Paulson, D. F.:   Isolation of a human prostate carcinoma cell line (DU 145).   Int. J. Cancer 21:274-281, 1978.

3.   Okada, K., Laudenbach, I., and Schroeder, F. H.:   Human prostatic epithelial cells in culture: Clonal selection and androgen   dependence   of   cell   line   EB   33.   J.   Urol. 115:164-167, 1976.

4. Chang, C. F. and Pollard, M.: _In vitro_ propagation of prostate adenocarcinoma cells from rats. Invest. Urol. 14:331-334, 1977.

5. Dunning, W. F.: Prostate cancer in the rat. Natl. Cancer Inst. Monogr. 12:351-369, 1963.

6. Pollard, M. and Luckert, P. H.: Transplantable metastasizing prostate adenocarcinomas in rats. J. Natl. Cancer Inst. 54:643-649, 1975.

7. Shain, S. A., McCullough, B., and Nitchuk, W. M.: Primary and transplantable adenocarcinomas of the A X C rat ventral prostate gland: Morphologic characterization and examination of C_{19}-steroid metabolism by early-passage tumors. J. Natl. Cancer Inst. 62:313-322, 1979.

8. Noble, R. L.: The development of prostatic adenocarcinoma in Nb rats following prolonged sex hormone administration. Cancer Res. 37:1929-1933, 1977.

9. Drago, J. R., Gershwin, M. E., Maurer, R. E., Ikeda, R. M., and Eckels, D. D.: Immunobiology and therapeutic manipulation of heterotransplanted Nb rat prostate adenocarcinoma into congenitally athymic (nude) mice. I. Hormone dependency and histopathology. J. Natl. Cancer Inst. 62:1057-1066, 1979.

10. Smolev, J. K., Heston, W.D.W., Scott, W. W., and Coffey, D. S.: Characterization of the Dunning R3327H prostatic adenocarcinoma: An appropriate animal model for prostatic cancer. Cancer Treat. Reports 61:273-287, 1977.

11. Shain, S. A., McCullough, B., Nitchuk, M., and Boesel, R. W.: Prostate carcinogenesis in the AXC rat. Oncology 34:114-122, 1977.

12. Shain, S. A., McCullough, B., and Segaloff, A.: Spontaneous adenocarcinomas of the ventral prostate of aged A X C rats. J. Natl. Cancer Inst. 55:177-180, 1975.

13. Weiss, S. A., Lester, T. L., Kalter, S. S., and Heberling, R. L.: Chemically defined serum free media for the cultivation of primary cells and their susceptibility to viruses. In Vitro 15:1980. In press.

14. Boesel, R. W., Klipper, R. W., and Shain, S. A.: Androgen regulation of androgen receptor content and distribution in the ventral and dorsolateral prostates of aging AXC rats. Steroids 35:February, 1980. In press.

15. Shain, S. A. and Boesel, R. W.: Androgen receptor content of
     the normal and hyperplastic canine prostate.   J. Clin.
     Invest. 61:654-660, 1978.

16. Shain, S. A., Boesel, R. W., Lamm, D. L., and Radwin, H. M.:
     Cytoplasmic and nuclear androgen receptor content of normal
     and neoplastic human prostate and lymph node metastases of
     human prostatic adenocarcinoma. J. Clin. Endocrinol. Metab.
     50:April, 1980. In press.

17. Hanlin, M. L. and Yount, A. P.: Prolactin binding in the rat
     ventral prostate. Endocrine Res. Commun. 2:489-502, 1975.

18. Kledzik, G. S., Marshall, S., Campbell, G. A., Gelato, M.,
     and Meites, J.: Effects of castration, testosterone, estra-
     diol, and prolactin on specific prolactin-binding activity in
     ventral prostate of male rats.   Endocrinology 98:373-379,
     1976.

19. Tabor, C. W. and Tabor, H.:   1,4-Diaminobutane (putrescine),
     spermidine, and spermine.   Annu. Rev. Biochem. 45:285-306,
     1976.

20. Williams-Ashman, H. G., Coppac, G. L., and Weber, G.: Imbal-
     ance in ornithine metabolism in hepatomas of different growth
     rates as expresed in formation of putrescine, spermidine, and
     spermine. Cancer Res. 32:1924-1932, 1972.

21. Pegg, A. E., Lockwood, D. H., and Williams-Ashman, H. G.:
     Concentrations of putrescine and polyamines and their enzymic
     synthesis during androgen-induced prostatic growth. Biochem.
     J. 117:17-31, 1970.

22. Helminen, H. J., Ericsson, J.L.E., Rytoluoto, R., and
     Vanha-Perttula, T.:   Acid phosphatases of the rat ventral
     prostate. IN: Symposium on the Normal and Abnormal Growth
     of the Prostate, San Antonio, Texas, 1973, M. Goland (ed.).
     Charles C. Thomas, Springfield, Ill. 1975, pp. 275-316.

POTENTIAL BIOCHEMICAL MARKERS IN THE DIAGNOSIS

AND MANAGEMENT OF HUMAN PROSTATE CARCINOMA

W. Ian P. Mainwaring

Department of Biochemistry
9 Hyde Terrace
Leeds LS2 9LS, U.K.

INTRODUCTION

Particularly during the last few years, the benefit of
accurate and early diagnosis in the successful arrest and management
of human cancer has been universally acknowledged. Many trials are
currently in progress worldwide, with several objectives in view:
(a) to screen large populations for potential cancer victims,
(b) to provide alternative criteria to clinical judgements alone in
selecting the most appropriate form of therapy for a given cancer
patient and finally (c) to devise simple but reliable tests for
monitoring the progress and efficacy of cancer therapy.

Throughout all urbanized, western-styled societies, benign
prostatic hyperplasia and invasive prostatic adenoma remain the
fourth most common manifestation of cancer among ageing human males.
With the onset of senescence, all Caucasian and Black males are
potential victims of abnormal prostatic growth and the incidence of
such disease shows no apparent correlation with social standing,
economic status, occupation or personal habit. Despite the large
numbers of patients involved, modern urological surgery is now
generally recognized as a safe, efficient and acceptable means for
combating benign prostatic hyperplasia. By contrast, prostatic
adenomata are seldom amenable to surgical ablation or anucleation
because such tumours metastasize frequently and widely, especially
into the spinal vertebrae, sacrum or pelvis. The present concensus
is that chemotherapy remains the most hopeful avenue to the successful control of this form of malignant disease in males. Based on
the classical observations of John Hunter over two hundred years
ago, and of Ramm[1] in Norway and of White[2] in the U.S.A. about the
turn of the last century, prostatic cancer is widely believed to be

a hormone-sensitive neoplasm, although this supposition still requires rigorous, incontestable validation. Nonetheless, the putative necessity for androgens in prostate tumour growth was exploited by Huggins and Hodges[3] when they advocated stilboestrol as a prostate antagonist. Subject to its necessary restriction to a "low-dose" regimen[4], this synthetic oestrogen often provides patients with prostate cancer with relief from bone pain and even long-term cure, despite the serious limitations and side effects of this chemotherapeutic agent[5].

As is the case with other forms of human cancer, urologists and oncologists urgently need markers in prostate adenomata, not only of the extent of dedifferentiation of the tumour[6], but also to indicate whether hormonal manipulation will be clinically effective[5]. The urgency for such prostatic markers is well reflected in recent international symposia on this topic[7]. Much is now known about the mode of action of androgens at the molecular level[8] and the present paper describes preliminary studies on potentially important, biochemical markers in the context of the diagnosis and prognosis of human prostatic carcinoma. The importance of androgen receptors in regulating normal prostate growth is now beyond dispute[8], but although some refined work on receptors in cancerous specimens of human prostate is available in the recent literature[9], other parameters of prostate growth were overlooked in this[9] and other studies[10]. Here, I attempt to correlate the androgen receptor content in specimens of human prostatic carcinomata with proven indicators of prostate growth and DNA replication, including ornithine decarboxylase[11].   DNA polymerase α (DNA replication enzyme)[12], thymidine kinase[12] and DNA-unwinding protein[13,14]. The components associated with DNA synthesis are particularly important, because Mainwaring et al.[15] have shown convincingly that, during ventral prostate growth evoked in castrated rats by testosterone in vivo, they are synthesized de novo precisely and only at the time of mitosis. A possible corollary in the clinical sense is that hormone-sensitive or rapidly-dividing prostate tumour cells will be particularly rich in the components necessary for DNA replication, whereas hormone-insensitive or slowly dividing tumour cells will not.

MATERIALS AND METHODS

Experimental Hepatectomies

Radical hepatectomy was performed according to Higgins and Anderson[16] on male Wistar rats (200 g body weight) under ether anaesthesia. As a routine, the medium and left lateral lobes were removed, resulting in a 65-70% reduction in the wet weight of the liver. During recovery, animals were given unrestricted access to rat chow and a 5% (w/v) solution of D-glucose. Survival was 95% or better.

Samples of Human Prostate Carcinomas

Over a period of four years, 23 such specimens were obtained with the considerate help of urological surgeons in London, the Home Counties and Yorkshire. During the early phase of this study, specimens were halved; one half was analyzed directly and the other after storage in liquid nitrogen for up to 6 months. The absolute consistency of these comparative analyses was such that specimens were quenched in liquid nitrogen on removal, transported to the laboratory and stored at -196° C. Several stored samples were then worked up concurrently. For every specimen, the presence of prostate carcinoma was verified at the hospital of origin by routine pathological examination.

Biochemical Studies on Regenerating Rat Liver

(a) Mitotic indices. At 2 h before sacrifice, rats were injected subcutaneously with colchicine (150 μg/100 g body weight) in 0.5 ml of 0.9% NaCl to arrest dividing cells in metaphase. Samples of regenerating liver were fixed in Carnoy's medium (ethanol- chloro-form-acetic acid, 6:3:1, v/v) for 2 h, embedded in paraffin wax and sections (2-4 nm thick) were cut in the standard histological procedure. After staining with haemotoxylin-eosin Y mixture, metaphase plates were counted under the microscope. At least 1000 were scanned and the mitotic index was calculated as the number of dividing cells per 1000 cells observed; a minimum of 6 slides was analyzed for each sample of liver.

(b) Incorporation of [^{3}H]thymidine into DNA. Rats were subdued by exposure to an atmosphere of 50% CO_2 - 50% air and 50 μCi of [methyl-^{3}H]thymidine (28 Ci/mmol; Radiochemical Centre, Amersham, U.K.) were injected in 0.5 ml of 0.9% NaCl into the tail vein. Exactly 1 h later, animals were killed by cervical dislocation and the incorporation of [^{3}H]thymidine into regenerating liver DNA was determined precisely as described by Coffey et al.[17].

(c) Biochemical Assays. Full details have already been published of the methods used for the assay or ornithine decarboxylase[11], DNA polymerase α[12], thymidine kinase[12] and DNA-unwinding protein[13,14]. Only the cytoplasmic form of thymidine kinase is assayed by the procedure for cell fractionation used here; DNA-unwinding activity was measured both by the retention of [^{3}H]thymidine-labelled, native DNA from Ehrlich ascites tumour cells on Millipore membranes[13] or the activation of native (helical) thymus DNA as a template for purified DNA polymerase α from ascites tumour cells[14]. Protein was measured by the Folin-Ciocalteu reagent[18], with crystalline bovine serum albumin as reference standard.

(d) Fractionation of Regenerating Liver. Pooled livers (up to

20 g wet weight) from at least 4 animals (often 6), were gently
but thoroughly homogenized in 5 volumes of 0.25 M sucrose containing 0.5% (v/v) Triton X-100, using a motor-driven, coaxial homogenizer (Silverson Machines Ltd., Chesham, U.K.; model E 25) at
500 rev/min for 1 min. Centrifugation at 1000 g for 10 min yielded
two fractions, a sediment containing nuclei and an opalescent
supernatant. The sediment was washed twice in sucrose-Triton
mixture and then extracted with 1 M NaCl and polyethylene glycol
6000 to release DNA-unwinding protein[13]; the assay of DNA-unwinding
activity was conducted after overnight dialysis of the active
nuclear extract to remove NaCl, other inhibitory materials and
cell-derived components of low molecular weight. The 1000 g supernatant fraction was clarified by ultracentrifugation at 150 000 g
for 1 h, and after overnight dialysis against medium R, i.e. 50 mM
Tris-HCl buffer, pH 7.4, containing 10% (v/v) glycerol, 0.5 mM
EDTA and 1.5 mM dithiothreitol, (with subsequent clarification by
centrifugation if necessary), the final soluble fraction or cytosol
was assayed for DNA-polymerase α and thymidine kinase activities.

(e) The Incorporation of [^{3}H]amino acids into specific proteins.
Mainwaring et al.[15] devised a scheme for labelling certain
components associated with DNA replication in vitro with subsequent
fractionation of the labelled cells such that the recovery of the
labelled but separated components gave a valid indication of their
synthesis in vivo. Essentially, the procedure depends on highly
selective separation of the components, with good recoveries
throughout. Tissue under investigation is coarsely minced in a
Latapie mincer (Baird and Tatlock Ltd., Chadwell Heath, U.K.) and
resuspended in Morton's minimal medium[19] (1 g/4 ml), supplemented
with a mixture of [^{3}H]L-amino acids (Radiochemical Centre, Amersham,
U.K.) at 50 μCi/ml. After incubation for 1 h in a Dubnoff
metabolic shaker, oscillating at 150 cyc/min, in an atmosphere of
5% CO_2 - 95% air at 37° C, the labelled tissue was drained and
rinsed three times in 0.25 M sucrose - 0.5% Triton X-100 (tritium-
free). Homogenization was then accomplished as described in
section (d), above, with centrifugation at 1000 g yielding labelled
nuclear and supernatant fractions. In the "work up" of each of
these fractions, the distinctive properties of the protein under
investigation are given in brackets. [^{3}H]DNA-unwinding protein
was separated from the nuclear sediment by sequential extraction
in 1 M-NaCl plus 20% polyethyleneglycol 6000 (extraction), chromatography on columns of Sepharose 4B containing immobilized
Cibacron Blue F3GA (adsorption; elution in 0.5 M-NaCl), dialysis
and isoelectric focussing in 5% polyacrylamide gels containing
ampholytes, pH range 3.5 - 10.0 (pI, 9.2). The [^{3}H] supernatant
was clarified by centrifugation at 100 000 g for 1 h and then used
for the separation of [^{3}H]DNA polymerase α and [^{3}H]thymidine
kinase. The [^{3}H] cytosol was loaded on to columns of Sepharose-CH,
containing covalently linked thymidine 3'-phosphate, yielding a

specifically absorbed protein fraction and a "flow-through" (non-adsorbed) fraction. After extensive washing of the columns, application of 1 mM thymidine selectively eluted [3H]thymidine kinase. The flow through peak was processed for [3H]DNA polymerase α by sequential adjustment of pH to 5.2 (precipitation), sucrose density gradients (9S), and electrophoresis in non-denaturing, 7.5% polyacrylamide gels at pH 8.9 (Rf 0.27, relative to the marker, bromophenol blue). Based on several criteria, all proteins were judged as active and homogeneous[15] with overall yields as follows: DNA-unwinding protein, 70%, thymidine kinase, 90%, and DNA polymerase α, 40%. [3H]Thymidine kinase was prepared in a homogeneous state directly. Where gel electrophoresis was the last step of the fractionation procedure, 50 µg of protein were separated and the radioactivity associated with the appropriate region of the gel was taken as a true indication of the recovery of [3H]DNA polymerase α or [3H]DNA-unwinding protein.

Biochemical Studies on Specimens of Human Prostatic Carcinomas

Frozen tissue was broken by tapping with a small hammer on a stainless steel plate, both previously cooled to -60° C in an acetone-solid CO_2 freezing mixture. The pulverized powder was suspended in medium R (1 g/3 ml) and blended in a Silverson homogenizer, operating at 500 rev/min for 1 min. Centrifugation at 100 000 g for 1 h provided a clear cytosol fraction. Aliquots were analyzed in triplicate for DNA-unwinding protein, ornithine decarboxylase, DNA polymerase α, thymidine kinase and specific androgen receptor proteins. The last procedure was accomplished by the exchange method of Davies et al.[20] for total receptor sites (i.e. free plus unoccupied sites), using both [3H]5α-dihydrotestosterone[20] or [3H]methyltrienolone[21] ([3H]-R1881) as model ligands.

RESULTS

In their recent paper, Mainwaring et al.[15] suggest that many of the essential components for DNA replication are synthesized de novo, precisely at the time of the S and M phases of the cell cycle. The experimental system employed[15] was the growth and regeneration of the ventral prostate gland promoted by the injection of testosterone in vivo into 7-day castrated rats. The concept of the de novo synthesis of the mitotic machinery is so important to the central theme of this present paper, that it was further corroborated in another experimental system, namely the regeneration of liver in the radically hepatectomized rat. Admittedly, liver regeneration has not been shown to be mediated by steroid hormones, but nevertheless, it does provide a dramatic and practically expedient system for monitoring the induction of mitosis under controlled experimental conditions. In addition, the abundance of actively-dividing liver cells makes the isolation and assay of specific components of DNA replication a relatively easy task.

The temporal features of the regeneration of rat liver are summarized in Table 1. Even within 12 hours of hepatectomy, mitotic activity is stimulated in the remaining liver parenchymal cells. This surge in cell division reaches a maximum 24 hours after hepatectomy and then gradually declines to the baseline levels of mitotic activity in normal, regenerating liver. What is particularly striking is that all the morphological and biochemical indicators of cell division are seen in close unison, indicating that whatever the molecular stimulus for liver regeneration really is, the overall process is rapidly accelerated yet closely controlled throughout.

Additional experiments, summarized in Table 2, indicate that many of the components required for DNA replication are synthesized at the time of maximal mitosis during regeneration of rat liver. Once this wave of mitotic activity is completed, the synthesis of all these components slows down to the maintenance levels found in normal, non-regenerating liver.

In a concluding series of experiments, performed intermittently over the last three years, several biochemical parameters were assayed quantitatively in the cytosol fraction prepared from 23 specimens of human prostatic adenoma. It should be emphasized that the fractionation of these surgical specimens was not as rigorous as that employed for regenerating liver (see Table 2). Because the prostate samples were necessarily frozen for long periods prior to analysis, it proved impossible to prepare intact prostate nuclei, retaining their full complement of DNA-unwinding protein. As a necessary alternative, homogenization conditions were deliberately selected, using a homogenization medium of low ionic strength such that nuclear lysis and complete cell destruction were encouraged, thus releasing all of the components under investigation into the prostate cytosol fraction[12,13]. These studies on prostatic carcinoma are presented in Table 3.

Irrespective of the model ligand used, the cytoplasmic androgen receptor content of these samples was remarkably similar, all the values falling within the narrow range of 17 - 27 f mol of specifically bound [3H]ligand/mg prostate cytosol protein. This similarity cannot be explained by experimental serendipity, because samples of the indefinitely stable receptor from rabbit uterus (with [3H]diethylstilboestrol as model ligand) were always run in parallel as a reliable internal control for our exchange assay system. In sharp contrast, all of the biochemical indicators of DNA replication, plus ornithine decarboxylase, a valid marker of prostate growth, presented an extremely wide spectrum of activities from one surgical specimen to another. Again, this wide range of results cannot be explained away by experimental errors and fluctuations. Considerably quality control was built into the assay scheme by including stable cytosol preparations derived from

Table 1. Time course of the changes evoked in rat liver by hepatectomy

Liver	Mitotic index$_a$	DNA synthesis$_b$	DNA polymerase α_c	Thymidine kinase$_d$	DNA-unwinding activity$_e$
(1) Normal	2 ± 0.1	1,610 ± 40	28.8 ± 4.1	9.2 ± 0.5	3.2 ± 0.3
(2) Regenerating					
12	14 ± 1	7,420 ± 200	47.2 ± 6.0	14.3 ± 0.8	8.4 ± 0.7
24	87 ± 3	29,440 ± 310	107.4 ± 8.9	31.7 ± 1.7	17.9 ± 1.7
36	76 ± 6	21,920 ± 170	99.1 ± 7.2	28.4 ± 1.1	16.4 ± 1.2
48	41 ± 4	13,100 ± 40	48.2 ± 5.4	21.2 ± 0.9	14.9 ± 1.4
72 hours after hepatectomy	13 ± 1	1,100 ± 20	30.1 ± 1.7	10.1 ± 0.6	4.6 ± 0.4

Footnotes: All results are given as the mean ± S.E.M. Enzyme assays were made on tissue pooled from at least 4 animals. DNA synthesis was measured in 2 animals. Mitotic indices were measured in 2 animals, with 6 slides being examined for mitotic figures for each specimen. a, Number of mitotic cells/1000 cells. b, Incorporation of [³H]thymidine into DNA (d.p.m./mg DNA). c, with heat-denatured DNA as template, p mol [³H]dGMP incorporated/mg protein/30 min at 37º C. d, p mol [³H]dTMP formed/mg protein/30 min at 37º C. e, μg [³H] native DNA retained on Millipore filters/ 100 μg protein.

Table 2. The synthesis of key components during the regeneration of rat liver

Liver	DNA-unwinding protein	DNA polymerase α	Thymidine kinase
(1) Normal	430 ± 20	240 ± 10	200 ± 20
(2) Regenerating			
12	620 ± 40	390 ± 40	370 ± 10
24	1,070 ± 90	890 ± 60	640 ± 40
36	820 ± 20	880 ± 10	680 ± 50
48	640 ± 70	740 ± 40	530 ± 30
72 hours after hepatectomy	400 ± 10	300 ± 10	240 ± 10

In each experiment, livers pooled from 4 animals were minced and incubated with a mixture of [^{3}H] amino acids in vitro for 1 h.   The labelled tissue was then processed as described in the Materials and Methods section, leading to the isolation of [^{3}H]-labelled protein. In every case, the last purification step was performed on replicates of 50 μg of [^{3}H]-labelled proteins and the radioactivity associated with the specific protein was determined. All results are the mean ± S.E.M. of assays performed in triplicate, as d.p.m./purified protein band recovered after gel electrophoresis. In the case of thymidine kinase, the protein was purified to a homogeneous state by the concluding step of affinity chromatography; these values are given, therefore, as d.p.m./ 50 μg recovered enzyme

Table 3. Biochemical assays conducted on cytosols from
23 samples of human prostatic adenomas

Androgen receptors (f mol/mg protein) (a) [^{3}H]5α-Dihydrotestosterone or (b) [^{3}H]R 1881 as model ligand	20.5 ± 1.1 22.0 ± 4.6
DNA polymerase α (p mol [^{3}H]GMP incorporated/mg protein/30 min at 37° C)	117 ± 98
Thymidine kinase (p mol [^{3}H]TMP formed/mg protein/30 min at 37° C)	76 ± 51
DNA-unwinding protein (μg [^{3}H] native DNA retained/100 μg protein)	14.2 ± 7.9
Ornithine decarboxylase (p mol [^{14}CO$_2$] released/mg protein/30 min at 37° C)	840 ± 490

Ehrlich ascites tumour cells as internal standards. Since these
components for growth and DNA replication are generally synthesized
only in actively-dividing cells (Tables 1 and 2), then it would
appear that these surgical specimens of prostate adenoma had a
markedly disparate potential in terms of mitosis and cell division.
Surprisingly, this diversity of mitotic potential was not reflected
in the androgen receptor contents of the samples.

DISCUSSION

Stemming from the original work of Chiu and Baril[22] on synchronized HeLa cells, there has been the suggestion that components
for DNA replication are temporally induced to coincide precisely
with the S phase of the cell cycle. This viewpoint has been
extended in recent reviews on DNA replication in eukaryotes (for
example)[23]. The work described here in Tables 1 and 2 indicates
that the temporal association between the S phase and component
induction is actually explained by the restricted synthesis of the
replication machinery during this particular phase of the cell
cycle only. This is an important concept, because it follows that
only actively dividing cells, including tumours, will be enriched
in these indicators of DNA replication, whereas slowly dividing
cells will not.

In attempting to establish valid and direct markers for the
state of dedifferentiation[6] or division rate of prostate carcinoma
cells, components for DNA replication appear to be prime candidates.
From the restricted evidence presented here (Table 3), prostate

carcinoma present a remarkably wide diversity in terms of growth
or replication potential. In one sense, this is not surprising,
as this form of human malignancy is known to present as a highly
invasive, rapidly dividing, dedifferentiated form of disease to a
less invasive, slower dividing, differentiated state of neoplasia.
What is very surprising, and indeed disappointing, is that all of
the tumours in this survey contained a remarkably similar content
of cytoplasmic androgen receptor protein. My own estimates of
receptor content are in excellent agreement with the data of Voigt
and Kreig[9], but in neither this latter[9] nor other studies[24] on
prostatic carcinoma, were additional biochemical parameters
measured at the same time. The sense of disappointment surrounding
the present data is that the measurement of androgen receptors had
been widely believed to be of importance in the diagnosis and
prognosis of human prostatic carcinoma; the success of oestrogen
receptor assays in the management of human breast cancer certainly
illustrates the potential value of such an approach. Nonetheless,
it may be that biochemical parameters other than receptors may be
more useful in the long term during the clinical management of
human prostatic carcinoma. Certainly, the components included in
the present survey are completely stable in frozen tissue and the
assays are extremely sensitive, reliable and reproducible. Clearly
a lot more work has yet to be done in providing urological surgeons
with sound techniques and tumour markers for improving the management and chemotherapy of human prostate carcinoma.

        This work was supported by the Yorkshire Cancer Research
Campaign.

        The help of Ms. Anne Turner in the preparation of the manu-
script is gratefully acknowledged.

REFERENCES

1.   F. Ramm, "Kastrationens betydning i prostata hypertropiens
          behandluig," H. Ascheong & Co., Kristiana (1894).
2.   J.W. White, The results of double castration in hypertrophy
          of the prostate, Ann. Surg. 22:1 (1895).
3.   C. Huggins and C.V. Hodges, Studies on prostatic cancer I.
          Effects of castration, of estrogen and of androgen on
          serum phosphatase in metastatic carcinoma of the prostate,
          Cancer Res. 1:293 (1941).
4.   Leader articles (a) Brit. Med. J. 8:520 (1974) and (b) N.Z.
          Med. J. 14:113 (1974).
5.   W.I.P. Mainwaring, The relevance of studies on androgen action
          to prostatic cancer, in: "Steroid Hormone Action and
          Cancer," K.M.J.Menon and J.R.Reel, eds., Plenum Press,
          New York (1976).

6. R.A. Willis, "Pathology of tumours" (Fourth Edition), Chapter 34, Butterworth, London (1967).

7. For example: IUCC Technical Report Series, Volume 28, Prostate Cancer, Union Internationale Contre le Cancer, Geneva (1979).

8. W.I.P. Mainwaring, "The Mechanism of Action of Androgens," Springer Verlag, New York (1977).

9. K.D. Voigt and M. Kreig, Biochemical endocrinology of prostatic tumours, Current Topics Exptl. Endocr. 3:173 (1978).

10. J. Geller, Androgen receptors in human prostate cancer, in: "Steroid Hormones and the Management of Cancer," E.B. Thompson and M. Lippmann, eds., CRC Press Inc., West Palm Beach (in press).

11. F.R. Mangan, A.E. Pegg and W.I.P. Mainwaring, A reappraisal of the effects of adenosine 3':5'-cyclic monophosphate on the function and morphology of the rat prostate gland, Biochem. J. 134:129 (1973).

12. P.S. Rennie, E.K. Symes and W.I.P. Mainwaring, The androgenic regulation of the activities of enzymes engaged in the synthesis of deoxyribonucleic acid in rat ventral prostate gland, Biochem. J. 152:1 (1975).

13. W.I.P. Mainwaring, P.S. Rennie and J. Keen, The androgenic regulation of prostate proteins with a high affinity for deoxyribonucleic acid, Biochem. J. 156:253 (1976).

14. W.I.P. Mainwaring, J. Keen and M.W. Stewart, Further studies on the DNA-unwinding protein of the rat ventral prostate: evidence for local areas of denaturation, J. Steroid Biochem. 7:1013 (1976).

15. W.I.P. Mainwaring, T.J. Hadlam and D.J. McIlreavy, The de novo synthesis of enzymes and factors for DNA replication during the S phase of the cell cycle, Biochem. J. (in press).

16. G.M. Higgins and R.M. Anderson, Experimental pathology of the liver. I. Restoration of the liver of the White rat following partial surgical removal, Arch. Path. 12:186 (1931).

17. D.S. Coffey, J. Shimazaki and H.G. Williams-Ashman, Polymerization of deoxyribonucleotides in relation to androgen-induced prostatic growth, Arch. Biochem. Biophys. 124:184 (1968).

18. O.H. Lowry, N.J. Rosebrough, A.L. Farr and R.J. Randall, Protein measurement with the Folin-Ciocalteu reagent, J. Biol. Chem. 193:265 (1951).

19. H.J. Morton, Improved media for tissue culture, In Vitro 6:89 (1970).

20. P. Davies, P. Thomas and K. Griffiths, Measurement of free and occupied cytoplasmic and nuclear androgen receptor sites in rat ventral prostate gland, J. Endocr. 74:393 (1977).

21. C. Bonne and J.-P. Raynaud, Methyltrienolone, a specific ligand for cellular androgen receptors, Steroids, 26:227 (1975).

22. R.W. Chiu and E.F. Baril, Nuclear DNA polymerases and the HeLa

cell cycle, J. Biol. Chem. 250:7951 (1975).

23. A. Weissbach, Eukaryotic DNA polymerases, Ann. Rev. Biochem.
     46:25 (1977).

24. B.G. Mobbs, I.E. Johnson, J.G. Connolly and A.F. Clark,
     Androgen receptor in human benign and malignant prostatic
     tumour cytosol using protamine sulphate precipitation,
     J. Steroid Biochem. 9:289 (1978).

EVALUATION OF IN VIVO AND IN VITRO RESPONSES OF ENDOMETRIAL

ADENOCARCINOMA TO PROGESTINS

C.F. Holinka, L. Deligdisch, G. Deppe, H. Fleming,
C. Namit, M.M. de la Pena, and E. Gurpide

Departments of Obstetrics and Gynecology and of
Pathology, Mount Sinai School of Medicine, New York
New York   10029

In vivo effects of progesterone and other progestins on normal
human endometrium have been evident histologically since the 1930's
(1,2). Histochemical procedures have been used to demonstrate the
influence of these compounds on glycogen accumulation and secretion
of proteins and carbohydrates (3). Correlation of changes in enzymatic activities and other biochemical parameters throughout the
menstrual cycle have suggested specific effects of progesterone on
the endometrium (4). In some cases, these putative effects could be
ascertained in vivo by administering progestins to women in the
follicular phase of their menstrual cycles and examining endometrial biopsies taken before the onset of the luteal phase. Experiments of this type showed that progestins increase the activity of
estradiol 17β dehydrogenase (E_2DH) (5) and reduce the levels of
estrogen receptors (R_E) in the tissue (6). The in vivo effect of
progestins on endometrial E_2DH activity was also noted when they
were administered to postmenopausal women (7).

In vitro effects of progestins were demonstrated histologically (8, 9) and also biochemically during incubations of fragments
of proliferative normal endometrium under organ culture conditions.
Hughes and coworkers (10, 11) and, more recently, Shapiro et al
(12), have shown that addition of progestins to the medium produced an increase in the glycogen content of the tissue. A similar
experimental design served to prove that progestins induce E_2DH by
direct action on the endometrium (5). No enhancement of this enzymatic activity by progestins was observed during incubations of
secretory endometrium, in which the levels of the enzyme are
already high. It has been emphasized elsewhere (13) that the influence of progestins on endometrial E_2DH and R_E levels are of
great importance since they contribute to the antiestrogenic

365

actions which can account for many of the physiologic and pharmacologic effects of progesterone and synthetic progestins on the
endometrium.

Extension of these studies to endometrial adenocarcinoma are
of considerable interest not only because of the information they
can yield on biologic differences between normal and transformed
endometrial cells but also because treatment with progestins is
the hormone-related therapy most commonly used for recurrent
endometrial cancer (14, 15).

In vivo effects of progestins on endometrial cancer

Effects of short term administration (2 to 10 days) of medroxy-
progesterone acetate (MPA) in the form of Provera[R] (Upjohn) tablets
(60 mg/day) to postmenopausal patients with endometrial adenocarcinoma were described in a recent publication (16). In some, but
not all of the patients, clear responses were noted by evaluating
histologic features, R_E levels and E_2DH activities in endometrial
tissue obtained before and after MPA administration. These results
indicated that the experimental protocol was capable of yielding
evidence of responsiveness of the neoplastic tissue to progestin
treatment. It was also of interest to note that even some undifferentiated adenocarcinomas could be affected histologically and biochemically by the progestin. Several other published reports have
described histologic changes (17-19), reduction of R_E levels (20-
22) and enhancement of E_2DH (7) in endometrial adenocarcinoma
after short-term treatment with progestins.

Accumulated information on the mode of action of steroid hormones (23) have suggested the likelihood that progesterone receptors
(R_P) are mediators of the pharmacologic effects of progestins in
endometrial cancer tissue. Since R_P levels decline with the loss
of differentiation of the tumor, it is not suprising that the responsiveness to progestins is lowest in patients with poorly differentiated or undifferentiated endometrial adenocarcinoma (24).
However, degree of differentiation is not an adequate predictive
index of responsiveness to progestin treatment since remissions
are noted in patients with grade 3 tumors (25) and some poorly-
differentiated tumors contain progesterone receptors (26).

Ehrlich and collaborators have measured R_P concentration in
accessible tumors derived from endometrial adenocarcinoma or stromal
sarcoma and found that those containing cytoplasmic receptor levels
below 50 fmol/mg protein did not respond to progestin therapy,
whereas remissions were noted in those with higher R_P levels (24).
It therefore appears that R_P levels may serve to identify patients
who might benefit from treatment with progestins. A program to
obtain further validation of this important conclusion has been
set up by the National Cancer Institute.

While the absence of receptors may preclude hormonal action, their presence does not assure responsiveness to the hormone since several steps, any of which may be altered in the neoplasm, intervene between the formation of the steroid-receptor complex and the final hormonal effect. We have therefore started a new series of short-term in vivo tests which involves the same protocol (60 mg/d Provera, 2-10 days) described above (16) but includes the measurement of Rp levels in the specimen obtained before the administration of MPA. The purpose of this study is to determine whether responsiveness to progestins, evaluated either histologically or biochemically, can be correlated to the presence and levels of Rp.

Methods for tissue collection, measurement of estradiol receptor levels and estimation of E_2DH activity have been previously described (5, 6). Progesterone receptor levels were determined by incubation of cytosol with 20nM tritiated progesterone plus 2 μM cortisol in the presence or absence of a 100-fold excess of unlabeled progesterone, followed by separation of unbound hormone with dextran-coated charcoal, according to the method described by Bayard et al (27). The tissue was assayed immediately after biopsy, with the exception of the specimen RM (Table 1), which was frozen in liquid nitrogen and kept at -80C for 1 day before analysis.

Although only 7 patients have been studied in this new series, we wish to comment on the histologic results so far obtained; effects of MPA treatment on E_2DH and estrogen receptor levels will not be discussed.

Correlation between Rp levels and histologic changes after MPA Administration

The formation of subnuclear vacuoles appears to be the most reliable histologic effect of progesterone on the endometrium. In the normal menstrual cycle, electron microscopy reveals accumulation of glycogen at a subnuclear location a few hours after ovulation (28) and light microscopy shows clear vacuoles, staining for glycogen, at 24-36 hours after ovulation. Similar changes can be seen in endometrial adenocarcinoma of some postmenopausal patients treated with progestins (Fig. 1).

The patients included in the present study were diagnosed as having endometrial adenocarcinoma, ranging from poorly- to well-differentiated. After treatment with Provera, the hysterectomy specimen revealed the presence of endometrial subnuclear vacuoles in 3 cases, 2 of grade 1-2 and 1 of grade 2-3. The other 4 cases, including 2 well-differentiated adenocarcinomas, did not show any subnuclear vacuoles. In the poorly-differentiated adenocarcinoma which responded to the Provera treatment (specimen RM, Table 1), the vacuoles had a subnuclear location in the part of the tumor where a glandular pattern was still present (Fig. 2). Subnuclear

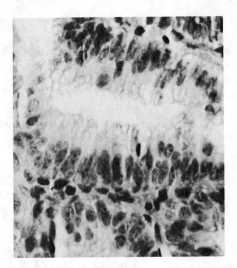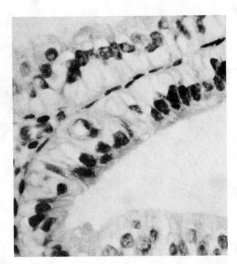

Fig.1 - Left. Endometrial carcinoma, well-differentiated, showing
back to back glands lined by pseudostratified epithelial cells with
pleomorphic nuclei. Right. Same patient after 6 day administration
of Provera (60 mg/d): there is marked subnuclear vacuolation and the
glandular epithelium is reminiscent of the normal early secretory
endometrium.

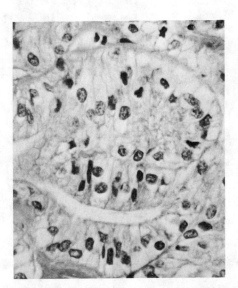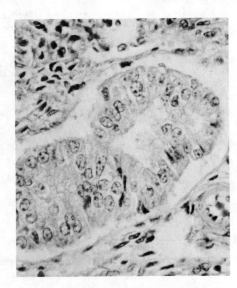

Fig.2 - Left. Endometrial carcinoma, poorly to moderately differentiated (patient RM), after Provera administration (3 d, 60 mg/d):
subnuclear vacuoles are present in almost all glandular structures.
Right. Same specimen, infiltrating adenocarcinoma into myometrium:
no subnuclear vacuoles are seen, the glandular structure is pseudostratified and shows a high nucleo-cytoplasmic ratio.

vacuoles were distinguished from randomly located cytoplasmic vacuoles, usually found in degenerating endometrial tumors. The latter were present in poorly preserved tissue, with pyknotic or disrupted nuclei; the former showed PAS positive granules in the cytoplasm and had well preserved nuclei. The histologic response to MPA, when present, was found in some areas of the adenocarcinoma, while other areas were unaffected or showed evidence of degenerative processes.

Table 1 illustrates a relationship between the presence and amount of progesterone receptors and the formation and intensity of subnuclear vacuoles. In a patient with high PR levels, the histologic pattern of the endometrial carcinoma was even reminiscent of that of the early normal secretory endometrium: not only were subnuclear vacuoles present in almost all the glands, but the epithelial cells had a quiescent appearance, displaying a low nucleo-cytoplasmic ratio.

Interestingly, the infiltrating adenocarcinoma of the endometrium into the myometrium did not reveal any subnuclear vacuolization (Fig. 2), even in the cases in which such a histologic response was present in the superficial adenocarcinoma. Whether the lack of histologic response to MPA of adenocarcinoma in the myometrium is related to the absence of endometrial stroma, to a relatively lower blood and hormonal supply to the myometrium or to other factors, remains to be further studied. A stromal-epithelial interaction in the endometrium has already been proposed (29).

Pertinent to discussions on in vivo endometrial responses to progestins is the known requirement of estrogens for the induction of progesterone receptors. It would seem logical to attempt priming the target tissue in postmenopausal patients before searching for the presence of progesterone receptors, or before treating with a progestin. Ethical considerations, however, prevent studies of this type since estrogen administration may be harmful to patients with endometrial cancer. As recently suggested (30), the difficulty may be avoided by the use of Tamoxifen, an antiestrogen widely used in the treatment of breast cancer, which has been shown to be a good inducer of progesterone receptors in the endometrium. Therefore, administration of Tamoxifen together with progestins, either for diagnosis or for treatment, makes for an interesting possibility.

In vitro effects of progestins on endometrial cancer

Responses of endometrial tissue to progestins can also be studied during in vitro incubations. Histologic changes similar to those observed in normal proliferative endometrium exposed in organ culture to progestins could be noted when fragments of endometrial adenocarcinoma were incubated with MPA (Fig. 3). Not all specimens responded, however, and many showed evidence of necrosis after the

Table 1. Effects of MPA on Endometrial Adenocarcinoma

Patient	Age	Histologic Grading	Progesterone Receptor Levels (fmol/mg prot)	Days of Therapy (60 mg/day)	Histologic Effects of MPA Administration	
					Superficial	Infiltrating
MJ	65	1	0	3	-	-
RM	84	2-3	360	3	++	-
RA	55	3	80	2	-	No infiltration
FB	52	3	160	3	-	-
RT	68	1-2	2400	2	+++	-
FE	59	1-2	380	3	++	-
PB	61	1	190	2	-	-

period of incubation, as reported by others (31).

Attempts to demonstrate significant increases of E_2DH activity in endometrial adenocarcinoma in organ culture by addition of MPA to the medium have not produced satisfactory results. Table 2 shows results from 15 experiments in which tissue fragments were kept from 1 to 3 days in Trowell T-8 or MEMα medium supplemented with 10% fetal bovine serum and insulin. As consistently found in specimens of endometrial cancer from postmenopausal patients, the levels of E_2DH in the tissue before incubation ("fresh" tissue) were low. The enzymatic activities of portions of the same specimens incubated in medium containing MPA were usually lower than those corresponding to fresh tissue, although increases of questionable significance were noted in some cases. In contrast, the enzymatic activities were often higher than those of "control" incubations, in which MPA was not added to the medium, and a 3-fold elevation was observed in one case. There were no instances, however, in which the enhancement of E_2DH activity relative to both control and fresh tissue could be documented or correlated to histologic changes.

It is our impression that the results obtained with cancer tissue do not allow us to propose at this time an _in vitro_ test for responsiveness to progestins based on E_2DH induction. Although not all of the specimens tested might have been responsive _in vivo_ (progestin treatment is effective in only about 1/3 of the treated patients), clear augmentation of E_2DH was expected to occur in some of the specimens since, under the same experimental conditions, the

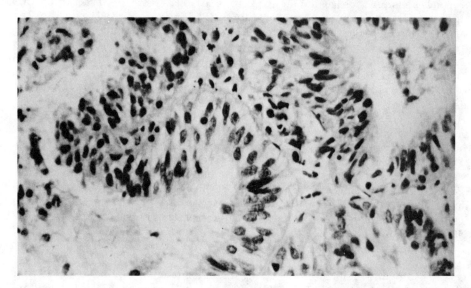

Fig. 3. Well-differentiated adenocarcinoma (patient NS) exposed in organ culture to MPA (0.5 µg/ml for 2 days): subnuclear vacuolation is present in major portions of the glandular structure.

enzymatic activity was increased several-fold in normal proliferative endometrium (5). Moreover, cancerous tissue deteriorated
during these incubations to a larger extent than normal endometrium,
as judged by both macroscopic and histologic appearances. Attempts
to improve viability and responsiveness by varying the length of the
incubation period, by using a richer medium (MEMα, which contains
nucleosides) or by adding to the medium protease inhibitors, cortisol or spermidine failed to produce significant effects (Table 2).

The concern about viability of the tissue in organ culture led
us to culture epithelial cells dispersed from specimens of endometrial adenocarcinoma and to attempt inducing E_2DH by addition of MPA
to the culture medium.

Monolayer cultures of epithelial cells from endometrial adenocarcinoma

Specimens of endometrial adenocarcinoma were treated with 0.25%
collagenase (Worthington, Type I) for 2 h at 37 C. After separation
of undigested tissue, the supension was filtered through a stainless
steel filter (38 μ pore size) in order to isolate glands, in cases
of well-differentiated tissue, or clumps of epithelial cells in less
differentiated adenocarcinomas (32). The material retained in the
filter was transferred to plastic Petri dishes with either McCoy 5a
or Ham F-10 medium and homogeneous monolayers of epithelial cells
were obtained. The effects of progestins on these cells were
studied in the primary cultures or, in some cases, after a first and
second passage, using concentrations of MPA ranging from 5 to 500
ng/ml, in the presence or absence of 2.5 ng/ml estradiol. The length
of the incubations ranged from 1 to 5 days. No increases in the
specific activity of E_2DH relative to the original tissue were noted
in 5 specimens of endometrial adenocarcinoma studied in this manner.
Increases relative to control cultures in which MPA was absent were
observed in some of the experiments but they were small and of
doubtful significance.

The possibility that these results reflect responses of the
adenocarcinoma to MPA is further diminished by the lack of response
of cultures of epithelial cells derived from specimens of normal
proliferative endometrium which responded to MPA in organ culture.
In a series of experiments involving 7 specimens of normal endometrium, an increase in E_2DH activity relative to the original tissue
(40%) was observed in 1 case. The activity in the cells exposed to
MPA was about equal to the activity in control incubations, but in
2 experiments the levels doubled.

We do not consider to have demonstrated by these experiments
inducibility by MPA of E_2DH activity in endometrial cells under the
culture conditions tested. However, Dr. Satyaswaroop, who parti-
cipated in the cell culture studies, expressed a different conclusion

Table 2. E$_2$DH Activity in Endometrial Adenocarcinoma in Organ Culture

Patient	Age	Histologic Grading	Medium*	MPA µg/ml	Days in Culture	E$_2$DH Act. [nmol E$_2$/mg prot.xh)] Fresh	MPA/Control	MPA/Fresh
GL	61	1	T-8	0.7	2	1.3	1.0	1.0
EP	49	1	T-8	0.3	2	1.0	0.6	0.5
NS	45	1	T-8	2.5	2	2.6	2.0	0.7
HZ	60	1	T-8	2.5	3	2.6	1.9	0.7
MM	54	1	T-8	0.5	1	-	2.4	-
			"	0.5	1	-	2.0	-
			MEMα	0.5	1	-	1.0	-
			" + Cortisol (3µM)	0.5	1	-	1.0	-
AH	52	1	MEMα	0.5	3	4.2	1.5	0.4
ED	73	1	MEMα	0.5	1	0.6	1.2	1.8
			" + TLCK (1mM)	0.5	1	0.6	0.7	1.2
LW	52	1	MEMα	0.5	2	0.7	1.1	1.6
			" + Spermidine (1mM)	0.5	2	0.7	1.2	1.6
VB	63	1	MEMα	0.5	1	1.0	1.5	0.9
CA	68	2	T-8	0.2	2	1.4	3.3	0.7
EW	60	2	MEMα	0.5	1	1.8	0.9	0.8
EDD	79	2	T-8 (no FBS)	0.5	1	1.8	1.3	0.5
			T-8	0.5	1	5.7	0.7	0.4
			" + Cortisol (3µM)	0.5	1	5.7	-	0.6
			MEMα	0.5	1	5.7	1.3	0.6
			" + Cortisol (3µM)	0.5	1	5.7	0.9	0.4
GG	61	3	T-8	1.3	2	1.1	1.0	1.0
JP	80	3	T-8	1.0	1	0.9	1.2	0.8
FM	64	3	MEMα	0.5	1	4.5	0.9	0.8

* Media were supplemented with 10% fetal bovine serum (FBS) and bovine insulin (10-40 µg/ml)

drawn from the same data.

It is possible, however, that induction of the enzyme in epithelial cells in monolayer may be achieved under proper culture conditions since autoradiographic studies have clearly demonstrated that E_2DH activity is increased in the glandular epithelium during the luteal phase of the cycle (33) and in vitro experiments have shown that progesterone is responsible for that stimulation (5).

In order to evaluate factors which might influence the responsiveness of epithelial cells in culture, a study of receptor levels was begun. The initial studies were conducted on estradiol receptors and revealed a surprising day-to-day variation in the receptor levels (34). Further studies of these phenomena, conducted on synchronized endometrial cells, have shown a clear pattern of variation of estrogen receptor levels during the cell cycle (Fleming et al, unpublished). Advances in our knowledge of the dynamics of steroid receptor levels and enzymatic activities may yield information pertinent to the design of in vitro tests for responsiveness of endometrial tissue to hormones.

REFERENCES

1. Wiesbader, H., Oral therapy with pregneninolone in functional uterine bleeding, Am. J. Obstet. Gynecol. 42:1013 (1941).
2. Noyes, R.H., Hertig, A.T., and Rock, J., Dating the endometrial biopsy, Fertil. Steril. 1:3 (1950.
3. Schmidt-Matthiesen, H., Histochemistry of the effects of gestagens on the human endometrium, in: "International Encyclopedia of Pharmacologic Therapy", Section 48, Vol. 1, Tausk, M., ed., Pergamon Press, Oxford, p. 457 (1971).
4. Boutselis, J.G., Histochemistry of the normal endometrium, in: "The Uterus", Norris, H.J., Hertig, A.T., and Abell, M.R., eds., The Williams and Wilkins Co., Baltimore, p. 175, (1973).
5. Tseng, L., and Gurpide, E., Induction of human endometrial estradiol dehydrogenase by progestins, Endocrinology 97:825 (1975).
6. Tseng, L., and Gurpide, E., Effects of progestins on estradiol receptor levels in human endometrium, J. Clin. Endocrinol. Metab. 41: 402 (1975).
7. Pollow, K., Schmidt-Gollwitzer, M., Boquoi, E., and Pollow, B., Influence of estrogens and gestagens on 17β-hydroxysteroid dehydrogenase in human endometrium and endometrial carcinoma, J. Molec. Med. 3:81 (1978).
8. Csermely, T., Demers, L.M., and Hughes, E.C., Organ culture of human endometrium. Effects of progesterone, Obstet. Gynecol. 34:252 (1969).
9. Kohorn, E.I., and Tchao, R.J., Conversion of proliferative endometrium to secretory endometrium by progesterone in

     organ culture, J. Endocrinol. 45:401 (1969).
10. Hughes, E.C., Demers, L.M., Csermely, T., and Jones, D.B.,
     Organ culture of human endometrium. Effect of ovarian
     steroids. Am. J. Obstet. Gynecol. 105:707 (1969).
11. Hughes, E.C., Csermely, T.V., Jacobs, R.D., and O'Hern, P.A.,
     Biochemical parameters of abnormal endometrium, Gynecol.
     Oncol. 2:205 (1974).
12. Shapiro, S.S., Dyer, R.D., and Colás, A.E., Progesterone-in-
     duced glycogen accumulation in human endometrium during
     organ culture, Am. J. Obstet. Gynecol. 136:419 (1980).
13. Gurpide, E., Enzymic modulation of hormonal action at the
     target tissue, J. Toxicol. Environ. Health 4:249 (1978).
14. Kelly, R.M., and Baker, W.H., The role of progesterone in
     human endometrial cancer, Cancer Res. 25:1190 (1965).
15. Reifenstein, E.C., The treatment of advanced endometrial
     cancer with hydroxyprogesterone caproate, Gynecol. Oncol.
     2:377 (1974).
16. Gurpide, E., Tseng, L., and Gusberg, S.B., Estrogen metabolism
     in normal and neoplastic endometrium, Am. J. Obstet. Gynecol.
     129:809 (1977).
17. Kistner, R.W., Griffiths, C.T., and Craig, J.M., The use of
     progestational agents in the management of endometrial cancer,
     Cancer 18:1563 (1965).
18. Anderson, D.G., Management of advanced endometrial adenocar-
     cinoma with medroxyprogesterone acetate, Amer. J. Obstet.
     Gynecol. 92:87 (1965).
19. Howard, J.A., Cornes, J.S., Jackson, W.D., and Bye, P., Effect
     of a systemically administered progestin on histopathology of
     endometrial carcinoma, J. Obstet. Gynaec. Brit. Cwlth. 81:786
     (1974).
20. Pollow, K., Boquoi, E., Lübbert, H., and Pollow, B., Effect of
     gestagen therapy upon 17β hydroxysteroid dehydrogenase in
     human endometrial adenocarcinoma, J. Endocrinol. 67:131
     (1975).
21. Syrjala, P., Kontula, K., Jänne, O., Kavppila, A., and Vihko,
     R., Steroid receptors in normal and neoplastic human uterine
     tissue, in: "Endometrial Cancer", Brush, M.G., King, R.J.B.,
     and Taylor, R.W., eds., Bailliere Tindall, London, p. 242
     (1978).
22. Martin, P.M., Rolland, P.H., Gammerre, M., Serment, H., and
     Toga, M., Estradiol and progesterone receptors in normal and
     neoplastic endometrium: correlations between receptors, histo-
     pathological examinations and clinical responses under pro-
     gestin therapy, Int. J. Cancer 23: 321 (1979).
23. Higgins, S.J., and Gehring, V., Molecular mechanism of steroid
     hormone action, Adv. Cancer Res. 28;313 (1978).
24. Ehrlich, C.E., Cleary, R.E., and Young, P.C.M., The use of pro-
     gesterone receptor assay in the management of a recurrent
     endometrial cancer, in: "Endometrial Cancer", Brush, M.G.,
     King, R.J.B., and Taylor, R.W., Baillere Tindall, London,

p. 258 (1978).

25. Bonte, J., Decoster, J.M., Ide, P., Wynants, P., and Billiet, G., Progesterone in endometrial cancer, in: "Recent Progress in Obstet. Gynaec.", Amsterdam, Excerpta Medica, p. 285 (1974).

26. McCarty, K.S., Jr., Barton, T.K., Fettler, B.F., Creasman, W.T., and McCarty, K.S., Sr., Correlation of estrogen and progesterone receptors with histologic differentiation in endometrial adenocarcinoma, Am. J. Pathol. 96:171 (1979).

27. Bayard, F., Damilano, S., Robel, P. and Baulieu, E.E., Cytoplasmic and nuclear estradiol and progesterone receptor in human endometrium, J. Clin. Endocrinol. Metab. 46:635 (1978).

28. Ferenczy, A., and Richart, R.M., "Female Reproductive System: Dynamics of Scan and Transmission Electron Microscopy", John Wiley and Sons, New York (1974).

29. Cunha, G.R., and Lung, B., The importance of stroma in morphogenesis and functional activity of urogenital epithelium, In Vitro 15:50 (1979).

30. Robel, P., Levy, C., Wolff, J.P., Nicolas, J.C., and Baulieu, E.E., Réponse à un anti-oestrogene comme critère d'hormonosensibilité du cancer de l'endomètre, C.R. Acad. Sci., Paris, Série D, 173, 27 Nov. (1978).

31. Kohorn, E.I., The limitations of progesterone sensitivity testing of endometrial carcinoma using organ culture, in: "Human Tumors in Short Term Culture", Dendy, P.P., ed., Academic Press, London-New York- San Francisco, p. 245 (1976).

32. Satyaswaroop, P.G., Fleming, H., Bressler, R.S., and Gurpide, E., Human endometrial cancer cells. Cultures for hormonal studies, Cancer Res. 38:4367 (1978).

33. Scublinsky, A., Marin, C., and Gurpide, E., Location of estradiol 17β dehydrogenase in human endometrium, J. Steroid Biochem. 7:745 (1976).

34. Fleming, H., Namit, C., and Gurpide, E., Estrogen receptors in epithelial and stromal cells of human endometrium in culture, J. Steroid Biochem., 12:169 (1980).

ACKNOWLEDGEMENT

This investigation was supported by Grant Number CA-15648, awarded by the National Cancer Institute, DHEW.

ESTROGEN RECEPTOR, A MARKER FOR HUMAN BREAST CANCER

DIFFERENTIATION AND PATIENT PROGNOSIS

C.K. Osborne, E. Fisher, C. Redmond, W.A. Knight, M. G. Yochmowitz, and W.L. McGuire

Department of Medicine, University of Texas Health Science Center, San Antonio, TX 78284 and Department of Pathology, Shadyside Hospital, University of Pittsburgh School of Medicine, Pittsburgh, PA 15244

INTRODUCTION

Breast cancer is the leading cause of cancer death in American women. Over the past 80 years this malignancy has been studied intensively not only because of its high incidence, but also because of interest generated by the original observation of Beatson demonstrating that some tumors are hormone dependent. Unfortunately, it has only been over the past decade that real advances have been made in the treatment of this disease, as well as in our understanding of breast tumor biology and natural history.

One of these advances has been the development of the estrogen receptor (ER) assay to predict tumor endocrine dependence. It had been known for many years that about one-third of human breast cancers would temporarily regress with an appropriate alteration in the hormonal milieu such as ovariectomy or hypophysectomy, or additive hormonal therapy. However, selection of patients likely to respond to these maneuvers by clinical criteria was not very successful[2], and, therefore, many patients were subjected to the risks of ablative endocrine therapy when the treatment was doomed to failure from the outset. The development of another effective approach to the treatment of women with advanced breast cancer, cytotoxic chemotherapy, reinforced the need for an accurate predictive index of hormonal responsiveness in order to select and individualize therapy. With the discovery that a protein (ER) was present in all normal estrogen target tissues such as the uterus or breast which was necessary for estrogenic activity, investigators asked whether some breast cancers might also contain ER, the measurement of which might serve as a marker for hormone dependence. This hypothesis has now been con-

377

firmed;[3] patients with ER negative tumors rarely respond to endocrine therapy, whereas about 60% of patients with ER positive tumors have an objective response. Patients with tumors containing very high ER concentrations or those also containing progesterone receptor have response rates approaching 80%.[4,5] Thus, steroid hormone receptor assays have proven very useful in helping clinicians select patients with endocrine-responsive tumors, enabling them to optimize the use of currently available modalities of treatment, as well as providing new areas of investigation.

Recent studies of ER in patients with primary breast cancer undergoing surgery for their disease have revealed another role for the ER assay as a prognostic factor for recurrence and ultimate survival. We and others have reported that patients with ER positive tumors have a lower recurrence rate and better survival than patients with ER negative tumors.[6-13]

These data are not surprising in light of the cell kinetic studies reported by Meyer et al.[14,15] and Silvistrini et al.[15] demonstrating that ER negative tumors have a more rapid proliferative potential. They used the thymidine labeling (TLI) index as a measure of the proportion of tumor cells engaged in DNA synthesis at a given point in time. A good correlation was found among several favorable morphological features, the presence of ER, and a low TLI, indicating that tumors with a lower proliferative potential are more likely to be endocrine dependent.

The relationship between ER and prognosis also is not surprising if one accepts the hypothesis that the presence of ER indicates a relative degree of tumor differentiation toward the normal or non-malignant state, and that well differentiated tumors generally tend to be more indolent in their clinical behavior. A recent report by Fisher et al.[17] suggests that ER does correlate directly with the presence of several morphological features indicative of tumor differentiation. In the present paper we will present results from a group of patients from San Antonio undergoing mastectomy for primary breast cancer, demonstrating that ER may be a biochemical

Table 1. Tumor Differentiation and Patient Prognosis
as a Function of Morphology

Characteristic	Favorable (Well Differentiated)	Unfavorable (Poorly Differentiated)
Lymphoid cell reaction	Absent	Marked
Necrosis	Absent	Marked
Elastica	Marked	Absent
Nuclear grade	Grade 3	Grade 1
Histologic grade	Grade 1	Grade 3

Table 2. Correlation of ER with Nuclear
and Histologic Grade

	% ER Positive	% ER Negative
Histologic Grade[a]		
1	100	0
2	93	7
3	61	39
Nuclear Grade[b]		
1	50	50
2	90	10
3	100	0

[a]As grade increases the degree of morphological differentiation decreases.
[b]As nuclear grade increases the degree of nuclear differentiation increases.

marker for tumor differentiation. Furthermore, we will update and expand our original study showing that ER is an important independent prognostic variable in patients with primary breast cancer.

ER AND BREAST CANCER HISTOPATHOLOGY

Several morphological variables are thought to correlate directly with the degree of tumor differentiation and indirectly with patient prognosis.[18] Some of these are listed in Table 1 and include lymphocyte infiltration into the tumor, evidence of tumor necrosis, the degree of elastosis, and the degree of nuclear and histologic atypia. In order to determine if there is a relationship between the presence of ER and morphological evidence of tumor differentiation we have studied 147 patients undergoing mastectomy for primary breast cancer in whom we had performed an ER assay.* Histopathologic review was performed by one of us (E.F.) without knowledge of the ER result or the patients clinical history.

The correlation of ER with nuclear and histologic grade is shown in Table 2. Traditionally low histologic grade and high nuclear grade correspond to the least morphological atypia or best differentiation. The characteristics of the grading system have been described previously.[18] A striking association between the presence of ER and a high degree of differentiation is evident. Tumors with histologic grade 1 or nuclear grade 3 (best differentiated) always contained the ER protein. In contrast,

*Fisher, E. et al., manuscript submitted for publication.

poorly differentiated tumors (histologic grade 3, nuclear grade 1) were ER positive in only 50 to 60 percent of cases. Tumors of intermediate grade had an intermediate rate of ER positivity. The association between well differentiated tumors, which have a relatively good prognosis,[18] and ER compliments the data discussed below purporting that ER has prognostic significance.

Tumor necrosis, the degree of elastosis, and lymphocyte cell reaction are also related to the degree of tumor differentiation and have prognostic significance.[18] Marked necrosis, marked cell reaction, and absent elastica are features of poorly differentiated breast cancers and are associated with the absence of ER (Table 3). In contrast the absence of necrosis, marked elastica, and absent lymphocyte infiltration were nearly always associated with a positive ER status.

Table 4 shows the cumulative data correlating ER with the absence or the presence of one or more of five unfavorable morphological characteristics. Tumors containing 3 or more of these variables were frequently ER negaive (70%). In contrast, 79% of tumors with only 1 or 2 of the unfavorable features were ER positive. A striking correlation was found for tumors displaying none of the 5 unfavorable characteristics; 98% of these tumors had a positive ER assay. These studies clearly demonstrate that the presence of ER is linked closely to the degree of breast cancer differentiation.

Table 3. Correlation of ER with Tumor Necrosis,
Elastica, and Lymphocyte Infiltration

	% ER Positive	% ER Negative
Tumor Necrosis		
Absent	88	12
Moderate	66	34
Marked	10	90
Elastica		
Absent	52	48
Moderate	75	25
Marked	92	8
Lymphocyte Infiltration		
Absent	94	6
Moderate	69	31
Marked	46	54

Table 4. Correlation of ER with Prognostically
Unfavorable Morphological Characteristics[a]

Characteristics	% ER Positive	% ER Negative
0 Unfavorable	98	2
1 or 2 Unfavorable	79	21
3 or More Unfavorable	30	70

[a]Unfavorable characteristics include marked lymph-ocyte infiltration, marked necrosis, no marked elas-tica, histologic grade 3, and nuclear grade 1.

ER AND THE PROGNOSIS OF PATIENTS WITH BREAST CANCER

The results of the kinetic studies showing that ER positive breast cancers have a low proliferative potential and the pathological studies correlating ER with tumor differentiation provide a rationale for the use of ER as a convenient prognostic indicator in patients with this disease.

Several years ago we were interested in determining the ER status in primary breast tumors at the time of mastectomy in patients with clinically localized disease (Stage I and II) as an aid in predicting endocrine responsiveness later at the time of recurrence. Analysis of these data revealed an interesting trend; patients with ER negative cancers had a higher rate of relapse than patients with ER positive tumors. Three years ago we first reported the results of 145 patients with primary disease treated by radical or modified radical mastectomy.[6] At a median followup of 18 months the recurrence rate for patients with ER negative tumors was twice that for patients with ER positive tumors, an observation which appeared to be independent of other prognostic variables such as age, lymph node involvement, or size and location of the primary. These data suggested that ER positive tumors are more indolent in their growth behavior than the ER negative group. However, this initial study is limited by small patient numbers, short patient followup, and by the fact that the patient population was heterogeneous with regard to the administration of post-operative adjuvant chemotherapy or endocrine therapy. We have recently updated the study including additional patients (288 total) and excluding all patients who had received any systemic adjuvant therapy. The median followup is now 28 months. The general pattern of results is identical to that observed in our initial study; ER negative patients are recurring at a significantly higher rate than ER positive patients (Fig. 1). Thirty-five percent of patients with ER negative tumors have developed recurrent disease compared to 21% of patients with ER positive tumors. The data shown in Table 5 suggest that ER is an independent prognostic

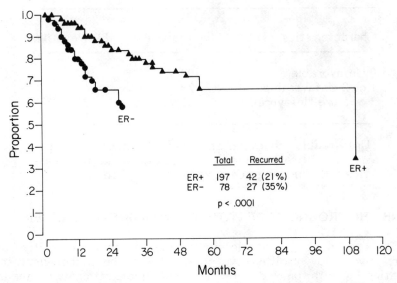

Fig. 1. Recurrence rates for all patients as a function of ER status.

variable. Regardless of menopausal status, the number of positive axillary nodes, or location of the primary in the breast, ER negative patients are recurring at a high rate. The differences are impressive when the patients are stratified by the most important prognostic factor, lymph node status. Only 8% of ER positive, node negative patients have recurred compared to more than one-fourth of the ER negative group. These data are important when one considers that node negative patients are usually excluded from adjuvant chemotherapy because of their "good prognosis" with surgery alone. ER negative patients with positive axillary nodes have a very bad prognosis; 43% of patients in this group with 1 to 3 positive nodes and 68% of those with more than 3 nodes have already recurred by 2 years.

These patients have now been followed long enough to begin to examine the effect of ER status on survival. Actual patient survival at the time of analysis is shown in Table 6. Fifteen percent of the entire group have died. However, significantly more ER negative patients (22%) have died compared to ER positive patients (12%). The survival advantage of patients with ER positive tumors holds even when the patients are stratified by nodal status (Table 7). As expected node negative patients have the best survival and to date only 10% have died. However, again

Table 5. Recurrence by ER Status and
Other Potential Prognostic Factors

Subgroup	Estimated Recurrence at 2 years (%)	
	ER Positive	ER Negative
Menopausal Status		
Pre	18	35
Post	15	38
Node Status		
0	8	26
1-3	16	43
>3	40	68
Tumor Location		
Outer	12	32
Inner + Central	12	50

more ER negative patients have died (14% compared to 8%), a difference which has nearly reached statistical significance. The difference becomes more apparent in the node positive group; 43% of ER negative patients have already died compared to only 19% of the ER positive group. In fact ER positive, node positive patients are dying at a rate very similar to ER negative patients with negative axillary nodes. The prognosis for ER negative patients is indeed poor.

Thus, these studies indicate that the ER status of a primary breast cancer is an important independent prognostic variable for recurrence and survival of patients with this neoplasm. Several other investigators have now confirmed these results,[7-13] but additional followup will be required to determine whether these patterns persist with time.

IMPLICATIONS FOR THERAPY OF PRIMARY BREAST CANCER

The results of our studies suggest that ER positive tumors tend to be well differentiated with a low proliferative capacity which is reflected by

Table 6. Patient Survival at 28 Months
by ER Status

ER Status	Mortality (%)	
Total	43/288	(15%)
Positive	25/207	(12%) p<.004
Negative	18/81	(22%)

Table 7. Patient Survival at 28 Months
by ER and Nodal Status

Status	Mortality (%)		
Node Negative			
ER positive	11/133	(8%)	p<.07
ER negative	8/58	(14%)	
Node Positive			
ER positive	14/74	(19%)	p<.004
ER negative	10/23	(43%)	

their indolent clinical behavior and favorable prognosis. Furthermore many of these tumors are responsive to endocrine therapy. ER negative tumors tend to be poorly differentiated with a high proliferative capacity and aggressive clinical behavior. The risk for recurrence of these tumors is relatiely high even when the axillary nodes are uninvolved with tumor. ER negative tumors rarely respond to endocrine therapy.

These findings form a framework for a new approach to the treatment of primary breast cancer. It is of obvious importance that clinical studies of new treatments should at least stratify patients by ER status just as is done for nodal status and other prognostic factors. Moreover, ER may also be used to design new treatment strategies. For instance, axillary node negative, ER positive patients have a good prognosis and can probably be managed with local modalities of therapy only. On the other hand, adjuvant chemotherapy (on a research basis only) should be considered in the ER negative subgroup because of the relatively higher rate of recurrence. Axillary node positive patients are at a greater risk for recurrence, especially the subgroup with ER negative tumors. Intensive chemotherapy should be considered for this subgroup in an attempt to control micrometastases and improve the dismal survival. ER positive patients with positive nodes also have a relatively high risk for recurrence, but the endocrine dependence of many of these tumors permits alternative treatment approaches. Endocrine therapy with or without cytotoxic chemotherapy might be studied in these patients, particularly the post-menopausal subgroup where adjuvant chemotherapy alone has not been uniformly beneficial. Clinical trials to answer these important questions are now underway.

REFERENCES

1.   G. T. Beatson, On treatment of inoperable cases of carcinoma of mamma. Suggestions for a new method of treatment with illustrative cases, Lancet 2:104 (1896).
2.   B. A. Stoll, "Hormonal Management in Breast Cancer," J. B. Lippincott, Philadelphia (1969).

3. W. L. McGuire, P. P. Carbone, and E. P. Vollmer, "Estrogen Recep-
    tors in Human Breast Cancer," Raven Press, New York (1975).
4. C. K. Osborne and W. L. McGuire, Current use of steroid hormone
    receptor assays in the treatment of breast cancer, Surg. Clinics N.
    Amer. 58:777 (1978).
5. K. B. Horwitz, W. L. McGuire, O. H. Pearson, and A. Segaloff,
    Predicting response to endocrine therapy in human breast cancer: A
    hypothesis, Science 189:726 (1975).
6. W. A. Knight, R. B. Livingston, E. J. Gregory, and W. L. McGuire,
    Estrogen receptor is an independent prognostic factor for early
    recurrence in breat cancer. Cancer Res. 37:4669 (1977).
7. E. R. DeSombre, G. L. Greene, and E. V. Jensen, in "Hormones,
    Receptors, and Breast Cancer" (W. L. McGuire, ed.), pp. 1-14, Raven
    Press, New York (1978).
8. M. A. Rich, P. Furmanski, and S. C. Brooks, Prognostic value of
    estrogen receptor determinations in patients with breast cancer,
    Cancer Res. 38:4296 (1978).
9. J. C. Allegra, M. E. Lippman, R. Simon, E. B. Thompson, A. Barlock,
    L. Green, K. K. Huff, H. M. T. Do, S. C. Aitken, and R. Warren,
    Association between steroid hormone receptor status and dis-
    ease-free interval in breast cancer, Cancer Treat. Rep. 63:1271
    (1979).
10. P. V. Maynard, R. W. Blamey, C. W. Elston, J. L. Haybittle, and K.
    Griffiths, Estrogen receptor assay in primary breast cancer and early
    recurrence of the disease, Cancer Res. 38:4292 (1978).
11. H. M. Bishop, C. W. Elston, R. W. Blamey, J. L. Haybittle, R.
    I.Nicholson, and K. Griffiths, Relationship of oestrogen-receptor
    status ot survival in breast cancer, Lancer 2:283 (1979).
12. T. Booke, R. Shields, D. George, P. Maynard, and K. Griffiths,
    Oestrogen receptors and prognosis in early breast cancer, Lancer
    2:995 (1979).
13. R. Hahnel, T. Woodings, A. B. Vivian, Prognostic value of estrogen
    receptors in primary breast cancer, Cancer 44:671 (1979).
14. J. S. Meyer, W. C. Bauer, and B. R. Rao, Subpopulations of breast
    caricnoma defined by S-phase fraction, morphology, and estrogen
    receptor content, Lab. Investig. 39:225 (1978).
15. J. S. Meyer, B. R. Rao, S. C. Stevens, and W. L. White, Low incidence
    of estrogen receptor in breast carcinomas with rapid rates of cellular
    replication, Cancer 40:2290 (1977).
16. R. Silvestrini, M.G. Daidone, and G. DiFronzo, Relationship between
    proliferative activity and estrogen receptors in breast cancer, Cancer
    44:665 (1979).
17. E. R. Fisher, C. K. Redmond, H. Lin, H. Rockette, and B. Fisher,
    Correlation of estrogen receptor and pathologic characteristics of
    invasive breast cancer, Cancer, in press, 1980.
18. E. R. Fisher, R. M. Gregorio, and B. Fisher, The pathology of invasive
    breast cancer. A syllabus derived from findings of the National
    Surgical Adjuvant Breast Project (Protocol No. 4), Cancer 36:1,
    (1975).

CLINICAL USEFULNESS OF MARKERS IN MONITORING PATIENTS WITH CANCER

Leonard M. Pogach and Judith L. Vaitukaitis

Section of Endocrinology and Metabolism
Thorndike Memorial Laboratory
Boston City Hospital
Department of Medicine
Boston University School of Medicine
Boston, Massachusetts

INTRODUCTION

In recent years there has been increasing interest in the identification and clinical application of tumor-associated antigens. Most antigens associated with tumors may be subclassified simply as hormonal or non-hormonal. Some of those markers may be found associated with some tumors as well as normal fetal fluids or tissues and, consequently, are termed oncofetal proteins. Those fetal antigens may be present in some tissues and serum of the fetus in large quantities, but circulate at considerably lower concentrations at the end of gestation and in the adult. Oncofetal proteins include alphafetoprotein and carcinoembryonic antigen. Some hormonal markers provide clues to occult carcinomas because of associated paraendocrine syndromes. In most cases, tumor production of hormonal or non-hormonal substances does not result in clinical syndromes. In selected cases, hormonal and non-hormonal markers may provide excellent markers to monitor tumor therapy and recurrence. The "ideal" tumor marker has never been realized in that a substance has not been identified for a specific tumor type and not found in sera of patients without tumor.

Almost every hormone known to be physiologically secreted by a normal endocrine cell has been associated with a tumor. Consequently, tumors may eutopically or ectopically secrete hormones. That definition is confounded by the hypothesis that all cells secrete those hormones, but some more efficiently than others. However, for our present discussion, the term "ectopic" will refer

to those hormones secreted by cells not normally associated with
secretion of readily detectable levels of that hormone. In addition to the above classes of tumor markers, others exist and include exocrine cell products such as lactoferrin and lactalbumin
and normal cell constituents such as enzymes and polyamines.
Since the latter group of tumor markers has not yet found wide ap-
plicability, it will not be included in the present discussion.

Since many tumor markers are present in picogram or nanogram
levels and are usually measured by radioimmunoassay, it is necessary for the practicing physician to have an understanding of the
limitations of that sensitive technique. It is imperative that
the antisera be specific and that the range of normal levels be
carefully defined for normal people and sick patients without
tumor. Moreover, that normal range will change with different
batches of specific antisera harvested from the same animal at
different times after immunization or from different animals.
Consequently, if radioimmunoassay kits are purchased commercially,
sufficient information should be available to allow the laboratory to ascertain whether the "normal range" of concentrations
need be redefined. The concentration of a marker may be monitored
serially. One should realize that concentrations determined on
separate assays have more "scatter" than if the two samples were
measured on the same assay.

The current discussion will be limited to the most commonly
used tumor markers which either provide clinical clues to occult
tumors or are commonly used to monitor patients with defined neoplasms.

CARCINOEMBRYONIC ANTIGEN (CEA)

In 1965 Gold and Freedman first described the presence of a
carcinoembryonic antigen in extracts of normal fetal gut and in
extracts of adenocarcinomas of the gastrointestinal tract. Although first thought to be specific for colorectal cancers, elevated concentrations have been observed in a number of benign
and other malignant conditions.[1] Moreover, CEA represents a heterogenous group of molecules and its detection may vary considerably with the laboratory technique utilized.[2] Rather than being
a single molecular entity, CEA is a heterogenous group of glycoproteins with a molecular weight of about 200,000. The measurement of CEA is most commonly performed using the "Z-gel" assay.
Since the concentration of CEA measured in a radioimmunoassay reflects the characteristics of the antiserum, it follows that it is
critical to carefully characterize the antisera and carefully define the normal range for CEA.

Utilizing both immunofluorescent antibody techniques and im-
munocytochemical staining, CEA has been localized both within the

lumen and on the surface (glycocalyx) of villi in adenocarcinomas of the colon.[3] However, a CEA-like substance has been detected in colonic mucosa remote from colonic neoplasms, as well as in benign colonic polyps, mucosal glands obtained from patients with ulcerative colitis, most epithelial cell tumors and perfusates of all levels of the normal human intestinal tract distal to the stomach.[4]

The metabolism of CEA has been partially elucidated by studies injecting radiolabeled CEA into laboratory animals. As much as 50% of the marker disappears from the circulation in 5 minutes and 70% in one hour, primarily due to liver uptake.[5] On the basis of these data, it has been hypothesized that increased serum concentrations among patients with benign liver disease or hepatic metastases may result from incomplete removal or degradation of CEA by the liver.[6] Although CEA has been found in hepatic metastases, it does not appear that hepatocytes synthesize CEA. Serum CEA levels are also elevated among patients with chronic renal failure, an observation consistent with animal studies in which 95% of the injected marker was ultimately excreted in the urine.[7]

Screening and Management

Multiple studies have indicated that the CEA is both too non-specific and too insensitive to be utilized in random screening of populations at risk for malignancy. The Busselton Population Studies Group, which included 2372 patients aged 40 or over, reported that the prevalence of positive tests, defined as a CEA level greater than 5 ng/ml, was 73 (3.5%).[8] However, abnormally high levels were observed among 9.5% of individuals smoking over 15 cigarettes daily. The yield of cancer from this gruop was small and also emphasizes careful definition of the "normal" range since 9.5% of smokers may have had false positive results. Nine patients with elevated CEA levels (13%) had a malignancy and in only two was the diagnosis the result of CEA testing. In the CEA negative group, 25 of 2299 patients (1%) were subsequently diagnosed as harboring a malignant tumor.

While 38 to 88% of patients with Laennec's cirrhosis may have "false positive" elevations of CEA levels (greater than 2.5 ng/ml), patients with any hepatic disorder may present with an elevated level.[6] Values higher than 20 ng/ml, while uncommon, have been reported. In patients at high risk for developing colonic carcinoma, including those with ulcerative colitis or colonic polyps, no correlation between CEA levels and foci of mucosal dysplasia or in situ carcinoma could be found.[9]

Monitoring CEA levels among patients with colorectal adenocarcinoma has been extensively used to detect recurrent tumor and to manage therapy among that patient group.[10] The incidence of

abnormally high CEA levels among patients with adenocarcinomas
staged by the Dukes classification has been reported as follows:
Type A: 0-40%; B: 35-76%; C: 61-100%; D: 79-100%. Although there
is a wide overlap among the stages and disparities among published
observations, there is a general trend toward increased concentrations with advanced disease.

It does seem, however, that levels which are persistently in
excess of 10-15 ng/ml are most likely correlated with disseminated
disease.[11] Elevated values are more frequently associated with
patients having hepatic metastases (52/73 patients) than nonhepatic metastases (17/37 patients). In a 1976 prospective study of
377 patients in which both CEA levels and liver spleen scans were
performed, the use of CEA levels increased the diagnostic yield of
metastatic liver disease from 78.9% with scan alone to 93.9% with
both forms of monitoring.[12] When the liver biopsy was initially
negative, in patients with rising CEA levels, a repeat biopsy often revealed metastatic disease. The latter observation probably
reflects a sampling error with biopsy.

The use of CEA titers after curative surgery for adenocarcinoma of the colon is controversial. Most investigators would
agree that CEA titers in the postoperative period are meaningless.
However, it would appear that a rising CEA level reflects recurrent or persistent disease.

ALPHAFETOPROTEIN

Alphafetoprotein (AFP) was found in the serum of mice bearing
transplantable hepatomas by Abelov in 1963, making this the first
protein to be widely studied as a tumor associated product. It is
a glycoprotein of 70,000 molecular weight with a carbohydrate composition of approximately 4%.[13] Synthesized by the fetal yolk
sac, liver and gastrointestinal tract in many species, alphafetoprotein has no known biologic activity in the human, although it
is thought to be an organization signal for liver lobule formation.[14]

Initially AFP was measured by an agar gel precipitation technique which had a lower limit of sensitivity of 3000 ng/ml.[15]
Subsequently, more sensitive quantitative immunodiffusion and
counter-immunoelectrophoresis techniques were developed with sensitivities of 400 ng/ml and 100 ng/ml, respectively. While simple to perform and thus applicable to many laboratories, their
relative insensitivity made them less desirable than radioimmunoassay. The latter technique is sufficiently sensitive to detect
1 ng/ml of AFP.

Using the above techniques, it was found that AFP, which
reaches levels up to 3,000,000 ng/ml by the 12-15th week of

gestation, declines to 10,000-150,000 ng/ml at birth. At one year
of age, levels have dropped to normal adult range. A normal adult
level has been defined as less than 40 ng/ml based on the observation that none of 190 normal control subjects and only one of 500
subjects with benign nonhepatic disease exceeded that value.[16]

Elevated levels of AFP have been found to be associated with
normal fetal development, liver regeneration, chemical hepatocar-
cinogenesis, ataxia-telangiectasia, visceral cell tumors, hepatomas and nonseminiferous germinal cell tumors. It is in regard
to the latter two tumors that AFP is most utilized clinically.

Hepatomas

The use of AFP in the diagnosis of hepatoma is complicated by
AFP elevation in a number of hepatic disorders. Using a rat model
of carbon tetrachloride induced liver injury, it was found that
3-5% of regenerating liver cells yielded increased concentrations
of AFP within 72 hours of injury.[17] It is thus not surprising
that AFP levels greater than 40 ng/ml are observed in as many as
27% of patients with classic viral hepatitis, 24% of patients with
postnecrotic cirrhosis, and 15% of patients with active Laennec's
cirrhosis.[18] Virtually every nonmalignant hepatic disease may be
associated with an elevated serum AFP level.

However, the degree of elevation is usually less than 400
ng/ml, a value above this level occurring only once in 200 patients
with benign hepatic disorders. In addition, the elevated AFP levels in patients with viral hepatitis return to normal rapidly with
resolution of the disease and the values in other hepatic disorders are usually stable or decrease.

In contrast, 72-95% of patients with hepatoma have an AFP
concentration greater than 40 ng/ml and those levels continue to
rise in contrast to patients with nonmalignant liver disease.[19]
Patients with hepatoma have levels above 400 ng/ml and a significant number have values greater than 3000 ng/ml. Thus, patients
with AFP levels above 400 ng/ml should be further evaluated for
harboring an occult hepatoma. Conversely, however, normal AFP
levels do not exclude the diagnosis, since between 5-25% of histologically confirmed hepatocellular carcinomas are not accompanied
by a rise in serum concentration of AFP. Some correlation exists
between the degree of differentiation of the tumor and the AFP
levels, with a lower frequency of elevated levels in either highly
differentiated or anaplastic tumors.[20]

Germinal Cell Tumors

As many as 75% of patients with nonseminomatous testicular
cell tumors have abnormally high AFP levels, usually in the range

of 40-3000 ng/ml[21]. Patients with seminomas do not have elevated
AFP levels. Thus, an elevation of serum AFP concentrations in a
patient with a testicular tumor implies that the patient should be
treated for a nonseminomatous tumor. Monitoring of both AFP and
hCG levels (see below) has proved invaluable for monitoring men
with germinal cell tumors of the testes. Moreover, by monitoring
those levels, therapy can be better adjusted and tumor recurrence
can be detected earlier than both clinical evaluation and conventional diagnostic techniques permit.

AFP levels are also elevated among patients with teratocarcinomas of the ovary and extragonadal teratocarcinomas such as those
of the mediastinum, retroperitoneum and sacrococcygeal region.[22]
Those patients with mature teratomas, as well as women with dys-
germinomas, analogous to seminomas, have normal AFP levels.

HUMAN CHORIONIC GONADOTROPIN

Human chorionic gonadotropin (hGC) is a glycoprotein hormone
of approximately 45,000 daltons and is secreted by the placenta
and is normally readily detectable in serum only during pregnancy.
It is composed of two different subunits, designated α and β.
Whereas the former is virtually identical with the α subunits of
LH, FSH, and TSH, the β subunit contains immunologic determinants
unique to hCG which confer immunologic specificity for specific
hCG assays.

Although initially determined by bioassay, agglutination inhibition and complement fixation techniques, hCG presently is measured almost exclusively by radioimmunoassay. As can be predicted
from the structural homology of hCG with other glycoprotein hormones from the anterior pituitary, antisera which are generated
against the whole molecule of purified hCG frequently cross react
with other glycoprotein hormones.[23] Using the isolated, highly
purified β subunit of hCG, some rabbits generate antisera sufficiently specific to selectively measure hCG in serum or plasma
samples containing high physiologic levels of LH.[24] That assay
is commonly termed the "β subunit" assay, but actually detects
the predominant circulating molecular species, hCG, rather than
hCG-β. The plasma half-life of hCG-β is less than 1% of that for
hCG. The specific radioimmunoassay is several hundred-fold more
sensitive than conventional pregnancy tests. Consequently, a patient may have a "negative"pregnancy test which has a lower limit
of detection equivalent to 300 to 500 mIU/ml, but that patient may
have abnormally high circulating levels of hCG detectable with the
specific hCG assay. The specific hCG assay has a lower limit of
sensitivity of approximately 5 mIU/ml.

Elevated levels of hCG have been observed among patients with
adenocarcinomas of the ovary, stomach, pancreas, as well as among

among patients with hepatomas and germinal cell neoplasms of the testis.[25] Its greatest use in clinical oncology has been in the management and followup of patients with gestational trophoblastic disease and patients with nonseminomatous germ cell tumors.

Gestational Tumors - Diagnostic

Gestational neoplasms are a group of morphologically related tumors arising from the placenta. Although they most commonly follow molar pregnancy, they may also develop as a consequence of an ectopic, aborted, or full term gestation. These tumors include hydatidiform moles, which are characterized histologically as excessive trophoblastic growth ranging from hyperplasia to anaplasia with maintenance of placental villous structure, as well as choriocarcinoma, which consists of sheets of pure cytotrophoblasts and syncytiotrophoblasts.[26]

Although diagnosis of molar pregnancy can usually be made by combined clinical and radiologic evaluation, followup of that patient group with serial serum hCG levels at weekly intervals after spontaneous or surgical abortion is essential to determine whether the patient is one of the 14-18% who will subsequently develop a trophoblastic tumor.[27] After hCG levels become normal for three consecutive weeks, hCG concentrations can be measured monthly for six months and then discontinued if hCG levels are normal. Using that approach, women who develop a trophoblastic malignancy will be diagnosed within several weeks and appropriate therapy can be instituted quickly. This tumor type is unusual in that even if metastases are present, a very high percentage of affected women can be cured with chemotherapy and subsequently undergo normal pregnancies.

Germinal Cell Testicular Neoplasms

Germinal cell testicular tumors are the leading nonaccidental form of death in young men. It is mandatory to distinguish seminoma from the other histologic subtypes, including embryonal carcinoma, endodermal sinus tumor, choriocarcinoma and teratocarcinoma because different forms of treatment are used. Seminomas are usually responsive to radiotherapy while the other forms of testicular neoplasms may require retroperitoneal lymph node dissection followed by chemotherapy if the disease is metastatic.[28]

Up to 80% of nonseminomatous tumors have an elevation of hCG and/or AFP, and up to 25% of tumors thought to be pure seminomas have an elevation of hCG.[29] An elevated alphafetoprotein level strongly suggests that the tumor has nonseminomatous elements and should be treated as such. The frequent discordant change in serum concentration of hCG and AFP with therapy led investigators to postulate that those tumor markers may be synthesized by different

cell lines.[30] Moreover, although a patient may be diagnosed as
having a seminoma, small clusters of cells of nonseminomatous tumor may be present but not observed histologically because of a
sampling error. Consequently, it is probably wise to monitor both
AFP and hCG levels in men diagnosed as having "pure" seminoma with
local extension requiring node dissection, radiotherapy, or both.

Utilizing immunohistochemical techniques, it is now possible
to localize tumor markers in individual cells.[31] Alphafetoprotein
is found in association with embryonal cell carcinomas, teratocarcinomas or endodermal sinus tumors, whereas hCG may be found in
cells of choriocarcinomas and occasionally in cells of embryonal
carcinoma and giant syncytiotrophoblastic cells of seminomas. In
those patients with elevated hCG levels and a diagnosis of seminoma, immunohistochemical studies have localized hCG production to
syncytial giant cells of the seminoma. Since these cells may be
few in number and widely distributed, it is necessary to perform
meticulous thin slice sectioning of the tumor, preferably with
immunochemical staining, to determine whether syncytiotrophoblasts or elements of a mixed tumor are present. Finally, since
testicular germ cell tumors may contain multiple cellular components with variable growth and response to chemotherapy, both markers should be monitored to determine the presence of metastatic
disease.[32]

False positive hCG titers determined by commercial β-subunit
kits have been reported in hypogonadal men with high LH levels,
illustrating once again the necessity of employing specific antisera and good quality control.[33] Short term administration of
testosterone prior to repeating the hCG titer may help resolve the
issue. In the case of a patient with a rising AFP titer, it is
necessary to ascertain that the patient has not developed an inter-
current hepatic disease. Finally, altered forms of hCG have been
used in at least one instance to localize metastatic disease.
Measurement of the α subunit of hCG in blood obtained with selective catheterization of the right ascending lumbar vein revealed
the site of a previously undetected lesion in a patient with an
elevated hCG level.[34] However, rarely can one identify small metastatic sites of hCG production, since the native molecule has
such a long half-life and rarely do those tumors produce sufficient quantities of altered forms of hCG with shorter half-lives
so that differential concentrations can be used.

AFP and hCG levels may be used clinically to help the clini-
cian with therapy of testicular cancer. In one series, 16 of 24
patients who subsequently relapsed had either an elevated hCG or
AFP level at a time when their tumor was clinically undetectable.[35]
Biochemical evidence may precede clinical confirmation of recurrent disease by as much as six months. Some authorities now ad-
vise that any patient in clinical remission with an elevated AFP

or hCG level and the former not attributed to liver dysfunction should be treated with chemotherapy.[28] Any patient with a prior history of a germinal cell testicular neoplasm should be followed with serial measurements of hCG and AFP even if their disease was stage I.

Non-trophoblastic Tumors

In addition to germ cell tumors, hCG has also been associated with non-trophoblastic neoplasms. Although almost every visceral neoplasm, as well as many hematopoietic malignancies, has been associated with elevated hCG levels, the strongest correlation is with epithelial ovarian tumors and gastrointestinal cancers, especially those of the stomach, liver and pancreas.[36] As many as 22-41% of those patients may have elevated hCG concentrations, sometimes attaining the level of hCG observed in the first trimester of pregnancy. Although some women may exhibit hyperthyroidism or may present with dysfunctional uterine bleeding and some men may present with isosexual precocious puberty or gynecomastia, most patients have no clinical manifestations. This can be ascribed to the fact that over 75% of patients have hCG levels less than 10 ng/ml (1 ng = 5 mIU) which are elevated for only a relatively short duration. Since hCG has intrinsic TSH activity, patients with high hCG levels may have chemically or clinically significant hyperthyroidism.[37] The hyperthyroidism resolves when hCG levels are significantly lowered with therapy.

Although it was first thought that if hCG was demonstrable in the plasma of a man or nonpregnant woman it was indicative of a tumor, subsequent studies have shown the presence of hCG in a small percentage of patients with benign disease. Patients with inflammatory gastrointestinal disorders, including regional enteritis and ulcerative colitis, have levels in excess of 1 ng/ml in approximately 2-3% of cases (unpublished observation). Approximately 5% of patients with duodenal ulcers may have low but significant elevation of hCG levels.[38] Thus, although the presence of serum hCG is not specific for a malignancy, high levels are suggestive in patients without inflammatory bowel disease.

PARAENDOCRINE SYNDROMES ASSOCIATED WITH TUMORS

A variety of hormones may be secreted by tumors of the lung and pancreas primarily and those tumors secreting biologically active substances may induce marked metabolic aberrations. Those abnormalities may constitute a more life-threatening problem to the patient than their underlying tumor. The hormones ectopically secreted associated with marked metabolic aberrations include parathormone, antidiuretic hormone (ADH) and ACTH. Each of these syndromes is briefly described below, along with signs and symptoms and accepted forms of treatment used to correct the marked aberrations.

Hypercalcemia

   Hypercalcemia is the most common metabolic abnormality associated with malignancy, occurring in approximately 9-43% of cases.[39] Tumors may produce a variety of substances which promote
bone resorption and result in elevated serum calcium levels. With
ectopic hyperparathyroidism, serum phosphate levels are usually
within the normal range or below normal. On the other hand, when
hypercalcemia results from bony tumor invasions, both calcium and
phosphate levels are abnormally elevated. Berson and Yalow first
reported elevations of parathormone (PTH) in 29% (8 of 28) of nor-
mocalcemic, nonuremic patients with bronchogenic carcinoma.[40] Several other substances, including prostaglandin and osteoclastic
activating factor, may be secreted by tumor tissue and induce
hypercalcemia.

   Although patients with ectopic PTH production usually have a
clinically evident tumor, it may be occult. The problem of differentiating these patients from those with primary hyperthyroidism is further confounded by the observation that as many as 10-
30% of patients with parathyroid adenomas may develop a malignancy,
most commonly an epithelial tumor.[41] The other side of the coin
need be considered as well. Specifically, older patients with
hypercalcemia and elevated PTH levels, suspected of having primary
hyperparathyroidism, should be screened with appropriate diagnostic tests to exclude ectopic PTH production. Although pseudohyper-
parathyroidism, another term for ectopic PTH production, is most
commonly associated with renal cell carcinoma or squamous cell
bronchogenic tumors, it has been reported with virtually every epithelial cell tumor as well as mesenchymal tumor.[39]

   Clinical presentation. The patient's initial clinical presentation is the same whether the hypercalcemia is a result of
ectopic production of a tumor which enhances bone resorption or
whether the hypercalcemia results from direct invasion of bone by
tumor. The signs and symptoms of hypercalcemia range from thirst,
weakness and lethargy to marked obtundation and marked metabolic
aberrations. Those signs and symptoms progress as the level of
hypercalcemia increases. In fact, the marked metabolic aberrations are more life-threatening to the patient than the underlying
tumor.

   Therapy of hypercalcemia. Initial therapy of the hypercalcemia is the same no matter what the underlying etiology.[42] Initially, patients should be rigorously hydrated with physiologic
saline to enhance renal calcium excretion. Loop diuretics are
added to enhance renal calcium excretion and prevent fluid overload. If the patient is not responding well initially or has a
compromised cardiac status but good renal function, then 50 mmole

of phosphate may be slowly infused. Other agents such as mithra-
mycin (single bolus of 25 μg/Kg), calcitonin by hydrocortisone,
and other prostaglandinal synthesis inhibitors such as aspirin or
indomethacin may be incorporated. Definitive hypercalcemia therapy
after the initial emergency maneuvers is directed to the tumor in
terms of surgery, radiotherapy, chemotherapy, or some combination
of the foregoing.

Ectopic ACTH Syndrome

     Ectopic ACTH secretion was probably the first ectopic hormone
syndrome suspected. However, although a case of Cushing's syndrome
in a patient with small cell carcinoma of the lung was described
in 1928, it was not until 1965 that Liddle and his colleagues published a study of a series of patients presenting with both
Cushing's syndrome and neoplasms, establishing the syndrome clinically.[43] It is now well appreciated that ectopic ACTH secretion
is commonly observed among patients with small cell carcinomas of
the lung, pancreas and thymomas as well as adrenal pheochromo-
cytomas. Although only a small percentage, ranging from 0.4% to
2%, of such patients have clinical evidence of increased ACTH production, as many as 72% of patients with bronchogenic carcinoma may
have elevated levels of ACTH or its precursors.[44]

     ACTH ectopically secreted by tumor cells may be indistinguish-
able from "native" ACTH, a polypeptide of 39 amino acids with a
molecular weight of 4500. More recently, larger forms of ectopic
ACTH, "big ACTH" and "big, big ACTH" (20,000 and 31,000 daltons)
have been found in peripheral blood and tumor extracts.[45] "Big"
ACTH is glycosylated and contains only 4% of the bioactivity of
native ACTH. In addition, both larger forms and smaller ACTH
species have been identified from both pituitary cell cultures and
tumor extracts.[46]

     The measurement of ACTH was first determined by a difficult
in vitro bioassay using isolated adrenal cells obtained from hypophysectomized rats. That has been supplanted by sensitive radioimmunoassays. A new technique based on the cytochemical staining
of adrenal tissue has been developed and is considerably more sensitive than radioimmunoassay, but is too cumbersome to be employed
clinically on a routine basis at the current time.[47]

     Clinical syndrome. ACTH ectopically secreted by tumors is
usually biologically inert, but when an active form is produced,
some signs of Cushing's syndrome may be observed. Classically,
patients with the "full blown" syndrome present with a marked hypo-
kalemic metabolic alkalosis, marked dependent edema, hypertension,
hyperglycemia and diffuse hyperpigmentation.[48] For poorly understood reasons, the hallmarks of classical Cushing's syndrome,

including truncal obesity, moon shaped facies, plethora and hirsu-
tism, are usually not evident.

The distinction between ectopic ACTH production and pituitary dependent Cushing's syndrome may be difficult from both a clinical and biochemical standpoint. Although the high dose dexamethasone (8 mg/day x 2 days) suppression test has been the one most
commonly used to distinguish the two causes, results may be misleading.[49] False positive suppression may occur because suppres-
sibility does occur with some tumors, some tumors may secrete
ACTH releasing factors or some patients may have periodic secretion
of ACTH ("periodic hormonogenesis").

Ectopic production of ACTH is suggested by concentrations of
ACTH in excess of 200 pg/ml, concentrations observed among 65% of
affected patients.[50] In contrast, patients with pituitary Cushing's
syndrome have ACTH levels in the "normal" range 50% of the time,
and only rarely have values above 200 pg/ml.

Therapy. Because the marked metabolic alkalosis, hyperglycemia
and fluid retention associated with this syndrome may be more life-
threatening than the tumor itself, appropriate therapy need be instituted as quickly as possible. In practice, these include using
drugs which interfere with adrenal steroidogenesis.[51] Combined
metyrapone and aminoglutethamide (Elipten) therapy effectively inhibits steroidogenesis within a few days and their combined effects
may be so complete that patients may require replacement steroid
therapy to prevent adrenal insufficiency. The adrenolytic agent,
1,1-dichloro-2(o-chlorophenyl)-2(p-chlorophenyl)ethane(o,p'-DDD)
may also be used, but its therapeutic effects are not manifest for
several weeks. After ascertaining the tumor responsible for ectopic
ACTH secretion, anti-tumor therapy should be instituted as quickly
as possible in order to minimize the amount of biologically active
ACTH secreted by that tumor and, consequently, minimize adrenal
stimulation.

Syndrome of Inappropriate Anti-Diuretic Hormone Secretion (SIADH)

Although almost four decades ago hyponatremia was recognized
among patients with cancer, it was not until the last decade that
patients with tumors who displayed hyponatremia and water retention
were thought to have inappropriate secretion of anti-diuretic hormone (ADH) by the tumor.[52] Radioimmunoassays have been developed
and are currently available to measure circulating ADH levels, corrected to serum osmolality. However, in any patient suspected of
having ectopic ADH syndrome, several other factors must be excluded
and these include abnormal thyroid, adrenal and pituitary function,
as well as the exclusion of several drugs known to be associated
with SIADH. Those drugs include amitryptilline, barbiturates,
chlorpropamide, clofibrate, Cytoxan, nicotine, phenothiazines,

Tegretol and Vincristine.[53] Obviously, some of those drugs are
used for specific anti-tumor therapy but unfortunately can actually
make the patient worse clinically in terms of contributing to water
intoxication.

Signs and symptoms. Those tumors most commonly associated with
ectopic ADH syndrome are tumors of the lung and pancreas.[54] Patients initially present with graded signs of water intoxication
and those include signs ranging from mild confusion, weakness and
lethargy to convulsions and coma. The rate of change in the
patients' clinical presentation reflects the rate at which the
patients become hypo-osmolar. All patients with serum osmolalities
below 240 mOsm become symptomatic. In addition, electrolyte abnormalities may be observed and those include hyponatremia, hypoka-
lemia and hypocalcemia. Interestingly, rarely do patients with
SIADH display any signs of fluid overload in terms of dependent
edema.

Therapy. No matter what the cause of water intoxication, be
it drug or ectopic ADH-induced, initial therapy is water restriction.[55] Use of hypertonic saline is rarely indicated and should
be reserved only to life-threatening situations. With careful
monitoring, loop diuretics may be used to enhance formation of isotonic urine which is replaced with hypertonic fluid (normal saline). Demeclocyline in doses of 600-1200 mg per day may effectively reverse the symptoms of SIADH by interfering with ADH action
on the collecting duct. Lithium carbonate is less effective and
more toxic.

REFERENCES

1. N. Zamcheck, T. L. Moore, P. Dhar, H. Z. Kupchick, and J. J.
    Sorokin, Carcinoembryonic antigen in benign and malignant
    diseases of the digestive tract, Natl. Cancer Inst. Monogr.
    35:433 (1972).
2. J. J. Sorokin, H. Z. Kupchik, N. Zamcheck, and P. Dhar, A clin-
    ical comparison of two radioimmunoassays for carcinoembryonic
    antigen, Immunol. Commun. 1:11 (1972).
3. P. Gold, J. Krupoy, and H. Ansari, Position of the carcinoem-
    bryonic antigen of the human digestive system in ultrastruc-
    ture of tumor cell surface, J. Natl. Cancer Inst. 45:219 (1970)
4. F. G. Elias, F. D. Holyoke, and T. M. Chu, Carcinoembryonic
    antigen (CEA) in feces and plasma of human subjects and
    patients with colo-rectal carcinoma, Dis. Colon Rectum 17:8
    (1974).
5. J. Shuster, M. Silverman, and P. Gold, Metabolism of human
    carcinoembryonic antigen in xenogenic animals, Cancer Res.
    33:65 (1973).
6. M. Loewenstein and N. Zamcheck, Carcinoembryonic antigen and
    the liver, Gastroenterology 72:161 (1977).

7. R. D. Brandstetter, V. A. Graziano, M. J. Wade, and S. D. Saal, Carcinoembryonic antigen elevation in renal failure, Ann. Intern. Med. 91:867 (1979).

8. K. J. Cullen, D. D. Stevens, M. A. Frost, and I. R. Mackay, Carcinoembryonic antigen (CEA), smoking and cancer in a longitudinal population study. Aust. NZ J. Med. 6:279 (1976).

9. W. G. Doos, W. I. Wolff, H. Shinya, A. DeChabon, R. J. Stenger, L. S. Gottlieb, and N. Zamcheck, CEA levels in patients with colorectal polyps, Cancer 36:1996 (1975).

10. G. Reynoso and M. Keane, Carcinoembryonic antigen in prognosis and monitoring of patients with cancer, in: "Immunodiagnosis of Cancer," R. B. Heberman and K. R. McIntire, eds., Marcel Dekker, New York (1979).

11. M. Ravry, C. G. Moertel, A. J. Schutt, and V. L. W. Go, Usefulness of serial serum carcinoembryonic antigen (CEA) determinations during anticancer therapy or long-term follow-up of gastrointestinal carcinoma, Cancer 34:1230 (1974).

12. W. H. McCartney and P. B. Hoffer, Carcinoembryonic antigen assay in hepatic metastases detection, JAMA 236:1023 (1976).

13. E. Ruoslahti and M. Seppala, Studies of carcinofetal proteins: Physical and chemical properties of human α-fetoprotein. Int. J. Cancer 7:218 (1971).

14. S. Sell, The biological and diagnostic significance of oncodevelopmental gene products, in: "The Handbook of Cancer Immunology," H. Waters, ed., Garland SIPM Press, New York (1978).

15. T. A. Waldmann and K. R. McIntire, The use of sensitive assays for alpha-fetoprotein in monitoring the treatment of malignancy, in: "Immunodiagnosis of Cancer," R. B. Herberman and K. R. McIntire, eds., Marcel Dekker, New York (1979).

16. T. A. Waldmann and K. R. McIntire, The use of a radioimmunoassay for alphafetoprotein in the diagnosis of malignancy, Cancer 34:1510 (1974).

17. N. V. Engelhardt, M. N. Lazareva, G. I. Abelev, I. V. Uryvaeva, V. M. Factor, and V. Y. Brodsky, Detection of α-fetoprotein in mouse liver differentiated hepatocytes before their progression through S phase, Nature 263:146 (1976).

18. J. R. Bloomer, T. A. Waldmann, K. R. McIntire, and G. Klatskin, Serum alpha-fetoprotein levels in patients with non-neoplastic liver disease, Gastroenterology 65:530 (1973).

19. D. S. Chen and J. L. Sung, Serum alphafetoprotein in hepatocellular carcinoma, Cancer 40:779 (1977).

20. L. R. Purves, I. Bersohn, E. W. Geados, Serum alphafetoprotein and primary cancer of the liver in man, Cancer 25:1261 (1970).

21. N. Javadpour, K. R. McIntire, T. A. Waldmann, et al., The role of alphafetoprotein and human chorionic gonadotropin in seminoma, J. Urol. 120:687 (1978).

22. C. Mawas, D. Buffe, O. Schweisgath, and P. Burtin, Alphafetoprotein and children's cancer review. Eur. Clin. Biol. 16:430 (1971).

23. J. L. Vaitukaitis and G. T. Ross, Antigenic similarities among the human glycoprotein hormones and their subunits, in: "Gonadotropins," B. Saxena and H. Gandy, eds., Wiley, New York (1972).

24. J. L. Vaitukaitis, G. D. Braunstein, and G. T. Ross, A radioimmunoassay which specifically measures human chorionic gonadotropin in the presence of human luteinizing hormone, Am. J. Obstet. Gynecol. 113: 751 (1972).

25. G. D. Braunstein, J. L. Vaitukaitis, P. P. Carbone, and G. T. Ross, Ectopic production of human chorionic gonadotropin by neoplasms, Ann. Intern. Med. 78:39 (1973).

26. A. T. Hertig and W. H. Sheldon, Hydatidiform mole - pathologicoclinical correlation of 200 cases, Am. J. Obstet. Gynecol. 53:1 (1947).

27. D. P. Goldstein, Gestational neoplasms, in: "Endocrinology," L. J. DeGroot, ed., Grune and Stratton, New York (1979).

28. E. E. Fraley, P. H. Lange, and B. J. Kennedy, Germ-cell testicular cancer in adults, N. Engl. J. Med. 301: 1370, 1420 (1979).

29. N. Javadpour, K. R. McIntire, and T. A. Waldmann, Human chorionic gonadotropin and alphafetoprotein in sera and tumor cells of patients with testicular seminoma, Cancer 42:2768 (1979).

30. G. D. Braunstein, R. McIntire, and T. A. Waldmann, Discordance of human chorionic gonadotropin and alphafetoprotein in testicular teratocarcinomas, Cancer 31:1065 (1973).

31. R. J. Kurman, P. T. Scardino, K. R. McIntire, T. A. Waldmann, and N. Javadpour, Cellular localization of alphafetoprotein and human chorionic gonadotropin in germ cell tumors of the testes using an indirect immunoperoxidase technique, Cancer 40:2137 (1977).

32. E. Perlin, J. E. Engeler, M. Edson, D. Karp, K. R. McIntire, and T. A. Waldmann, The value of both human chorionic gonadotropin and alphafetoprotein for monitoring germinal cell tumors, Cancer 37:215 (1976).

33. W. Catalona, J. L. Vaitukaitis, and W. R. Fair, Falsely positive specific human chorionic gonadotropin assays in patients with testicular tumors: Conversion to negative with testosterone administration, J. Urol. 122:126 (1979).

34. N. Javadpour, K. R. McIntire, T. A. Waldmann, P. T. Scardino, S. Bergman, and T. Anderson, The role of radioimmunoassay of serum alphafetoprotein and human chorionic gonadotropin in the intensive chemotherapy and surgery of metastatic testicular tumors, J. Urol. 119:759 (1978).

35. P. T. Scardino, H. D. Cox, T. A. Waldmann, K. R. McIntire, B. Mittemeyer, and N. Javadpour, The value of serum tumor markers in the staging and prognosis of germ cell tumors of the testis, J. Urol., 118:994 (1977).

36. J. L. Vaitukaitis, G. T. Ross, G. D. Braunstein, and P. L. Rayford, Gonadotropin and their subunits: Basic and clinical studies, Recent Prog. Horm. Res. 32:289 (1976).

37. W. T. Cave and J. T. Dunn, CHoriocarcinoma with hyperthyroidism:
    probable identity of the thyrotropin with human chorionic gona-
    dotropin, Ann. Intern. Med. 85: 60 (1976).

38. G. D. Braunstein, Use of human chorionic gonadotropin as a
    tumor marker in cancer, in: "Immunodiagnosis of Cancer,"
    R. B. Herberman and K. R. McIntire, eds., Marcel Dekker, New
    York (1979).

39. D. A. Heath, Hypercalcemia and malignancy, Ann. Clin. Biochem.
    13:555 (1976).

40. S. A. Berson and R. S. Yalow, Parathyroid hormone in plasma
    in adenomatous hyperparathyroidism, uremia and bronchogenic
    carcinoma, Science 154:907 (1966).

41. H. W. Farr, T. J. Fahey, A. G. Nash, and C. M. Farr, Primary
    hyperparathyroidism and cancer, Am. J. Surg. 126, 539 (1973).

42. E. L. Mazzaferri, T. M. O'Dorisio, and A. F. LaBuglio, Treat-
    ment of hypercalcemia associated with malignancy, Sem. Oncology
    5:141 (1978).

43. C. K. Meador, G. W. Liddle, D. P. Island, W. E. Nicholson,
    C. P. Lucas, J. G. Nickton, and Luetscher, J., Cause of
    Cushing's syndrome in patients with tumors arising from "non-
    endocrine" tissue, J. Clin. Endocrinol. Metab. 22:693 (1962).

44. A. R. Wolfsen and W. D. Odell, ProACTH: Use for early detec-
    tion of lung cancer, Am. J. Med. 66:765 (1979).

45. B. A. Eipper, R. E. Mains, and D. Guenzi, High molecular
    weight forms of adrenocorticotrophic hormone are glycoproteins,
    J. Biol. Chem. 251:4121 (1976).

46. R. E. Mains and B. A. Eipper, Biosynthesis of adrenocortico-
    tropic hormone in mouse pituitary tumor cells, J. Biol. Chem.
    251:4115 (1976).

47. L. H. Rees, I. M. Holdaway, G. M. Besser, R. Kraner, J.
    Landon, J. Chayen, Comparison of the redox assay for ACTH with
    previous assays, Nature (London) 241:84 (1973).

48. H. Imura, S. Matsukura, H. Yamamoto, Y. Hirata, Y. Nakai, J.
    Endo, et al., Studies on ectopic ACTH-producing tumors.
    II. Clinical and biochemical features of 30 cases, Cancer
    35:1430 (1975).

49. E. M. Gold, The Cushing syndromes: Changing views of diagnosis
    and treatment, Ann. Intern. Med. 90: 829 (1979).

50. J. G. Ratcliffe, R. A. Knight, G. M. Besser, J. Landon, and
    A. G. Stansfield, Tumor and plasma ACTH concentrations in
    patients with and without the ectopic ACTH syndrome. Clin.
    Endocrinol. 1:27 (1972)

51. T. E. Temple and G. W. Liddle, Inhibitors of the adrenal
    steroid biosynthesis, Ann. Rev. Pharmacol. 10:199 (1970).

52. F. C. Bartter and W. B. Schwartz, The syndrome of inappropri-
    ate secretion of antidiuretic hormone, Am. J. Med. 42:806
    (1967).

53. A. M. Moses and M. Miller, Drug-induced dilutional hyponatre-
    mia, N. Engl. J. Med. 291:1234 (1974).

54. H. Vorherr, U. F. Vorherr, T. S. McConnell, N. M. Goldberg,
    M. Kornfeld, and S. W. Jordan, Localization and origin of
    antidiuretic principle in paraendocrine active malignant
    tumors, Oncology 29:201 (1974).
55. A. M. Moses, M. Miller, and D. H. P. Streeten, Pathophysiologic
    and pharmacologic alterations in the release and action of
    ADH, Metabolism 25:697 (1976).

CHORIONIC GONADOTROPIN SYNTHESIS AND GENE ASSIGNMENT

IN HUMAN:MOUSE HYBRID CELLS

Peter O. Kohler[*], Mary Riser[+], James Hardin[*],
Mark Boothby[**], Irving Boime[**], James Norris[*], and
Michael J. Siciliano[++]

[*]Department of Medicine
University of Arkansas
Little Rock, Arkansas

[+]Department of Cell Biology
Baylor College of Medicine
Houston, Texas

[**]Department of Pharmacology
Washington School of Medicine
St. Louis, Missouri

[++]Biology Department
The University of Texas System Cancer Center
Houston, Texas

INTRODUCTION

Chorionic gonadotropin (hCG) is a hormone of special interest
in the field of human tumor biology. This glycoprotein hormone
is secreted in vast quantities by the syncytiotrophoblast of the
placenta during normal pregnancy. However, ectopic or inappropriate secretion of either or both subunits of hCG is a relatively
common occurrence in tumors of non-placental origin[1-4]. Clearly,
an appreciation of the control of hCG synthesis would be useful
in determining the reason for the high frequency of ectopic synthesis of this tumor marker.

Structurally, hCG is similar to the pituitary glycoprotein
hormones: luteinizing hormone (hLH), follicle stimulating hormone (hFSH), and thyrotropin (hTSH). Each of these is a protein
heterodimer consisting of concovalently bound α and β subunits.[5]

The α subunits of these four hormones in humans are immunologically identical, while the unique β subunits of these proteins confer specific biological activity.[6] The gene frequency or dosage for the α subunit and the possible unique β subunits has not been determined. hCG has proved a unique system for studying this problem. Specifically, it has not been determined whether there is a single α subunit gene whose product is assembled with the various unique β subunits or if each glycoprotein hormone has an independent α-β linkage group. Knowledge of the relationship of the structural genes for the α and β subunits to hCG synthesis should provide insight into the deranged control of gene expression in the malignant state as well as the possible relationship between the α and β genes for other glycoprotein hormones.

We have utilized hybridization of somatic cells as a technique for mapping the structural genes for hCG. This cellular fusion allows genetic information from different cell types and different species to be combined into a single cell. Interspecific hybrids such as the human:mouse hybrid cells used in these studies also have the characteristic of preferential chromosome loss from one species, in this case human. Loss of chromosomes in these hybrids simplifies the correlation of hCG production with retention of certain human chromosomes.

The JEG-3 line of human choriocarcinoma cells[7,8] which produce complete steroid and protein hormones that are immunologically and biologically active were used for these studies.[9-11] These cells produce characteristic levels of chorionic gonadotropin (hCG), placental lactogen and progesterone as well as aromatizing the appropriate 19-carbon steroid precursors to estrogens. Several mouse fibroblast-like cell lines were used as the other parent cell for the fusion studies.

Analysis of hybrid clones producing hCG and correlation with the retention of certain human chromosomes has permitted localization of the hCG genes. The confirmation of this mapping was made possible with the recent isolation and cloning of the α and β hCG genes.[12] Because DNA hybridization does not require expression of a gene product for mapping, these hybrid cells now permit analysis of the relationship between retention of genetic information and expression for many normal placental functions present in the JEG-3 cells.

MATERIALS AND METHODS

Culture Methods

The JEG-3 line of human choriocarcinoma cells is one of

several clones originally isolated in 1967 in our laboratory[1] from a tumor metastasis which Hertz had earlier adapted to transfer in the hamster cheek pouch system.[13] These epithelioid cells exhibit a high plating efficiency and retain multiple placental functions including the production of biologically active hCG in vitro.[9]

Somatic Cell Hybridization

The JEG-3 cells have been fused with cells from several mouse lines deficient in either thymidine kinase (TK) or hypoxanthine guanine phosphoribosyltransferase (HGPRTase). These parent mouse lines are unable to survive in HAT (hypoxanthine-aminopterin-thymidine) selective medium in which the aminopterin blocks de novo synthesis of nucleotides and forces utilization of thymidine and hypoxanthine for synthesis of nucleotides through salvage pathways.[14,15]

The fibroblast mouse cells used included the LMTK⁻Clone 1D and the 3T3-4EF lines which are deficient in thymidine kinase and the A9 line which is deficient in HGPRTase.[16,17] The parent lines were treated with trypsin and 10^6 of both JEG-3 and mouse cells were fused in suspension using 2000 hemagglutination units of β-propiolactone inactivated Sendai virus or alternatively polyethylene glycol. After incubation for 2 hours at 37⁰ the fused cells were dispersed into 100 mm plastic culture dishes containing GIBCO F-12 medium as modified by Bordelon with 13% horse serum, 2.5% fetal bovine serum, 100 units/ml penicillin, and 100 μg/ml streptomycin. After 48 hours this medium was exchanged for the same medium containing HAT in order to kill non-fused mouse parent cells. Since HAT medium does not inhibit JEG-3 cells, hybrid colonies were selected on the basis of morphology and removed by a cloning ring technique. Hybrid cells selected thereafter appeared more fibroblast-like than the epithelioid JEG-3 parent line, but were resistant to HAT.

Hybrid Identification

The hybrid nature of the clones selected and removed with cloning rings was confirmed by chromosome morphology and isozyme analysis. The chromosome analysis was performed by both the Q and C banding techniques.[18] Quinicrine mustard dihydrochloride was used for the fluorescent Q bands and sequential 65⁰ salt treatment with Giemsa staining was utilized for the C band analysis.

Enzyme Marker Analysis

Starch gel electrophoresis of isozymes was utilized as another means of identifying human genetic components in the hybrid cell clones. After starch gel electrophoresis of homogenates of the hybrids, histochemical staining was performed to detect 28 enzyme loci for which the human and mouse products have different mobilities. These enzymes have been assigned to specific human chromosomes and therefore serve as markers for the chromosomes. The following enzymes have been examined: acid phosphatase (ACP), adenosine deaminase (ADA), adenylate kinase (AK), enolase (ENO), esterases (ESD), galactokinase (GALK), glucose-6-phosphate dehydrogenase (G6PD), glucosephophate isomerase (GPI), glutamate oxaloacetate transaminase (GOT-1), glyceraldehyde-3-phosphate dehydrogenase (GAPD), hexoseaminidases HEXA; HEXB), isocitrate dehydrogenases (IDH-1), lactate dehydrogenases (LDH-A; LDH-B), malate dehydrogenases (MDH), mannosephosphate isomerase, nucleoside phosphorylase (NP), peptidases (PEPA; PEPB; PEPC), phosphoglucomutases (PGM-1; PGM-2; PGM-3), superoxide dismutase (SOD-1), and triosephophate isomerase (TPI). This technique confirms both the hybrid nature of the clones and the human chromosomal content determined by chromosome morphology.[17] A radiometric assay for adenosine deaminase (ADA) was also utilized.[19]

Hormone Assays

We have measured the hCG produced by the cultured cells by radioimmunoassay.[9] Specific subunit assays have been performed in collaboration with Dr. Judith Vaitukaitis. Progesterone has been assayed by a saturation assay using corticosteroid-binding globulin.[21] This assay is sensitive to 0.1 ng progesterone per ml medium. Estradiol was measured by radioimmunoassay utilizing the technique of Loriaux et al.[22]

Nucleic Acid Hybridization Techniques

The nucleic acid hybridization studies were performed on DNA from the parent cells and hybrid clones. Cells were grown to confluency, washed once with phosphate buffered saline and DNA isolated by the procedure of Gross-Bellard et al.[23] The final DNA concentration was determined by absorbance at 260 nM. DNA was stored in 10 mM Tris-HCl, pH 7.8, 1 mM EDTA. The restriction endonuclease digestion of the DNA utilized endonucleases obtained from Bethesda Research Laboratories. These were used according to the conditions recommended by the supplier. Reactions generally contained 5 to 10 μg of DNA. Reactions were terminated by the addition of sodium dodecyl sulfate, EDTA, glycerol and bromphenol blue to final concentrations of 1%, 2.5 mM, 10%, and 0.005% respectively.

Agarose electrophoresis was performed with slab gels containing 0.8 to 1% agarose prepared and run in a buffer containing 50
mM Tris pH 8.0, 20 mM Na acetate, 18 mM NaCl and 2 mM EDTA. At
the end of the electrophoresis, gels were stained in ethidium
bromide, destained in H2O and photographed with U.V. trans-
illumination. Gels were treated and transferred to nitrocellulose using the conditions described by Southern.[24]

Hybridization probes were prepared by nick translation of
cloned doubled stranded DNA of the mRNA for α hCG using DNA
polymerase I and α ^{32}P-dATP essentially as described by Maniatis
et al.[25] Filters were prehybridized for 2 hours at 68° in sealed
plastic bags which contained 5xSSC (1xSSC, 0.15 M NaCl, 0.015 M
Na citrate, pH 7.0), 5x Denhardt's reagent[26], 20 µgs/ml of
denatured salmon sperm DNA, 20 mM NaPO4, pH 6.5, 1% glycine and
10% dextran sulfate.[27,28] Hybridizations were for 16 hours at
68° in a solution which contained 5xSSC, 2x Denhardt's reagent
20 mM NaPO4, 50 µg/ml of denatured salmon sperm DNA, 50 µg/ml E.
coli tRNA, 25 µg/ml poly A, 20 µg/ml poly C, 10% dextran sulfate
and 5 x 10^6 cpm of ^{32}P labeled DNA probe. At the end of the
hybridization period, filters were washed 5 times with 0.1xSSC
containing 0.05% SDS and 3 times with 0.1xSSC all at 55°. Filters were dried and subjected to autoradiography with DuPont
lightning-plus itensifying screens at -70° C.

RESULTS

Hybrid Formation

Over two hundred human:mouse hybrid clones have been developed
as the result of multiple separate choriocarcinoma:mouse fibroblast fusion studies. The cellular morphology of most of the
clones has been intermediate between the epithelioid JEG-3 and
fibroblast-like mouse parental cells. However, the appearance of
the hybrid has not been useful in predicting which of the hybrids
would synthesize hCG.

Correlation of hCG Synthesis with Human Chromosomes

Since "luxury" functions such as hormone synthesis are not
absolutely necessary for cell growth in culture, these are often
extinguished in somatic cell hybrids.[29] This loss of gene
function may depend on gene dosage. Therefore, we were interested
to find that hCG was synthesized by 20% of hybrid clones isolated
from the JEG-3/Clone ID cross. The frequency of expression was
less than 10% in clones from the JEG-3/3T3-4EF fusions, and none
of the JEG-3/A9 hybrids produced hCG. Previous studies in our
laboratory[16] indicated that the frequency of hCG-producing clones
was 75-80% in human:human hybrids. The synthesis of hCG by the
positive human:mouse hybrids was always less than 5% of the

JEG-3 parent line which produced hCG at the rate of about one
IU/ml medium/24-hour period. The production of isolated subunits
has not been extensively analyzed to date. However, large amounts
of isolated α and β subunits have not been detected in any of the
hybrid clones. The presence of measurable quantities of either
subunit appears to have occurred only in association with complete
hCG synthesis.

The correlation of hCG synthesis in the hybrids with the content of chromosomes determined by isozyme analysis is shown in
Table 1. A similar analysis utilizing chromosome identification
by morphology is shown in Table 2. The chromosomes from hybrid
clone 124c were analyzed by karyology at passage 9 when it was
producing hCG and again at passage 37 when it no longer produced
detectible levels of hCG. Several chromosomes had been lost
during the intervening passages. Hybrid 124c-1 which retained
hCG synthesis was also examined at passages 10 and 36.

Table 1 Enzymatic Chromosome Markers in Hybrid Clones

		hCG Positive		hCG Negative			
		114a	124c-1	112b	123b-2	130g	137a
Chromosome Enzymes							
1	PEPC, PGM-1, ENO-1	+	NC	−	−	+	−
2	ACP-1, MDH-1, IDH-1	−	−	−	−	+	−
4	PGM2	−	−	−	−	+	−
5	HEXB	+	−	−	−	+	+
6	GLO-1, PGM-3, ME-1	+	−	NC	+	−	−
8	GSR	−	−	−	−	+	−
9	AK1	−	−	−	−	−	−
10	GOT-1, ADK	+	+	−	−	−	+
11	LDH-A	+	+	±	−	+	−
12	LDH-B, PEPB, TP1	+	+	+	+	+	+
13	ESD	+	+	+	+	+	−
14	NP	+	+	+	−	+	+
15	PKM$_2$, HEXA	+	+	+	−	+	−
16	APRT	+	+	+	+	+	−
17	TK, GALK	+	+	+	+	+	−
18	PEPA	+	+	+	−	+	−
19	GPI, PEPD	+	+	+	−	+	−
20	ADA, ITP	+	+	+	−	+	−
21	SOD1	+	+	+	−	+	−
X	G6PD, HPRT	−	+	−	+	+	+

NC = Non-concordance of assay. There were no useful enzyme
    marker on chromosomes 3, 7, or Y in our system. hCG
    positive indicated presence of detectable quantities of
    hCG by radioimmunoassay in the medium.

Table 2 Percentage of Cells Retaining Each Human Chromosome by Morphology

Clone	hCG Positive				hCG Negative				
	114a	124c-1 (early passage)	124c-1 (late passage)	124c (early passage)	124c (late passage)	112b	123b-2	130g	137a
Chromosome									
1	9	0	0	8	0	0	0	0	0
2	4	0	0	19	0	0	0	53	0
3	13	0	0	8	0	0	0	20	0
4	0	0	0	27	0	0	0	43	17
5	39	4	0	8	0	13	6	57	0
6	17	0	0	0	0	0	0	50	0
7	9	0	0	0	0	3	9	57	42
8	17	39	53	27	4	9	3	40	0
9	0	0	0	8	0	0	0	0	33
10	35	30	73	35	4	3	6	7	0
11	26	0	0	23	0	13	0	53	17
12	9	0	0	27	0	0	18	0	33
13	13	0	0	0	0	0	15	0	0
14	65	83	93	81	22	16	3	67	0
15	4	0	0	15	0	0	0	17	0
16	26	0	0	58	0	0	0	80	0
17	43	91	93	81	52	31	44	77	17
18	83	74	60	46	0	9	3	50	0
19	30	30	20	27	0	6	3	63	0
20	43	35	60	42	22	31	0	53	8
21	91	61	87	54	0	34	3	63	0
22	83	26	53	46	35	19	12	87	0
X	4	65	40	42	0	25	44	80	42
Y	0	0	0	4	0	13	9	43	0

Assignment of the genes for hCG by segregation to a single human chromosome was not possible from these data.[17] The results appear to indicate that a combination of two human chromosomes, 10 and 18, were both present with a high frequency in the clones which synthesized hCG. The combination of chromosomes 10 and 18 were also uniformly absent or present at very low frequencies in the hCG negative clones. To further analyze the segregation of hCG synthesis with chromosomes 10 and 18, the hCG producing clone 124c-1 was recloned and the correlation of hCG production with presence of chromosomes 10 and 18 by isozyme analysis was determined.

Table 3 Relationship of hCG Synthesis to Chromosomes 10 and 18
in Subclones of 124c-1

	hCG	Chromosome 10 (GOT-1 and ADK)	Chromosome 18 (PEPA)
Clone 124c-1	+	+	+
Subclones			
1	+	+	+
2	−	+	−
3	−	−	+
4	−	−	+
5	+	+	+
7	−	−	+
8	−	−	+
9	−	−	+
10	+	+	+

Again, hCG synthesis occurred only in the subclones 1, 5, and 10 which contained both chromosomes 10 and 18. Subclones with only 10 or 18 did not produce detectible quantities of hCG. We therefore initiated the studies described below to determine the relationship between the presence of the structural genes for the α and β subunits and expression of hCG synthesis.

Nucleic Acid Hybridization Studies

We performed the initial hybridization studies utilizing the ^{32}P-labeled cloned cDNA prepared from α glycoprotein subunit mRNA and placental lactogen (hPL) mRNA as probes hybridized to DNA isolated from the 130g hybrid and DNA from term placenta. Clone 130g has negligible quantities of human chromosome 10, a high frequency of chromosome 18, and does not synthesize detectible quantities of hCG. The molecular hybridization experiments were designed to determine if the structural gene for α subunit were present in this clone which contains chromosome 18, but fails to produce hCG.

As indicated in Fig. 1 the hybridization patterns obtained with DNA isolated from clone 130g and human placental DNA and cleaved with EcoR1 were essentially identical when ^{32}P α hCG cDNA was used as a probe. This pattern was characterized by a single band in the 5 kilobase area of the gel and a double band in the 10 kilobase area of the gel. The hybridization pattern was also identical for the two DNA's when ^{32}P-hPL probe was used. The gene for hPL previously has been assigned to chromosome 17[32] which was retained in clone 130g. Control mouse DNA has not been fully cleaved by our endonuclease digestions to date. Since a true mouse chorionic gonadotropin remains questionable, it is not clear whether there will be any detectable homology of the pure mouse DNA with our α hCG probe. This control is necessary before assignment of α hCG to a particular chromosome can be made. We interpreted the present studies to indicate that the α subunit gene was present in the non-producing 130g clone of human:mouse hybrid cells and may therefore be associated with human chromosome 18. However, since multiple copies of the α gene may be present, additional analyses of the hybrids and mouse control DNA are necessary prior to final assignment.

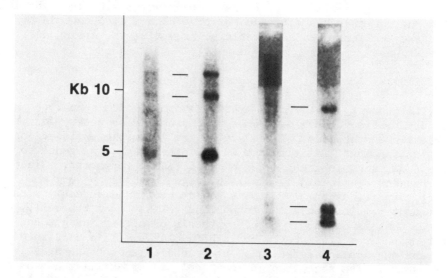

Fig. 1 Nucleic acid hybridization with ^{32}P-labeled cDNA for α glycoprotein subunit and placental lactogen with DNA isolated from hybrid 130g and term placenta.

DNA was isolated from either clone 130g or human term placenta. The DNA was digested with EcoRI, electrophoresed on 0.8% agarose slab gels, and transferred to nitrocellulose by the method of Southern. The DNA containing filters were subsequently hybridized to ^{32}P-cDNA for either the α glycoprotein subunit or for hPL. Lanes 1 and 3 contain 130g DNA, lanes 2 and 4 contain term placenta DNA. Lanes 1 and 2 were hybridized with α hCG DNA, lanes 3 and 4 with hPL DNA. Similar hybridization patterns were noted for the 130g clone and term placenta DNA.

Steroid Synthesis

Progesterone production by the JEG-3 parent line was measured
at levels of 21.0 $g.cell^{-1}.10^{-15}$. No progesterone was detected
in Cl ID or 3T3-4EF cells. None of the hybrid clones had detectible progesterone secreted into the medium immediately after
fusion or after being cultured for one year.

Production of estrogen as measured by radioimmunoassay was
3000 pg of estradiol per milliliter of culture medium for JEG-3,
100 pg/ml for 3T3-4EF, and non-detectible for Cl ID cells. In
5 of 13 JEG-3.3T3-4EF, hybrids estrone levels of 100-200 pg/ml
were found, but other hybrids had no detectible estrogen in the
medium.[16] The 24-hour measurement of conversion of labeled precursors revealed the parent JEG-3 cells could aromatize the A
ring of weak androgens in a manner analagous to the placenta.[8]
Conversion rates of dehydroepiandrosterone sulfate were 5.7% to
estrone and 34% to estradiol. The 3T3-4EF parent cells showed
conversion of 7.47% of estrone sulfate to estradiol, but no
conversion from earlier precursors. The results with the hybrid
cells suggest that the estrogen positive clones also contain a
sulfatase activity, but are unable to aromatize the A ring of
the androgens.

DISCUSSION

The present somatic cell hybridization studies appear to
indicate that more than one human chromosome is necessary for
complete hCG synthesis. There are several possible explanations
for this finding. The simplest is that the structural genes for
the α and β subunit are located on different chromosomes. Since
the subunits are joined by simple hydrogen bonding to form the
intact hormone, synthesis of each could occur independently with
subsequent combination prior to hormone release from the cell.
However, unbalanced or isolated synthesis of either subunit has
not been observed to date in our hybrid clones. This certainly
does not exclude localization of the subunit genes to separate
chromosomes. The fact that an identical or very similar α subunit is found in hCG, hLH, hFSH and hTSH raises the question of
whether there are single or multiple copies of the genes for the
α subunit. Although an hCG-like material is found in low levels
in many human tissues,[30] the frequent secretion of α subunit
ectopically by tumors increases the suspicion that multiple
copies of this gene might be present in the human genome. There
also may be only one copy of the α gene which may be linked to
the genes for the several β chains, or each hormone may have a
separate α-β genetic linkage and regulation. Information from
the correlation of gene mapping with the β hCG probe and the in
vitro production of hCG should answer these questions with regard
to hCG.

The lack of α subunit synthesis in clone 130g which appears to retain a gene for this peptide by our nucleic acid hybridization studies, but does not produce active subunits, suggests that other control factors might be involved in the regulation of its production. The assembly process of the subunits into active hCG including the addition of sialic acid and carbohydrate moieties is also not known. This could provide another type of control in the expression of the hCG genes. The choriocarcinoma hybrids have the advantage of permitting evaluation of gene expression as well as gene localization of the type recently reported assigning insulin to chromosome 11[31] and growth hormone and placental lactogen to chromosome 17.[32]

The finding that progesterone production was not retained in the hybrid cells is not surprising in view of the multiple enzymatic steps necessary for steroid synthesis. However, these hybrids should allow mapping of the sulfatase which converts estrone sulfate to estrone. In addition, specific steps in the steroid synthetic pathways may be evaluated in the future utilizing specific labeled steroid precursors. Presumably, human ectopic steroid hormone secretion does not occur because the synthetic pathway is more complicated, but selected steroid converting enzymes can be studied.

The current studies will primarily provide basic information regarding the genetic and cellular mechanisms regulating human glycoprotein and steroid hormone synthesis. For example, α glycoprotein hormone subunit deficiency presumably would represent a lethal mutation in vivo, and therefore can be studied only in culture. Appreciation of the cellular control of hormone synthesis should ultimately provide a basis for efforts to modify production of specific hormones by endocrine cells. Knowledge of the cellular control may also help to elucidate the lack of negative control in the instance of ectopic protein hormone production by tumors of non-endocrine tissue such as lung. Assignment of specific endocrine functions to specific human chromosomes will have multiple advantages in the future. Protein hormone and subunits may provide markers for specific chromosomes in the same manner as enzymes. Linkage groups are now being established and with the mapping of the human genome and rapid developments in molecular techniques, gene replacement may ultimately become a reality.

REFERENCES

1. G. D. Braunstein, J. L. Vaitukaitis, P. P. Carbone, and G. T. Ross, Ectopic production of human chorionic gonadotropin by neoplasms, Ann. Int. Med. 78:39 (1973).

2. B. D. Weintraub and S. W. Rosen, Ectopic production of the isolated beta subunit of human chorionic gonadotropin. J. Clin. Invest. 52:3135 (1973)

3. S. W. Rosen and B. D. Weintraub, Ectopic production of the isolated alpha subunit of the glycoprotein hormones: A quantitative marker in certain cases of cancer, N. Engl. J. Med. 290:1441 (1974).

4. M. R. Blackman, B. D. Weintraub, S. W. Rosen, I. A. Kourides, K. Steinwascher, and M. H. Gail, Human placental and pituitary glycoprotein hormones and their subunits as tumor markers: A quantitative assessment, J. Nat. Canc. Inst. 65:81 (1980).

5. L. C. Giudice and J. G. Pierce, Glycoprotein hormones: Some aspects of studies of secondary and tertiary structure, in: "Structure and Function of Gonadotropins," K. W. McKerns, ed., Plenum Press, New York, 1978.

6. J. L. Vaitukaitis, Glycoprotein hormones and their subunits – immunological and biological characterization, in: "Structure and Function of Gonadotropins," K. W. McKerns, ed., Plenum Press, New York (1978).

7. P. O. Kohler and W. E. Bridson, Isolation of hormone-producing clonal lines of human choriocarcinoma, J. Clin. Endocr. Metab. 32:683 (1971).

8. P. O. Kohler, W. E. Bridson, J. M. Hammond, B. D. Weintraub, and D. H. Van Thiel, Clonal lines of human choriocarcinoma cells in culture. Acta Endocr. Supp. 153:137 (1971).

9. W. E. Bridson, G. T. Ross, and P. O. Kohler, Immunological and biological activity of chorionic gonadotropin synthesized by cloned choriocarcinoma cells in culture, J. Clin. Endocr. Metab. 33:145 (1971).

10. J. M. Hammond, W. E. Bridson, P. O. Kohler, and A. Chrambach, Physical characteristics of chorionic gonadotropin produced in cell culture, Endocrinology, 89:801 (1971).

11. J. M. Hammond, W. E. Bridson, A. Chrambach, and P. O. Kohler, Isohormones of chorionic gonadotropin produced by cloned cell lines in cultures, J. Clin. Endocr. 34:185 (1972)

12. M. Boothby, S. Daniels-McQueen, D. McWilliams, M. Zernik, and I. Boime, Human chorionic gonadotropin α and β mRNA's; Translatable levels during pregnancy and molecular cloning of DNA sequences complementary to hCG, in: "The Chorionic Gonadotropin Molecule," S. Segal, ed., Plenum Press, New York (in press).

13. R. Hertz, Choriocarcinoma of women maintained in serial passage in hamster and rat, Proc. Soc. Exper. Biol. Med. 102:77 (1959).

14. J. Littlefield, Selection of hybrids from matings of fibroblasts in vitro and their presumed recombinants, Science 145:709 (1964).

15. P. O. Kohler, Isolation, cloning and hybridization of endocrine cell-lines, in: "Methods in Enzymology," B. W.

O'Malley and J. G. Hardman, eds., Academic Press, New York (1975).

16. M. R. Bordelon, H. G. Coon, and P. O. Kohler, Human glyco-protein hormone production in human-human and human-mouse somatic cell hybrids, Exp. Cell Res. 103:303 (1976).

17. M. R. Bordelon-Riser, M. J. Siciliano, and P. O. Kohler, Necessity for two human chromosomes for human chorionic gonadotropin production in human-mouse hybrids, Somatic Cell Genetics 5:597 (1979).

18. M. R. Bordelon, Staining and photography for quinicrine mustard and Hoechst 33258, Tissue Culture Assn. Manual 3:587 (1977).

19. M. J. Siciliano, M. R. Bordelon, and P. O. Kohler, Expression of human adenosine deaminase after fusion of adenosine deaminase-deficient cells with mouse fibroblasts, Proc. Natl. Acad. Sci. (USA) 75:936 (1978).

20. M. J. Siciliano, M. E. Bordelon-Riser, R. S. Freedman, and P. O. Kohler, A human trophoblastic isoenzyme (lactate dehydrogenase-Z) associated with choriocarcinoma, Canc. Res. 40:283 (1980).

21. M. Lipsett, P. Doerr, and J. A. Bermudez, Saturation assays for plasma progesterone and 17-hydroxyprogesterone, Acta Endocr. Supp. 147:155 (1970).

22. D. L. Loriaux, H. J. Ruder, and M. B. Lipsett, The measure-ment of estrone sulfate in plasma, Steroids 18:463 (1971).

23. M. Gross-Bellard, P. Ouslet, and P. Chambon, Isolation of high molecular weight DNA from mammalian cells, European J. Biochem. 36:32 (1973).

24. E. M. Southern, Detection of specific sequences among DNA fragments separated by gel electrophoresis, J. Mol. Biol. 98:503 (1975)

25. T. Maniatis, A. Jeffrey, and D. G. Kleid, Nucleotide sequence of the rightward operation of phage λ, Proc. Natl. Acad. Sci. (USA) 72:1184 (1975).

26. D. T. Denhardt, A membrane-filter technique for the detection of complementary DNA, Biochem. Biophys. Res. Comm. 23:641 (1966).

27. G. M. Wahl, M. Stern, and G. R. Stark, Efficient transfer of large DNA fragments from agarose gels to diazobenzyloxymethyl-paper and rapid hybridization by using dextran sulfate, Proc. Natl. Acad. Sci. (USA) 76:3683 (1979).

28. L. H. T. Van der Ploeg, A. Konings, M. Oort, D. Roos, L. Bernini, and R. A. Flavell, γ-β-Thalassaemia studies showing that deletion of the γ and δ-genes influences β-globin gene expression in man, Nature 283:637 (1980).

29. R. L. Davidson, Regulation of melanin synthesis in mammalian cells: Effect of gene dosage on the expression of differentiation, Proc. Natl. Acad. Sci. (USA) 69:951 (1972).

30. G. D. Braunstein, V. Kamdar, J. Rasor, N. Swaminathan, and M. E. Wade, Widespread distribution of a chorionic gonado-

tropin-like substance in normal human tissues, J. Clin.
Endocrinol. Metab. 49:917 (1979).

31. D. Owerbach, G. I. Bell, W. J. Rutter and T. B. Shows,
The insulin gene is located on chromosome 11 in humans,
Nature 286:82 (1980).

32. D. Owerbach, W. J. Rutter, J. A. Martial, J. D. Baxter, and
T. B. Shows, Genes for growth hormone, chorionic somato-
mammotropin, and growth hormone-like gene on chromosome 17
in humans, Science 209:289 (1980).

ACKNOWLEDGMENTS

These studies were supported in part by NIH grants AM17307
and AM21458. We are grateful to Dr. Judith Vaitukaitis for the
subunit assays.

INDEX